Immunochemistry

Immunochemistry

Editor:

Pam Wang, Ph.D.

Delve Publishing
www.delvepublishing.com

Immunochemistry

Editor: Pam Wang, Ph.D.

708 3rd Avenue, 6th Floor

New York, NY 10017

United States of America

www.delvepublishing.com

ISBN: 978-1-68095-900-0

Library of Congress Control Number: 2016951758

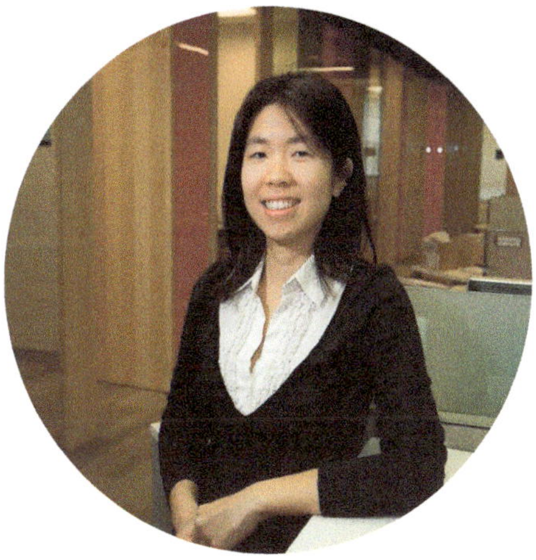

About the Editor

Pam Wang, Ph.D.

Pam Wang is a chemical biologist by training who has research experience in a variety of interdisciplinary fields. She received her PhD in 2014 studying artificial proteins and is now an industrial postdoc working on bacterial genome engineering. Her interests lie primarily in the application of biophysical, biochemical, and molecular engineering techniques to biotechnology and the pharmaceutical sciences.

Contents

List of Contributors

Tamara Aleksic
Department of Oncology, Old Road Campus Research Building, Roosevelt Drive, Oxford OX3 7DQ, UK

Andrew Ross Worrall
Department of Oncology, Old Road Campus Research Building, Roosevelt Drive, Oxford OX3 7DQ, UK

Clare Verrill
Department of Cellular Pathology, Oxford University Hospitals NHS Foundation Trust, John Radcliffe Hospital, Oxford OX3 9DU, UK

Helen Turley
Department of Cellular Pathology, Oxford University Hospitals NHS Foundation Trust, John Radcliffe Hospital, Oxford OX3 9DU, UK

Leticia Campo
Department of Oncology, Old Road Campus Research Building, Roosevelt Drive, Oxford OX3 7DQ, UK

Valentine M Macaulay
Department of Oncology, Old Road Campus Research Building, Roosevelt Drive, Oxford OX3 7DQ, UK
Oxford Cancer and Haematology Centre, Oxford University Hospitals NHS Foundation Trust, Churchill Hospital, Oxford OX3 7LJ, UK

Wilson IB Onuigbo
Department of Pathology, Medical Foundation and Clinic, Enugu 40001, Nigeria

Danielle E. Green
Division of Surgical Oncology, Department of Surgery, Medical College of Wisconsin, Milwaukee, WI, USA

Thejus T. Jayakrishnan
Division of Surgical Oncology, Department of Surgery, Medical College of Wisconsin, Milwaukee, WI, USA

Michael Hwang
Division of Surgical Oncology, Department of Surgery, Medical College of Wisconsin, Milwaukee, WI, USA

Sam G. Pappas
Division of Surgical Oncology, Department of Surgery, Loyola University Medical Center, Maywood, IL, USA

T. Clark Gamblin
Division of Surgical Oncology, Department of Surgery, Medical College of Wisconsin, Milwaukee, WI, USA

Kiran K. Turaga
Division of Surgical Oncology, Department of Surgery, Medical College of Wisconsin, Milwaukee, WI, USA

Naoya Maekawa
Department of Disease Control, Graduate School of Veterinary Medicine, Hokkaido University, Sapporo, Japan,

Satoru Konnai
Department of Disease Control, Graduate School of Veterinary Medicine, Hokkaido University, Sapporo, Japan,

Tomohiro Okagawa
Department of Disease Control, Graduate School of Veterinary Medicine, Hokkaido University, Sapporo, Japan,

Asami Nishimori
Department of Disease Control, Graduate School of Veterinary Medicine, Hokkaido University, Sapporo, Japan,

Ryoyo Ikebuchi
Department of Disease Control, Graduate School of Veterinary Medicine, Hokkaido University, Sapporo, Japan,

Yusuke Izumi
Veterinary Teaching Hospital, Graduate School of Veterinary Medicine, Hokkaido University, Sapporo, Japan,

Satoshi Takagi
Veterinary Teaching Hospital, Graduate School of Veterinary Medicine, Hokkaido University, Sapporo, Japan,

Yumiko Kagawa
North Lab, Sapporo, Japan
Department of Diagnostic Pathology, Graduate School of Veterinary Medicine, Hokkaido University, Sapporo, Japan,

Chie Nakajima
Research Center for Zoonosis Control, Hokkaido University, Sapporo, Japan,

Yasuhiko Suzuki
Research Center for Zoonosis Control, Hokkaido University, Sapporo, Japan,

Yukinari Kato
Department of Regional Innovation, Graduate School of Medicine, Tohoku University, Sendai, Japan

Shiro Murata
Department of Disease Control, Graduate School of Veterinary Medicine, Hokkaido University, Sapporo, Japan,

Kazuhiko Ohashi
Department of Disease Control, Graduate School of Veterinary Medicine, Hokkaido University, Sapporo, Japan,

Nicolás Cuenca
Department of Physiology, Genetics and Microbiology, University of Alicante, Alicante, Spain

Laura Fernández-Sánchez
Department of Physiology, Genetics and Microbiology, University of Alicante, Alicante, Spain

Yves Sauvé
Departments of Ophthalmology and Physiology, University of Alberta, Edmonton, AB, Canada

Francisco J. Segura
Aragon Health Science Institute, IIS Aragon, Zaragoza, Aragon, Spain
Department of Surgery, School of Medicine, University of Zaragoza, Zaragoza, Aragon, Spain

Gema Martínez-Navarrete
Bioengineering Institute, Miguel Hernandez University, Elche, Alicante, Spain

José Manuel Tamarit
Bloss Group Company, Spain and Heidelberg Engineering Gmbh, Heidelberg, Germany

Lorena Fuentes-Broto
Aragon Health Science Institute, IIS Aragon, Zaragoza, Aragon, Spain
Department of Physiology, University of Zaragoza, Zaragoza, Aragon, Spain

Ana Sanchez-Cano
Aragon Health Science Institute, IIS Aragon, Zaragoza, Aragon, Spain
Department of Applied Physics, University of Zaragoza, Zaragoza, Aragon, Spain

Isabel Pinilla
Aragon Health Science Institute, IIS Aragon, Zaragoza, Aragon, Spain
Department of Surgery, School of Medicine, University of Zaragoza, Zaragoza, Aragon, Spain
Department of Ophthalmology, Lozano Blesa University Hospital, Zaragoza, Aragon, Spain

Priscilla Logerot
Department of Anatomy with Radiology, Faculty of Medical and Health Sciences, and Centre for Brain Research, University of Auckland, Auckland, New Zealand

Nils O. E. Kru¨tzfeldt
Department of Anatomy with Radiology, Faculty of Medical and Health Sciences, and Centre for Brain Research, University of Auckland, Auckland, New Zealand

J. Martin Wild
Department of Anatomy with Radiology, Faculty of Medical and Health Sciences, and Centre for Brain Research, University of Auckland, Auckland, New Zealand

M. Fabiana Kubke
Department of Anatomy with Radiology, Faculty of Medical and Health Sciences, and Centre for Brain Research, University of Auckland, Auckland, New Zealand

Alex D. Rygg
Department of Mechanical and Nuclear Engineering, The Pennsylvania State University, University Park, Pennsylvania, United States of America,
Applied Research Laboratory, The Pennsylvania State University, University Park, Pennsylvania, United States of America,

Adri C. T. van Duin
Department of Mechanical and Nuclear Engineering, The Pennsylvania State University, University Park, Pennsylvania, United States of America,

Brent A. Craven
Department of Mechanical and Nuclear Engineering, The Pennsylvania State University, University Park, Pennsylvania, United States of America,
Applied Research Laboratory, The Pennsylvania State University, University Park, Pennsylvania, United States of America,
Department of Bioengineering, The Pennsylvania State University, University Park, Pennsylvania, United States of America

Marleen H. van Coevorden-Hameete
Department of Biology, Division of Cell Biology, Faculty of Science, Utrecht University, Utrecht, Netherlands ,
Department of Neurology, Erasmus Medical Center, Rotterdam, Netherlands,

Maarten J. Titulaer
Department of Neurology, Erasmus Medical Center, Rotterdam, Netherlands,

Marco W. J. Schreurs
Department of Immunology, Erasmus Medical Center, Rotterdam, Netherlands

Esther de Graaff
Department of Biology, Division of Cell Biology, Faculty of Science, Utrecht University, Utrecht, Netherlands ,

Peter A. E. Sillevis Smitt
Department of Neurology, Erasmus Medical Center, Rotterdam, Netherlands,

Casper C. Hoogenraad
Department of Biology, Division of Cell Biology, Faculty of Science, Utrecht University, Utrecht, Netherlands

Minyong Kang
Graduate Schools of Medical Science and Engineering, KAIST, Daejeon, Republic of Korea,

Yong-Mahn Han
Graduate Schools of Medical Science and Engineering, KAIST, Daejeon, Republic of Korea,
Department of Biological Sciences, KAIST, Daejeon, Republic of Korea

Katrin Bomans
Pharma Development, Roche Diagnostics GmbH, Penzberg, Germany,

Antje Lang
Pharma Biotech, Roche Diagnostics GmbH, Penzberg, Germany,

Veronika Roedl
Pharma Biotech, Roche Diagnostics GmbH, Penzberg, Germany,

Lisa Adolf
Pharma Development, Roche Diagnostics GmbH, Penzberg, Germany,

Kyrillos Kyriosoglou
Pharma Development, Roche Diagnostics GmbH, Penzberg, Germany,

Katharina Diepold
Pharma Development, Roche Diagnostics GmbH, Penzberg, Germany,

Gabriele Eberl
Pharma Biotech, Roche Diagnostics GmbH, Penzberg, Germany,

Michael Mølhøj
Pharma Development, Roche Diagnostics GmbH, Penzberg, Germany,

Ulrike Strauss
Pharma Biotech, Roche Diagnostics GmbH, Penzberg, Germany,

Christian Schmalz
Pharma Biotech, Roche Diagnostics GmbH, Penzberg, Germany,

Rudolf Vogel
Professional Diagnostics, Roche Diagnostics GmbH, Penzberg, Germany

Dietmar Reusch
Pharma Development, Roche Diagnostics GmbH, Penzberg, Germany,

Harald Wegele
Pharma Development, Roche Diagnostics GmbH, Penzberg, Germany,

Michael Wiedmann
Pharma Development, Roche Diagnostics GmbH, Penzberg, Germany,

Patrick Bulau
Pharma Development, Roche Diagnostics GmbH, Penzberg, Germany,

Jean-Marc Collombet
De´partement de Toxicologie, Institut de Recherche Biome´dicale des Arme´es, Centre de Recherche du Service de Sante´ des Arme´es, La Tronche, France,

Mikael Elias
Architecture et Fonction des Macromole´cules Biologiques, Centre National de la Recherche Scientifique-Aix Marseille Universite´, Marseille, France,

Guillaume Gotthard
Architecture et Fonction des Macromole´cules Biologiques, Centre National de la Recherche Scientifique-Aix Marseille Universite´, Marseille, France,

Elise Four
De´partement de Toxicologie, Institut de Recherche Biome´dicale des Arme´es, Centre de Recherche du Service de Sante´ des Arme´es, La Tronche, France,

Fre´de´ rique Renault
De´partement de Toxicologie, Institut de Recherche Biome´dicale des Arme´es, Centre de Recherche du Service de Sante´ des Arme´es, La Tronche, France,

Aure´lie Joffre
Service de Microscopie et d'Imagerie Me´dicale, Institut de Recherche Biome´dicale des Arme´es, Centre de Recherche du Service de Sante´ des Arme´es, La Tronche, France

Dominique Baubichon
De´partement de Toxicologie, Institut de Recherche Biome´dicale des Arme´es, Centre de Recherche du Service de Sante´ des Arme´es, La Tronche, France,

Daniel Rochu
De´partement de Toxicologie, Institut de Recherche Biome´dicale des Arme´es, Centre de Recherche du Service de Sante´ des Arme´es, La Tronche, France,

Eric Chabrie` re
Architecture et Fonction des Macromole´cules Biologiques, Centre National de la Recherche Scientifique-Aix Marseille Universite´, Marseille, France,

Gabriela Gremel
Science for Life Laboratory, Department of Immunology, Genetics and Pathology, Uppsala University, Uppsala, Sweden

Karin Grannas
Science for Life Laboratory, Department of Immunology, Genetics and Pathology, Uppsala University, Uppsala, Sweden

Lesley Ann Sutton
Science for Life Laboratory, Department of Immunology, Genetics and Pathology, Uppsala University, Uppsala, Sweden

Fredrik Pontén
Science for Life Laboratory, Department of Immunology, Genetics and Pathology, Uppsala University, Uppsala, Sweden

Agata Zieba
Science for Life Laboratory, Department of Immunology, Genetics and Pathology, Uppsala University, Uppsala, Sweden

Science for Life Laboratory
Science for Life Laboratory, Department of Immunology, Genetics and Pathology, Uppsala University, Uppsala, Sweden

Huanhuan Xu
Key Laboratory of Pu-er Tea Science, Ministry of Education, Yunnan Agricultural University, Kunming, China,

Tea Research Center of Yunnan, Kunming, China
College of Food Science and Technology, Yunnan Agricultural University, Kunming, China

Ya Wang
Key Laboratory of Pu-er Tea Science, Ministry of Education, Yunnan Agricultural University, Kunming, China,
Tea Research Center of Yunnan, Kunming, China
College of Food Science and Technology, Yunnan Agricultural University, Kunming, China

Yana Chen
Key Laboratory of Pu-er Tea Science, Ministry of Education, Yunnan Agricultural University, Kunming, China,
Tea Research Center of Yunnan, Kunming, China

Pan Zhang
Key Laboratory of Pu-er Tea Science, Ministry of Education, Yunnan Agricultural University, Kunming, China,
Tea Research Center of Yunnan, Kunming, China

Yi Zhao
Key Laboratory of Pu-er Tea Science, Ministry of Education, Yunnan Agricultural University, Kunming, China,
Tea Research Center of Yunnan, Kunming, China

Yewei Huang
Key Laboratory of Pu-er Tea Science, Ministry of Education, Yunnan Agricultural University, Kunming, China,
Tea Research Center of Yunnan, Kunming, China
College of Food Science and Technology, Yunnan Agricultural University, Kunming, China

Xuanjun Wang
Key Laboratory of Pu-er Tea Science, Ministry of Education, Yunnan Agricultural University, Kunming, China,
Tea Research Center of Yunnan, Kunming, China
College of Pu-er Tea, Yunnan Agricultural University, Kunming, China,
State Key Laboratory for Conservation and Utilization of Bio-Resources in Yunnan, Kunming, China

Jun Sheng
Key Laboratory of Pu-er Tea Science, Ministry of Education, Yunnan Agricultural University, Kunming, China,
Tea Research Center of Yunnan, Kunming, China
State Key Laboratory for Conservation and Utilization of Bio-Resources in Yunnan, Kunming, China

Ryoma Morigaki
Department of Neurodegenerative Disorders Research, Institute of Biomedical Sciences, Graduate School of Medical Sciences, Tokushima University, Tokushima, Japan,
Parkinson's Disease and Dystonia Research Center, Tokushima University Hospital, Tokushima University, Tokushima, Japan,
Department of Neurosurgery, Institute of Biomedical Sciences, Graduate School of Medical Sciences, Tokushima University, Tokushima, Japan

Satoshi Goto
Department of Neurodegenerative Disorders Research, Institute of Biomedical Sciences, Graduate School of Medical Sciences, Tokushima University, Tokushima, Japan,
Parkinson's Disease and Dystonia Research Center, Tokushima University Hospital, Tokushima University, Tokushima, Japan,

Christopher W. Toon
Cancer Diagnosis and Pathology Group, Kolling Institute of Medical Research, Sydney, Australia,
Histopath Pathology, North Ryde, Australia,

Angela Chou
Cancer Diagnosis and Pathology Group, Kolling Institute of Medical Research, Sydney, Australia,
Dept of Anatomical Pathology, SYDPATH, St Vincents Hospital, Darlinghurst, Australia,

Adele Clarkson
Cancer Diagnosis and Pathology Group, Kolling Institute of Medical Research, Sydney, Australia,
Dept of Anatomical Pathology, Royal North Shore Hospital, St Leonards, Australia,

Keshani DeSilva
Dept of Anatomical Pathology, Royal North Shore Hospital, St Leonards, Australia,

Michelle Houang
Cancer Diagnosis and Pathology Group, Kolling Institute of Medical Research, Sydney, Australia,
Dept of Anatomical Pathology, Royal North Shore Hospital, St Leonards, Australia,

Joseph C. Y. Chan
University of Sydney, Camperdown, Australia,
Bill Walsh Cancer Research Laboratory, Kolling Institute of Medical Research, Sydney, Australia

Loretta L. Sioson
Cancer Diagnosis and Pathology Group, Kolling Institute of Medical Research, Sydney, Australia,
Dept of Anatomical Pathology, Royal North Shore Hospital, St Leonards, Australia,

Lucy Jankova
University of Sydney, Camperdown, Australia,
Bill Walsh Cancer Research Laboratory, Kolling Institute of Medical Research, Sydney, Australia

Anthony J. Gill
Cancer Diagnosis and Pathology Group, Kolling Institute of Medical Research, Sydney, Australia,
Dept of Anatomical Pathology, Royal North Shore Hospital, St Leonards, Australia,
University of Sydney, Camperdown, Australia,

Michael J. Kluk
Department of Pathology, Brigham and Women's Hospital and Harvard Medical School, Boston, Massachusetts, United States of America,

Todd Ashworth
Department of Pathology, Brigham and Women's Hospital and Harvard Medical School, Boston, Massachusetts, United States of America,

Hongfang Wang
Department of Pathology, Brigham and Women's Hospital and Harvard Medical School, Boston, Massachusetts, United States of America,

Birgit Knoechel
Departments of Pediatric Hematology/Oncology and Medical Oncology, Dana Farber Cancer Institute, Boston, Massachusetts, United States of America,

Emily F. Mason
Department of Pathology, Brigham and Women's Hospital and Harvard Medical School, Boston, Massachusetts, United States of America,

Elizabeth A. Morgan
Department of Pathology, Brigham and Women's Hospital and Harvard Medical School, Boston, Massachusetts, United States of America,

David Dorfman
Department of Pathology, Brigham and Women's Hospital and Harvard Medical School, Boston, Massachusetts, United States of America,

Geraldine Pinkus
Department of Pathology, Brigham and Women's Hospital and Harvard Medical School, Boston, Massachusetts, United States of America,

Oliver Weigert
Departments of Pediatric Hematology/Oncology and Medical Oncology, Dana Farber Cancer Institute, Boston, Massachusetts, United States of America,

Jason L. Hornick
Department of Pathology, Brigham and Women's Hospital and Harvard Medical School, Boston, Massachusetts, United States of America,

Lucian R. Chirieac
Department of Pathology, Brigham and Women's Hospital and Harvard Medical School, Boston, Massachusetts, United States of America,

Michelle Hirsch
Department of Pathology, Brigham and Women's Hospital and Harvard Medical School, Boston, Massachusetts, United States of America,

David J. Oh
Department of Pathology, Brigham and Women's Hospital and Harvard Medical School, Boston, Massachusetts, United States of America,

Andrew P. South
Division of Cancer Research and Genetics Core Services Unit, Medical Research Institute, Ninewells Hospital and Medical School, University of Dundee, Dundee, United Kingdom,

Irene M. Leigh
Division of Cancer Research and Genetics Core Services Unit, Medical Research Institute, Ninewells Hospital and Medical School, University of Dundee, Dundee, United Kingdom,

Celine Pourreyron
Division of Cancer Research and Genetics Core Services Unit, Medical Research Institute, Ninewells Hospital and Medical School, University of Dundee, Dundee, United Kingdom,

Andrew J. Cassidy
Division of Cancer Research and Genetics Core Services Unit, Medical Research Institute, Ninewells Hospital and Medical School, University of Dundee, Dundee, United Kingdom,

Daniel J. DeAngelo
Departments of Pediatric Hematology/Oncology and Medical Oncology, Dana Farber Cancer Institute, Boston, Massachusetts, United States of America,

David M. Weinstock
Departments of Pediatric Hematology/Oncology and Medical Oncology, Dana Farber Cancer Institute, Boston, Massachusetts, United States of America,

Ian E. Krop
Departments of Pediatric Hematology/Oncology and Medical Oncology, Dana Farber Cancer Institute, Boston, Massachusetts, United States of America,

Deborah Dillon
Department of Pathology, Brigham and Women's Hospital and Harvard Medical School, Boston, Massachusetts, United States of America,

Jane E. Brock
Department of Pathology, Brigham and Women's Hospital and Harvard Medical School, Boston, Massachusetts, United States of America,

Alexander J. F. Lazar
Department of Pathology, M. D. Anderson Cancer Center, Houston, Texas, United States of America,

Myron Peto
Knight Cancer Institute, Oregon Health & Science University, Portland, Oregon, United States of America,

Raymond J. Cho
Department of Dermatology, University of California, San Francisco, San Francisco, California, United States of America,

Alexander Stoeck
Merck Oncology, Boston, Massachusetts, United States of America

Brian B. Haines
Merck Oncology, Boston, Massachusetts, United States of America

Sriram Sathayanrayanan
Merck Oncology, Boston, Massachusetts, United States of America

Scott Rodig
Department of Pathology, Brigham and Women's Hospital and Harvard Medical School, Boston, Massachusetts, United States of America,

Jon C. Aster
Department of Pathology, Brigham and Women's Hospital and Harvard Medical School, Boston, Massachusetts, United States of America,

Giovanni Anthony
Department of Biological and Biomedical Sciences, North Carolina Central University, BBRI 215, 700 George Street, Durham, NC, 27707, United States of America

Ju-Ahng Lee
Department of Biological and Biomedical Sciences, North Carolina Central University, BBRI 215, 700 George Street, Durham, NC, 27707, United States of America

Yiping Du
Department of Oncology, First Affiliated Hospital of Nanjing Medical University, Nanjing, China,

Xin Zhou
Department of Oncology, First Affiliated Hospital of Nanjing Medical University, Nanjing, China,

Zebo Huang
Department of Oncology, First Affiliated Hospital of Nanjing Medical University, Nanjing, China,

Tianzhu Qiu
Department of Oncology, First Affiliated Hospital of Nanjing Medical University, Nanjing, China,

Jian Wang
Department of Oncology, First Affiliated Hospital of Nanjing Medical University, Nanjing, China,

Wei Zhu
Department of Oncology, First Affiliated Hospital of Nanjing Medical University, Nanjing, China,

Tongshan Wang
Department of Oncology, First Affiliated Hospital of Nanjing Medical University, Nanjing, China,

Ping Liu
Department of Oncology, First Affiliated Hospital of Nanjing Medical University, Nanjing, China,
Cancer Center of Nanjing Medical University, Nanjing, China

Preface

Immunochemistry is a sub-discipline of chemistry that focuses on the interactions between antibodies and antigens, which relate directly to the function of the immune system. Broadly speaking, immunochemistry is divided into two main areas of study: immunocytochemistry and immunohistochemistry.

In immunocytochemistry, an antibody is used to label a specific protein (or antigen) to determine its expression and localization within a cell. Typically, a fluorescence-based method is employed, wherein a primary antibody (that is known to bind to the protein of interest) is added to cells, followed by a reporter-coupled secondary antibody. This method allows for visualization of the protein under a fluorescence microscope, and bypasses the need for introducing fluorescent tags (e.g. green fluorescent protein, or GFP) which may interfere with the protein's structure or function. One common method of preparing samples for immunocytochemical analysis involves growing adherent cells on plastic support, then fixing and permeabilizing them (with organic solvent and detergent) to allow for antibody uptake. Alternatively, samples can also be analyzed in the form of cellular smears, swabs, aspirates, and suspensions. In certain cases, enzyme-coupled antibodies (such as horseradish peroxidase) or biospecific small molecules are used instead of a fluorescently labeled antibody. Although a two-antibody system (primary followed by a reporter-coupled secondary) is generally more sensitive and therefore preferred, immunostaining can be performed with a single antibody reporter in cases where the protein of interest is particularly abundant, or exhibits a strong affinity towards the antibody. On the other hand, immunohistochemistry refers to an antibody-assisted method of visualizing cellular components within complex tissues. This technique has important applications in medicine and underlies many diagnostic procedures, allowing for a direct comparison between healthy and diseased tissues on a subcellular level. Tissues for immunohistochemical analysis are fixed, embedded in paraffin blocks, then sectioned before protein detection. Similar to immunocytochemistry, the detection step involves a primary antibody that binds specifically to the protein of interest, followed by a reporter-coupled secondary antibody. However, in immunohistochemistry, enzymatic reactions that generate a colored deposit are more commonly used for detection than fluorescent methods; colored precipitates (usually blue or brown) are easily visualized with a light microscope and are stable over extended time periods. Nevertheless, fluorescent antibody reporters offer the advantage of labeling multiple protein targets in a single assay, and are employed in certain cases. Often, a counterstain is also used to enhance contrast between the tissue background and stained proteins. Overall, immunocytochemistry and immunohistochemistry are complementary techniques that both rely on the detection of specific interactions between a protein and a binding partner (most often an antibody) within the cellular context.

Editor
Pam Wang, Ph.D.

INTRODUCTION

Introduction

Immunochemistry is a branch of chemistry that studies the immune system. This includes the body's cellular and chemical responses to bacterial, fungal, and viral organisms. In the early 1900s, scientists Karl Landsteiner and Svante Arrhenius developed chemical methods of studying antibodies and their antitoxin response to toxins. These studies eventually led to the tests used to detect specific diseases and methods of treating different maladies.

Throughout human history, it has been understood that when an illness subsides, the individual who was ill is less likely to have a recurrence. In 1798, the English physician, Edward Jenner, tested a means of creating smallpox immunity by injecting another person with the contents of a cowpox lesion. The result was immunization against smallpox. Later scientists would discover the actions and components of the immune system.

During the early phases of immunochemistry, researchers formulated methods of observing immune responses outside of the body. These pioneers concluded that chemical reactions occurred but were unsure what exactly triggered a reaction or how to reproduce this reaction. Laboratory research revealed haptens, which are parts of antigens. Researchers eventually discovered that an immune response reaction occurred when antibodies contacted haptens that were attached to specific proteins. Using the combined substance, further testing indicated that an antigen reaction generally included the formation of a precipitate.

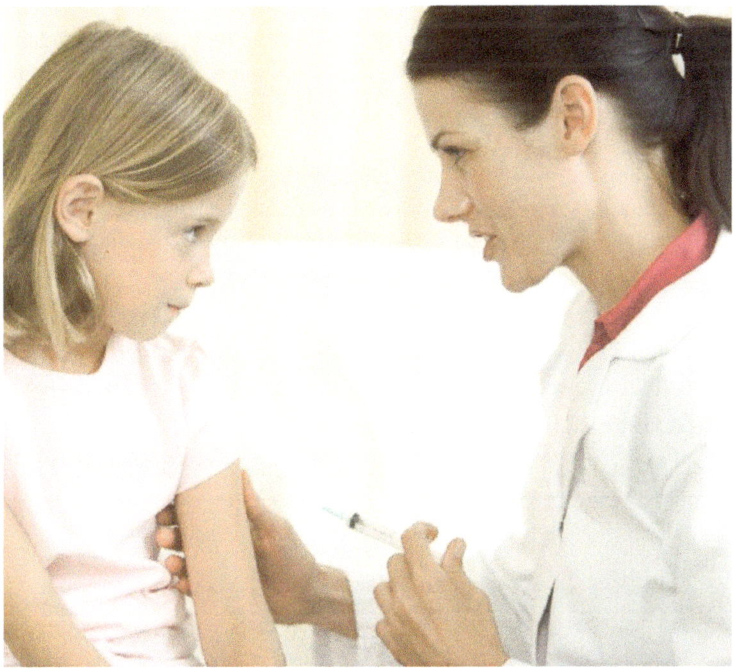

Continued evaluation of antibodies and reactants revealed that these immune system components distinguished between molecular structures with even the slightest difference. Certain substances produced a greater reaction than others. As an example, compounds containing a carboxylic group elicited a smaller response than substances containing a sulfuonic group. Advancements in immunochemistry eventually allowed researchers to study antibody binding and reacting properties by using luminescent molecules. Later research techniques usually involved electrophoresis. At the beginning of the 20th century, scientists also developed the Wasserman test for syphilis. The test was commonly performed by combining a sample of blood or cerebrospinal fluid with a lipid from sheep. The antibodies combined with the lipid exhibited varying degrees of reaction, depending on the severity of the condition. This type of test was also effective for detecting malaria and tuberculosis. The tests were not fool proof, and false positives or negatives sometimes occurred. Currently laboratory technicians use more sophisticated methods of testing. Virology, or the study of viruses, is also a branch of immunochemistry that classifies viruses, analyzes how infections are acquired, and develops methods of treatment. Molecular evolution usually involves the study microbiology at the level of deoxyribonucleic acid (DNA), ribonucleic acid (RNA) and proteins. This includes immunochemistry when the study concerns disease processes and infection.

Top 7 Types of Immunochemical Techniques Used in Biochemistry

Top seven types of immunochemical techniques used in biochemistry for various purposes such as:

(1) Immunoassay: a biochemical technique that measures the concentration of a substance in a biological liquid;

(2) Radioimmunoassay: a technique for detecting antigen or antibody;

(3) Enzyme-Linked Immunosorbent Assay: a technique used for both determining serum antibody concentrations and detecting the presence of antigen or antibody;

(4) Immunoprecipitation: a technique for detecting a particular antigen in a given cell or tissue type;

(5) Immunoelectrophoresis: a technique used in clinical laboratories to detect the presence or absence of proteins in the serum;

(6) Immunofluorescence: a technique used for labelling the antibodies and

(7) Immunohistochemistry: a technique used for localizing the proteins in cells of a tissue section.

1. Immunoassay

An immunoassay is a biochemical test that measures the concentration of a substance in a biological liquid, typically serum or urine, using the reaction of an antibody or antibodies to its antigen. The assay takes advantage of the specific binding of an antibody to its antigen.

Monoclonal antibodies are often used as they only usually bind to one site of a particular molecule, and therefore, provide a more specific and accurate test, which is less easily confused by the presence of other molecules. The antibodies selected must have a high affinity for the antigen (if there is antigen available, a very high proportion of it must bind to the antibody).

The presence of both antigen and antibody can be measured. For instance, when detecting infection the presence of antibody against the pathogen is measured. For measuring hormones such as insulin, the insulin acts as the antigen.

For numerical results, the response of the fluid being measured must be compared to standards of a known concentration. This is usually done through the plotting of a standard curve on a graph, the position of the curve at response of the unknown is then examined, and so the quantity of the unknown is found.

Detecting the quantity of antibody or antigen can be achieved by a variety of methods. One of the most common is to label either the antigen or antibody. The label may consist of an enzyme (see enzyme-linked immunosorbent assay (ELISA)), radioisotopes such as 1-125 Radioimmunoassay (RIA) or fluorescence. Other techniques include agglutination, nephelometry, turbidimetry and Western Blot. Immunoassays have a particularly important role in the diagnosis of HIV through the HIV test.

Types:

Immunoassays can be divided into those that involve labelled reagents and those which involve non-labelled reagents. Those which involve labelled reagents are divided into homogenous and heterogenous (which involved a separation step) immunoassays.

Heterogenous immunoassays can be competitive or non-competitive:

In a competitive immunoassay, the antigen in the unknown sample competes with labelled antigen to bind with antibodies. The amount of labelled antigen bound to the antibody site is then measured. In this method, the response will be inversely proportional to the concentration of antigen in the unknown. This is because the greater the response, the less antigen in the unknown was available to compete with the labelled antigen.

In noncompetitive immunoassays, also referred to as the "sandwich assay," antigen in the unknown is bound to the antibody site, and then labelled antibody is bound to the antigen. The amount of labelled antibody on the site is then measured. Unlike the competitive method, the results of the noncompetitive method will be directly proportional to the concentration of the antigen. This is because labelled antibody will not bind if the antigen is not present in the unknown sample.

Immunoassays can be homogeneous or heterogeneous

- A heterogeneous immunoassay will require an extra step to remove unbound antibody or antigen from the site, usually using a solid phase reagent.
- Because homogeneous assays do not require this step, they are typically faster and easier to perform.

Radioimmunoassay (RIA)

One of the most sensitive techniques for detecting antigen or antibody is radioimmunoassay (RIA). The technique was first developed in 1960 by two endocrinologists, S. A. Berson and Rosalyn Yalow, to determine levels of insulin-anti-insulin complexes in diabetics. Although their technique encountered some skepticism, it soon proved its value for measuring hormones, serum proteins, drugs, and vitamins at concentrations of 0.001 micrograms per millilitre or less.

In 1977, some years after Berson's death, the significance of the technique was acknowledged by the award of a Nobel Prize to Yalow. The principle of RIA involves competitive binding of radiolabelled antigen and un-labelled antigen to a high-affinity antibody. The labelled antigen is mixed with antibody at a concentration that saturates the antigen-binding sites of the antibody.

Then test samples of un-labelled antigen of unknown concentration are added in progressively larger amounts. The antibody does not distinguish labelled antigen from un-labelled antigen, so the two kinds of antigen compete for available binding sites on the antibody. As the concentration of un-labelled antigen increases, more labelled antigen will be displaced from the binding sites.

The decrease in the amount of radiolabelled antigen bound to specific antibody in the presence of the test sample is measured in order to determine the amount of antigen present in the test sample. The antigen is generally labeled with a gamma-emitting isotope such as 1251, but beta-emitting isotopes such as tritium (3H) are also routinely used as labels.

The radiolabelled antigen is part of the assay mixture; the test sample may be a complex mixture, such as serum or other body fluids, that contains the un-labelled antigen. The first step in setting up an RIA is to determine the amount of antibody needed to bind 50%— 70% of a fixed quantity of radioactive antigen (Ag*) in the assay mixture.

This ratio of antibody to Ag* is chosen to ensure that the number of epitopes presented by the labelled antigen always exceeds the total number of antibody binding sites. Consequently, un-labelled antigen added to the sample mixture will compete with radiolabelled antigen for the limited supply of antibody.

Even a small amount of un-labelled antigen added to the assay mixture of labelled antigen and antibody will cause a decrease in the amount of radioactive antigen bound, and this decrease will be proportional to the amount of un-labelled antigen added. To determine the amount of labelled antigen bound, the Ag-Ab complex is precipitated to separate it from free antigen (antigen not bound to Ab), and the radioactivity in the precipitate is measured.

A standard curve can be generated using un-labelled antigen samples of known concentration (in place of the test sample), and from this plot the amount of antigen in the test mixture may be precisely determined. Several methods have been developed for separating the bound antigen from the free antigen in RIA. One method involves precipitating the Ag-Ab complex with a secondary anti-isotype antiserum.

For example, if the Ag- Ab complex contains rabbit IgG antibody, then goat anti-rabbit IgG will bind to the rabbit IgG and precipitate the complex. Another method makes use of the fact that protein A of Staphylococcus aureus has high affinity for IgG. If the Ag-Ab complex contains an IgG antibody, the complex can be precipitated by mixing with formalin-killed S. aureus.

After removal of the complex by either of these methods, the amount of free labelled antigen remaining in the supernatant can be measured in a radiation counter; subtracting this value from the total amount of labelled antigen added yields the amount of labelled antigen bound. Various solid-phase RIAs have been developed that make it easier to separate the Ag-Ab complex from the unbound antigen.

In some cases, the antibody is covalently cross-linked to Sepharose beads. The amount of radiolabelled antigen bound to the beads can be measured after the beads have been centrifuged and washed. Alternatively, the antibody can be immobilized on polystyrene or polyvinylchloride wells and the amount of free labelled antigen in the supernatant can be determined in a radiation counter.

In another approach, the antibody is immobilized on the walls of microtiter wells and the amount of bound antigen is determined. Because the procedure requires only small amount of sample and can be conducted in small 96-well microtiter plates, this procedure is well suited for determining the concentration of a particular antigen in large numbers of samples.

For example, a microtiter RIA has been widely used to screen for the presence of the hepatitis B virus. RIA screening of donor blood has sharply reduced the incidence of hepatitis B infections in recipients of blood transfusions.

Transplant Immunology

Transplant immunology is the study of immune responses to transplantation of organs and other donor material, for the purpose of preventing rejection and increasing transplant success. This field includes researchers working in lab settings on transplant medicine, as well as doctors who interact directly with patients and perform transplants. People with a variety of medical and scientific backgrounds can pursue careers in transplant immunology, with many research centers using interdisciplinary teams for research. The risk of rejection is one of the key obstacles with transplanting donor tissue and other materials. If the recipient's immune system identifies the transplanted material as foreign and dangerous, it will attack, degrading the material. This can lead to death or severe illness for the recipient. Transplant immunologists study how the immune system responds to transplants with the goal of finding a way to interrupt it and encourage the body to accept the donor tissue. One aspect of transplant immunology involves screening donors and recipients to identify good matches. In addition to matching by blood type, researchers can also check for a number of other characteristics, searching for things like proteins in the donor material that the recipient's body will attack. Matching can take time if someone has an unusual blood type or other characteristics. By matching donors and recipients as precisely as possible, people can reduce the risk of rejection.

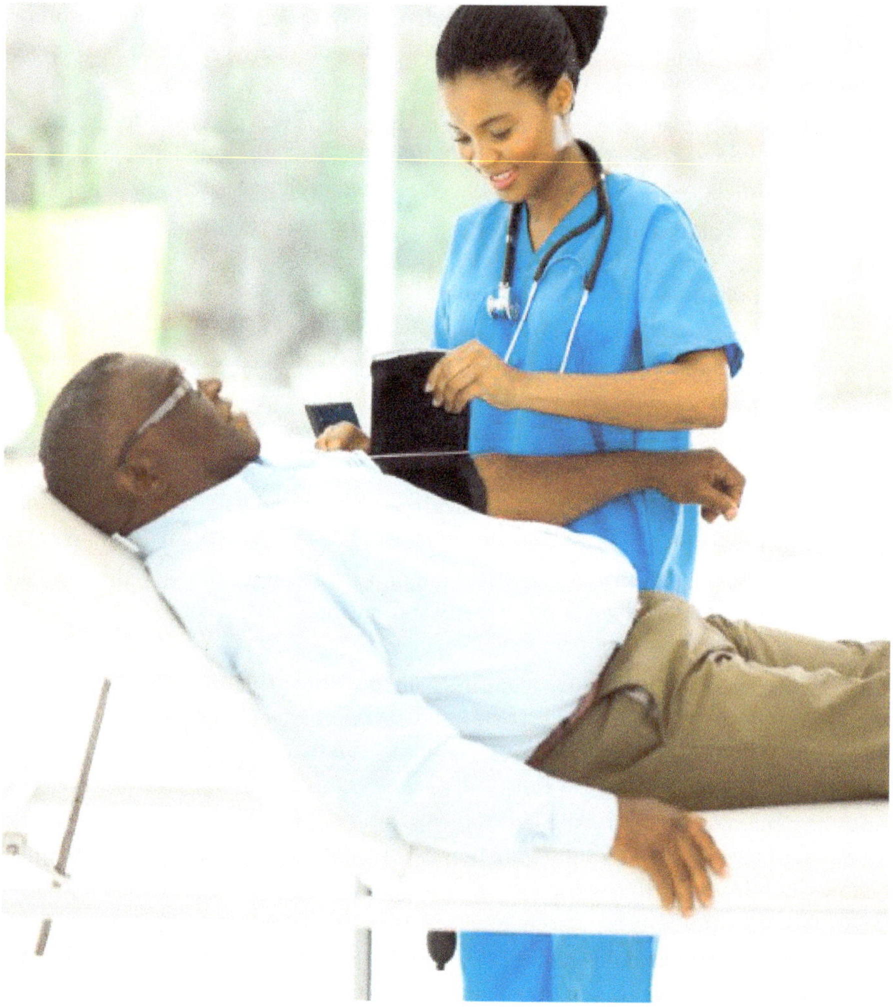

Another area of interest involves the development of anti-rejection drugs. Many of these work by suppressing immune responses so the recipient's body cannot start to attack the donor material. Developing drugs to suppress rejection without interfering with the immune system's ability to fight off actual infections is of interest to many researchers. Researchers develop drug regimens, study potential candidates for anti-rejection drugs, and follow up on patients to see how well they tolerate specific drugs. Transplant immunology is also a topic of interest for people developing artificial transplant materials, such as heart valves made from plastics and metals, grafts cultured in a lab using donor cells, or grafts of animal origin. The body usually responds to foreign objects by rejecting them, and developing effective transplants requires understanding how and where the body tags foreign materials to see if it is possible to develop artificial transplant materials that will not trigger a rejection response. People interested in transplant immunology careers will need to go to medical school or pursue graduate work in the sciences with a focus on immunology and related topics. Education for people in these fields can last 12 years or more.

Molecular Immunology

Molecular immunology is a subfield of immunology that aims to examine immune processes at a molecular level. The immune system is the bodily system that responds to foreign entities, such as bacteria or other infectious agents in the body. The immune response that such a foreign entity triggers tends to be highly specific. The body produces antibodies that are specifically designed to target a particular antigen, or foreign body that triggers an immune response, just as a single lock tends to be matched to a single key. The field of molecular immunology exists to examine this and other aspects of immune response that are controlled at a molecular level.

The goals of molecular immunology are varied, and various techniques in the field are used in both laboratory and clinical settings. Greater understanding of the molecular basis of immune function has allowed for more targeted and effective diagnostic and treatment methods for some illnesses. It has also provided many new experimental methods to be used in molecular biology and molecular immunology laboratories. The high degree of specificity of antibodies is particularly important, as antibodies can be produced to target almost any biological component of interest. They can, therefore, be used to "tag" certain cellular components or to determine if a particular substance is present in a sample because they will bind specifically to the antigen of interest.

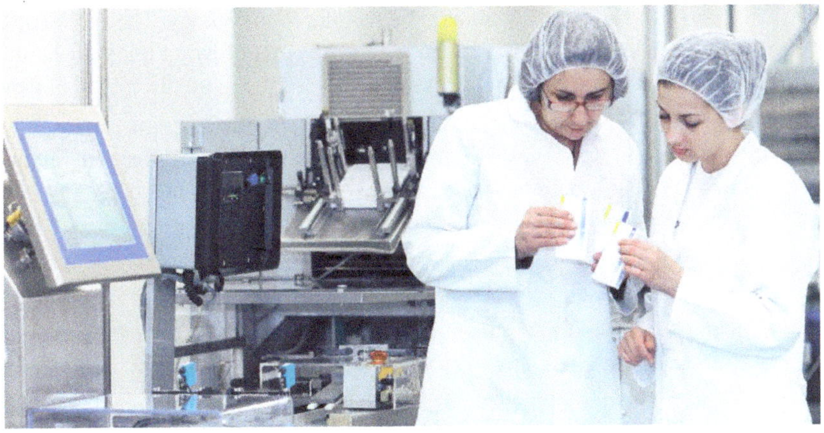

The interactions between antibodies and antigens are central to molecular immunology and to immunology as a whole. Various immune system cells have receptors that bind to antigens in the body and trigger an immune response. Antibodies are produced with molecular binding regions tailored specifically to the antigen of interest; they tend not to bind non-specifically to anything aside from the antigen they were made to target. Components of the immune system are also able to identify and attack cells that have been compromised, as in the case of viruses.

In addition to diseases that the immune system fights, the field of molecular immunology is also interested in diseases and disorders that affect the immune system itself. In the case of autoimmune diseases, for instance, the immune system targets "self" cells instead of antigens. In certain other disorders and diseases, the effectiveness of the immune system is reduced, thereby causing a state of immunodeficiency. Antigen recognition is driven by specific molecular mechanisms and even slight changes in the conformations of the structures of antigens can have significant effects on immune response. Scientists working in molecular immunology hope that greater understanding of the molecular basis of immunology will help them to better fight these and other diseases and disorders.

Cellular Immunology

Cellular immunology is the study of the cells and molecules of an organism's immune system. The field involves studying how those different cells and molecules work together to provide a defense against different types of pathogens. To better understand cellular immunology, researchers study both healthy immune systems and those that are actively fighting off pathogens, comparing the differences and similarities of how the immune system's cellular physiology operates.

The poor functioning or malfunctioning of an immune system at the cellular level is also a topic of study in cellular immunology. Topics of study include cellular deficiencies in the immune system, including patients who have diseases that lower immune system response such as HIV or AIDS. Cellular immunologists also study immune system hypersensitivities to environmental factors, like allergies or asthma. How autoimmune disease — when a body's immune system attacks various tissue cells in conditions such as diabetes — works is another topic of study in cellular immunology. Researchers also study on the cellular level why some organ transplants are rejected by people's immune systems.

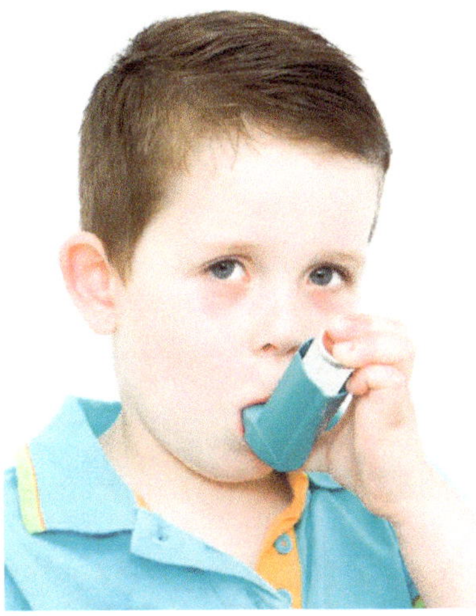

Those who study cellular immunology look at both innate immune system responses as well as adaptive immune system responses. Innate immune system responses are the body's first line of defense against infection, with defense mechanisms that are employed for all types of infections. Adaptive immune system responses are the body's second line of immune system defenses, and use cells that perform specific functions to rid the body of infections. These specific functions of these immune system cells, such as T cells and B cells, involve the defense-oriented cells remembering past infections so it can respond with faster and stronger measures later.

Cancer and how it grows in a person's body is also covered by cellular immunology. The spread of cancer through a person's body occurs at a cellular level, since cancer entails different body tissues' cells growing uncontrollably. Cellular immunologists look for ways to harness the functions of the body's immune system to prevent or stop the spread of cancer through body tissues.

Factors that affect cellular immunology are also studied by researchers. For example, the age of a person can affect his immune system's functionality on the cellular level. Researchers study how environmental factors affect immune system response at a cellular level, such as whether a patient was exposed to certain pathogens early versus later in life, the effect of sanitary conditions on a person's immune system and how genetics affect the immune system's functionality at the cellular level.

Systems Immunology

Systems immunology is generally the scientific study of the different types of cells, biological signals, and molecules that interact as part of the body's immune system. Researchers attempt to mathematically model how each of these function and react to new vaccines and drugs, for example. General knowledge of how each cell type normally interacts with another, and with many different proteins and enzymes, is typically essential as well. The field is often considered part of the field of systems biology, in which scientists study the interaction and function of every part of the body.

In addition to mathematics, scientists who specialize in systems immunology often use computers to analyze various biological components. Microchips can be used to analyze molecules, while a variety of other laboratory equipment is often applied to mix in different compounds and monitor the reactions that take place. Researchers sometimes use such techniques to pick out drugs to study. People in clinical trials can also be monitored with sophisticated equipment to detect the response of the immune system to drugs in development.

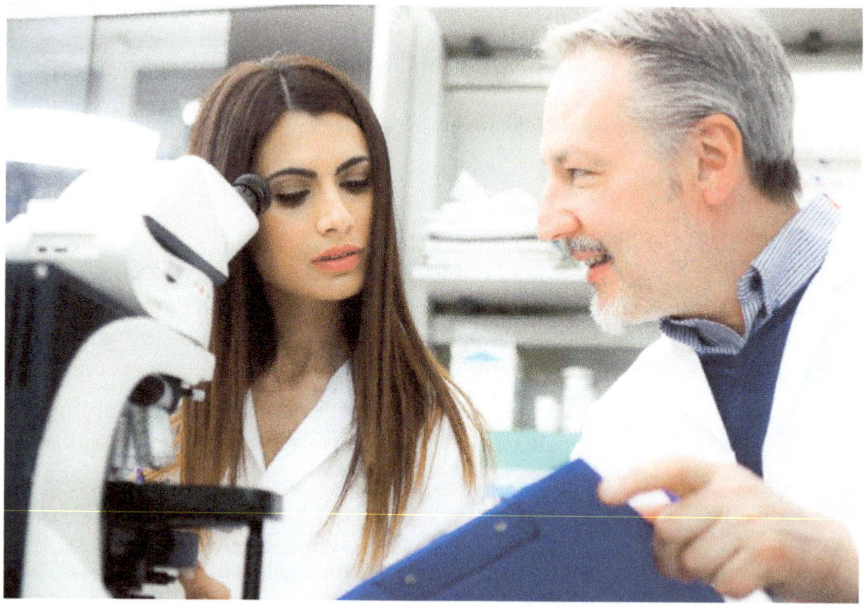

Laboratories around the world study systems immunology, often to find drugs effective against various infections and diseases, such as malaria, tuberculosis, and Human Immunodeficiency Virus (HIV). Such facilities often depend on local and regional funding to operate. To work in the field, one often requires advanced academic experience, typically at the post doctorate level. Knowledge of thousands of genes that code for proteins, as well as the responses that occur at a systemic and cellular level, is generally necessary.

The immune system consists of cells that attack foreign organisms, called phagocytes, as well as those that can remember the molecular signature of previous invading subjects, called lymphocytes. Some of these look for viruses and bacteria, for example, while others respond after an infection has been identified. The responses are typically dependent on proteins called antibodies. An assortment of enzymes and other proteins are normally involved in the signaling between cells, and the starting and stopping of an immune response.

Computers are often used to model the interaction of genes, cells, proteins, and foreign substances, as well as predict how the immune system will respond. Systems immunology can be applied to treating a patient as well as diagnosing him or her with a disease. Research scientists who perform systems immunology work often collaborate with experts in pharmacology, chemistry, and clinical trial design, while specialists in computers and biology are often familiar with concepts in both fields.

Mucosal Immunology

Mucosal immunology represents a branch of biomedicine that studies toxins entering the body through the respiratory, gastrointestinal, or reproductive tract. These cavities provide pathways where viruses, bacteria, or harmful pathogens enter the body from the outside environment. Mucus found in these tracts represents the first line of defense as part of the human immune system by creating barriers to toxic substances.

Researchers involved in mucosal immunology study how mucus membranes trap foreign substances called antigens and send messages to lymph nodes to begin attacking these invaders. Scientists working in this branch of bioscience hope to discover new medicines and vaccines that improve the functioning of the immune system to fight illness and cure disease. They also research how these mucus membranes are breached by specific viruses, bacteria, or chemicals.

An example of the body's mucosal immunology response occurs through coughing or sneezing, when tiny hairs called cilia trap antigens in the respiratory system. Diarrhea or vomiting typically occurs when gastrointestinal antibodies attempt to rid the body of harmful substances that enter the body from food or beverages. Tears, urine, sweat, and vaginal secretions also are part of the mucosal immunology system.

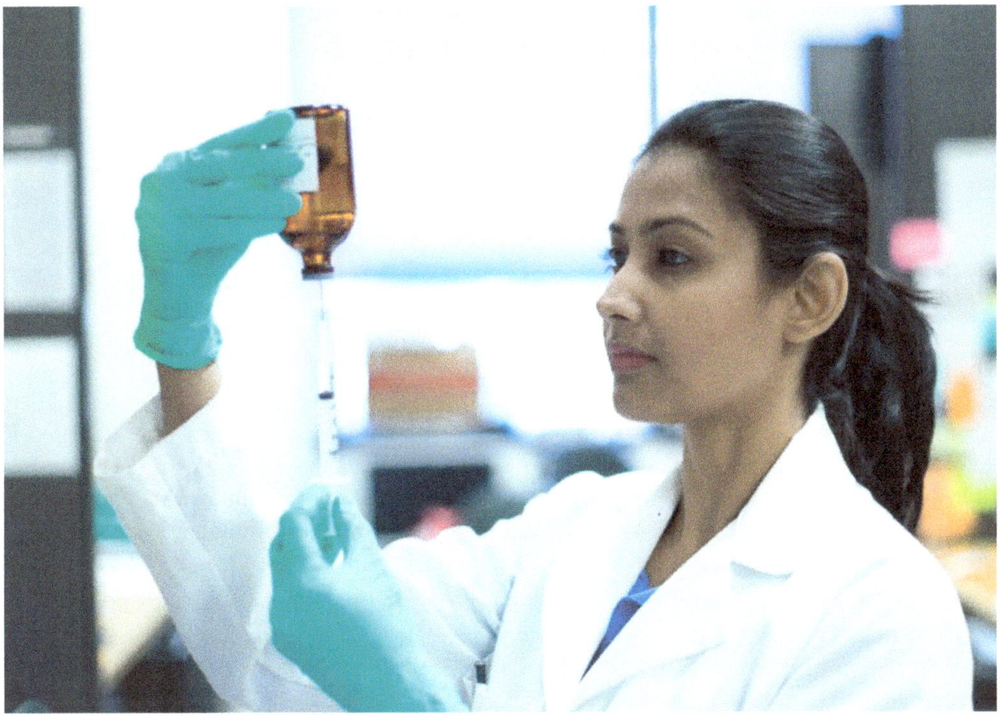

The human body produces immune cells called lymphocytes in bone marrow to attack different types of antigens, with the highest concentration of lymphocytes found in mucus. When these cells mature, they enter the bloodstream, lymph nodes, and spleen. These lymphocytes trigger the secretion of antibodies to destroy antigens and protect mucous membranes as part of a complex defense system against illness.

Mucous membranes are rich in dendritic cells, which are innate immune cells that can distinguish between benign and harmful substances that enter the body. If a bacterium or virus invades, dendritic cells stimulate production of white blood cells, or T cells, to attack the foreign antigen. B cells, considered helper cells, also become activated and bind to specific antigens. During this process, memory cells are also created that can activate a rapid response if the same foreign substance attacks the body again. Vaccines work by creating memory cells to protect against disease.

If the immune system malfunctions, antibodies attack healthy cells along with foreign invaders, leading to autoimmune diseases such as lupus, arthritis, multiple sclerosis, and allergies. The study of mucosal immunology looks at how antigens pass through mucus barriers and produce antibodies that destroy healthy tissue. This field of medicine also researches ways to strengthen the immune system and develop new vaccines to create memory cells.

Allergy Immunology

Allergy immunology is a subspecialty of medicine. Physicians in this field treat diseases of the immune system such as allergic reactions, anaphylactic shock, asthma, autoimmune disorders and transplant rejection. Allergy immunology is important to other fields of clinical medicine and research, especially dermatology, pulmonology, infectious diseases and transplant surgery. Some physicians in this specialty are called allergists, and they mostly work in allergy clinics. Research topics in immunology are robust and range widely, from the study of plant- and animal-induced allergies to the development of better treatments for immunodeficiency.

Clinically, allergy immunology specialists diagnose and treat patients for many conditions, including allergic reactions that are caused by other, non-immune diseases. As with most specialties, patients usually arrive by referral from primary care providers or hospital admitting physicians. Allergists provide extensive allergy testing, screen for food or substance sensitivity and provide treatments such as oral anti-inflammatories and steroid injections. Allergy clinics also develop personal treatment regimens for patient allergies, with specialized diets designed to avoid offending foods.

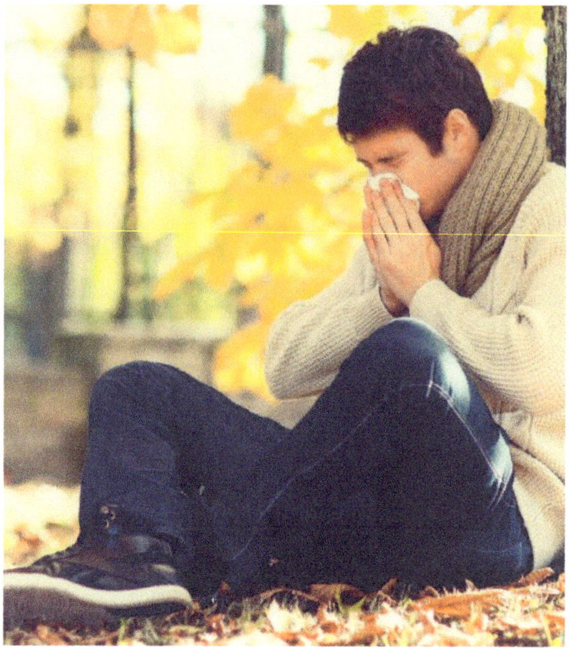

Allergy immunology includes the hospital care of patients with anaphylactic shock, systemic food allergies and severe cases of asthma that have become life-threatening. Research suggests that asthmatic patients who are cared for by allergists/ immunologists have fewer breathing problems and respond better to therapy than those receiving more generalized medical care. Hospital care also includes treatment of those suffering with immunosuppression, from human immunodeficiency virus (HIV) patients to recipients of organ transplants who require constant treatment to prevent their immune systems from rejecting the new tissue that they have received. Without this field, organ transplantation would not be possible.

Major priorities in allergy and immunology research reflect the challenges of treating a biological system with very diverse cellular and systemic functions. One key interest is in the development of better drugs to reduce immunosuppression in HIV. Work on preventing transplant rejection without complete suppression of T-cell response also receives much funding and intellectual dedication. Some researchers have tried to improve immunization efficacy or develop new vaccines, often in conjunction with virologists. Immunologists also pursue research into lupus and other autoimmune diseases with no known cures, incorporating techniques from genetics and molecular biology into their inquiry.

Physicians who specialize in allergy immunology must first complete an internship and residency in internal medicine or pediatrics. They then pursue a two- to three-year fellowship. Education involves adult and pediatric consultation and comprehensive training in laboratory medicine. Additional clinical learning might include rotations in allergy clinics, HIV care, transplantation immunology, pediatric and adult asthma centers, otolaryngology and hematology. Many fellows perform their own clinical or basic science research in these fields before taking a certification test.

CHAPTER 1

IMPROVED IMMUNOHISTOCHEMICAL DETECTION

Tamara Aleksic, Andrew Ross Worrall, Clare Verrill, Helen Turley, Leticia Campo and Valentine M Macaulay

Keywords: Cancer, Insulin-like growth factor, Type 1 IGF receptor, IGF-1R, Nuclear IGF-1R, Immunohistochemistry, FFPE, Antigen retrieval

INTRODUCTION

The contribution of insulin-like growth factors (IGFs) to cancer biology has been extensively studied in cell lines, revealing that IGFs activate type 1 IGF receptors (IGF-1Rs) to promote cell cycle progression, cell survival, motility and invasion [1,2]. These findings provoked interest in studying IGF-1R expression in clinical cancers, and in development of drugs that block IGF signaling. However, there has been striking variation in reported IGF-1R expression in tumors and normal tissues when detected by immunohistochemistry (IHC). For example IGF-1R was reported to be unchanged or down -regulated in prostate cancer compared with benign prostate [3,4], although since our report of IGF-1R up-regulation at the mRNA and protein level [5] most publications support up-regulation [6-8].

This lack of consensus also confounds attempts to interpret results of clinical trials of novel IGF inhibitory drugs. Early trials reported striking clinical responses to IGF-1R inhibition e.g., Ref. [9], but later trials showed very limited activity in unselected patients (reviewed in Ref. [10]. This raises the question as to whether tumor IGF-1R expression correlates with sensitivity to IGF-1R inhibition. Preclinical reports supporting such a link include studies in non-small cell lung cancer (NSCLC), breast and colorectal cancer, rhabdomyosarcoma,Ewing family tumours and neuroblastoma [11-14]. However, other preclinical and some clinical studies found IGF-1R expression not to associate with response to IGF-1R inhibition in breast cancer, NSCLC and sarcomas [15-17]. While it is possible that IGF-1R is predictive of response in some tumor types but not others, it is also likely that technical differences in IHC protocols contribute to the apparent variation in significance of IGF-1R expression. Notably, the study conducted by Schwartz and colleagues found no difference in clinical activity of IGF-1R antibody cixutumumab with temsirolimus in patients whose tumors were IGF-1R 'positive' or 'negative' by IHC using the automated Ventana platform [17]. This trial also assessed tumor IGF-1R in a subset of patients by western blotting of fresh tumor lysates, resulting in detection of IGF-1R in all 'IGF-1R negative' tumors that were tested.

Further complicating interpretation of IGF-1R IHC is the phenomenon of IGF-1R nuclear translocation, reported by several groups including ours [18-21]. In FFPE samples of human tumors, nuclear IGF-1R has been shown to associate with adverse prognosis in renal cancer [19], and with response to IGF-1R antibody in patients with sarcoma [21]. Lack of detection of nuclear IGF-1R prior to adoption of heat-based antigen retrieval [5,19] suggests that this also is influenced by technical variation in IHC methods.

These findings highlight the insensitivity of some IHC protocols, and the difficulties inherent in assessing the biological and clinical significance of IGF-1R expression and subcellular localization. Likely sources of variation include use of different antigen retrieval protocols and IGF-1R antibodies, and lot-to-lot variation in polyclonal antibodies. These technical factors may confound attempts to understand the role of IGF-1R in tumor biology, and the assessment of IGF-1R as a candidate prognostic and predictive biomarker. The aim here was to develop a robust IGF-1R IHC staining protocol that can be used to address these questions.

MATERIALS AND METHODS

We used formalin-fixed paraffin-embedded (FFPE) human tumors that were surplus to diagnostic need, available in the Department of Cellular Pathology, Oxford University Hospitals NHS Foundation Trust, John Radcliffe Hospital, Oxford, and accessed under National Research Ethics approved study

Citation: Aleksic T, Worrall AR, Verrill C, Turley H, Campo L, et al. (2016) Improved Immunohistochemical Detection. Immunochem Immunopathol 2:114. doi: 10.4172/2469-9756.1000114.

07/H0606/120. As cell line controls, we used human MCF7 breast cancer, SKUT-1 leiomyosarcoma, PC3 prostate cancer, and A375M melanoma. IGF-1R depletion was induced by transfection with IGF-1R siRNA (Hs_IGF1R_1, Qiagen), with Allstars siRNA (Qiagen) as non-silencing control, as described [22]. Subconfluent cultures were scraped into ice-cold phosphate buffered saline (PBS), pelleted by centrifugation (1250 rpm for 5 minutes, 4°C) and resuspended in 10% neutral buffered formalin (NBF) for 1 hour at 23°C or overnight at 4°C. After centrifugation (1250 rpm, 5 min) the cell pellet was resuspended in 2% w/v formalin-agarose (Sigma A9414 agarose, melting temperature 87°C, gelling temperature 36°C, in NBF) equilibrated to 60-65°C. After chilling on ice for 5-10 min the cell pellet was embedded in paraffin, from which 1 mm cores were removed and inserted into a recipient block using a tissue microarrayer (Beecher Instruments, Sun Prairie, WI, US), and annealed at 45-50°C for 20 min. Parallel cultures were lysed for western blotting using IGF- 1R antibodies and β-tubulin antibody (Sigma-Aldrich), as described [19]. IGF-1R IHC was performed on freshly-cut 4 μm tissue and tissue microarray (TMA) sections using #3027, #9750 and #14534 antibodies (Cell Signaling Technology). Table 1 shows the manual IHC protocol, which used methods based on Ref. [19,23], and Table 2 the automated protocol.

Table 1: Protocol for preferred manual IGF-1R IHC. This is a modification of the protocol reported in Ref. [19,23] using IGF-1R antibody #9750, and detecting bound antibody with reagents from MP-531-M3R25, Menarini Diagnostics (Winnersh-Wokingham, Berkshire UK).

Step	Protocol
Dewax, rehydrate	Incubate for 8 min in Citroclear (TCS Biosciences Ltd, UK), 8 min Citroclear, 2 min 100% ethanol, 2 min 95% ethanol, 2 min 80% ethanol, 2 min 70% ethanol, 2 min 50% ethanol, 10 min distilled water (dH_2O)
Antigen retrieval	Buffer: 50mM Tris-Cl, 2 mM EDTA pH 9 Use Decloaking chamber (DC2002, Biocare Medical, USA or similar) at 125°C for 2 min, 85°C for 10 min. Cool to room temperature (~23°C) by placing slide chamber on ice for 10-15 min.
Wash	Wash slides in PBS 3 × 5 min
Block endogenous peroxidase	Incubate slides in 3% H_2O_2 in dH_2O at 23 °C for 10 min
Wash	Wash slides in PBS 3 × 5 min
Block	Incubate slides in 5% BSA/5% goat serum in PBS 1 hr at 23°C. Drain blocking solution with Kimwipe (do not wash away)
Primary antibody	Mark around tissue area with PAP pen. Place slides in humidified chamber, incubate with IGF-1R-β antibody #9750 (Cell Signaling Technology), diluted 1:50 in blocking solution (5% BSA/5% goat serum in PBS), using 200-500 μl antibody solution per slide depending on tissue area. Incubate on level surface at +4°C overnight.
Wash	Wash slides in PBS 3 × 5 min
Detection of bound antibody	Use MP-531-M3R25, Menarini Diagnostics (Winnersh-Wokingham, Berkshire UK). Add 1-3 drops (depending on area to cover) of rabbit probe (neat as supplied) for 15 min (=5 min to come to ~23°C plus recommended 10 min). Wash in PBS 3 × 5 min, incubate with rabbit HRP polymer (neat as suplied) for 15 min at 23°C.
Wash	Wash slides in PBS 3 × 5 min
Color development	Incubate with DAB substrate (Envision) for 5-7 min
Wash	Wash slides in tap water 3 × 2 min
Counterstain	Counterstain with Mayer's haematoxylin (Vector Laboratories, USA) for 40 sec
Wash	Wash slides in copious tap water until water runs clear
Dehydrate	Incubate slides for 2 min in 50% ethanol, 2 min 70% ethanol, 2 min 80% ethanol, 2 min 95% ethanol, 2 min 100% ethanol, 5 min in Citroclear
Mount	Mount using DePex reagent (VWR International, UK)

Table 2: Automated IGF-1R IHC protocol. This protocol was tested on a Leica Bondmax autostainer to evaluate antibodies #9750 and #14534. The method produced acceptable specificity and sensitivity in cell controls (Figure 1D) but generated very weak staining in FFPE tissue (see Figure 2A) and is not recommended for future studies.

Step	Protocol
Bake, Dewax, rehydrate	Leica Bondmax autostainer standard bake at 60°C for 30 min, followed by standard dewax and rehydrate program using Leica Dewax solution (Cat no. AR9222), 100% ethanol and deionized water.
Antigen retrieval	Leica ER2 buffer pH 9 20 min 100°C
Wash	Bondmax standard wash protocol with Bond wash solution (Cat no. AR9590)
Block endogenous peroxidase	Peroxidase block at 23°C for 5 min with Bond Polymer Refine kit (Cat no. DS9800)
Wash	Bondmax standard wash protocol with Bond wash solution
Primary antibody	Diluted 1:50 in Bond antibody diluent (Cat no. AR9352) for 1 hr at 23°C
Wash	Bondmax standard wash protocol with Bond wash solution
Detection of bound antibody	Post Primary Antibody (8 min at 23°C) followed by standard wash and polymer from Bond Polymer Refine kit (Cat no. DS9800) for 8 min at 23°C
Wash	Bondmax standard wash protocol with Bond wash solution
Color development	DAB 10 min at 23°C from Bond Polymer Refine kit (Cat no. DS9800)
Wash	Standard Bond wash with distilled water.
Counterstain	Haematoxylin 5 min from Bond Polymer Refine kit (Cat no. DS9800)
Wash	Standard Bond wash with distilled water.
Mount	Aquatex aqueous mountant (Cat no 3631235, VWR).

RESULTS AND DISCUSSION

In our initial study of IGF-1R expression in prostate cancer, we had used polyclonal antibody sc713 (Santa Cruz) [5]. In a later study [24], sc713 was insufficiently specific, and we re-optimized our IHC protocol to another polyclonal, #3027 (Cell Signaling Technology) [19,24]. This antibody performed acceptably in western blotting (e.g., Ref. [19,25], but we recently questioned the specificity of current lots of this antibody in IHC. Therefore, we tested currently available lots of #3027 in IHC using FFPE sections of MCF7 and SKUT-1 cells, which express high and low IGF-1R respectively. Using the manual IHC protocol, there was detectable IGF-1R staining in both MCF7 and SKUT-1 cells, signal in the latter suggesting lack of specificity (Figure 1A). In comparison, monoclonal antibody #9750 showed greater differentiation between SKUT-1 and MCF7 cells. We also compared #3027 and #9750 by western blotting of cancer cell lysates (Figure 1B). Probing of duplicate membranes confirmed that both antibodies detected immunoreactive IGF-1R of the predicted size: mature IGF-1R beta subunit of 98 kDa and IGF-1R pro-receptor of 220 kDa. We noted that #3027 generated stronger signal than #9750, paralleling differences seen in IHC (Figure 1A). IGF-1R expression was relatively high in MCF7, lower but clearly detectable in A375M melanoma cells, and low/undetectable in SKUT- 1, PC3 and A375M cells in which IGF-1R was depleted by siRNA transfection (Figure 1B). These relative expression levels correspond to findings of our previous studies [19,25,26]. Comparable differences in signal were detected when we stained the control TMA with #9750 (Figure 1C). The close parallels between the relative intensity of IGF- 1R signal on western blot and IHC suggest that this antibody was sufficiently sensitive to detect differences in endogenous IGF-1R expression and changes induced by IGF-1R gene silencing. We then tested #9750 in parallel with a more recently-available IGF-1R rabbit monoclonal, #14534, comparing manual IHC with automated IHC on a Leica-Bond auto-stainer. Both antibodies showed clear discrimination between high IGF-1R MCF7 cells and IGF-1R-deficient SKUT-1 cells, with generally lower signal in the auto-stained samples (Figure 1D).

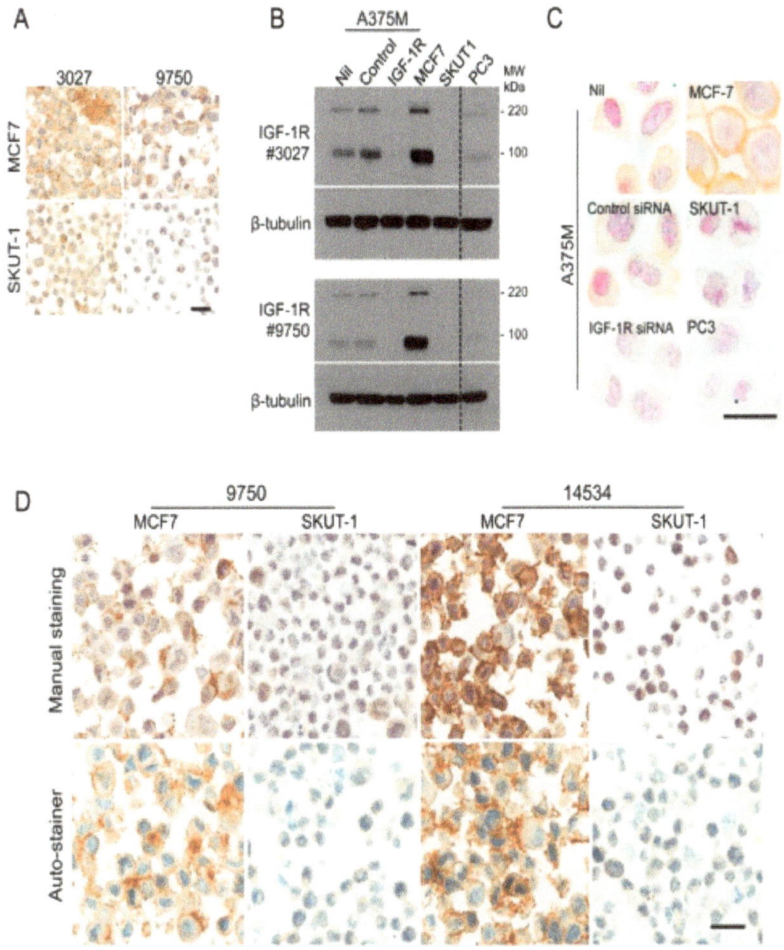

Figure 1: IGF-1R detection using polyclonal and monoclonal IGF-1R antibodies in human cancer cells. A. Manual IHC was performed on IGF-1R expressing MCF7 and IGF-1R deficient SKUT-1 cells using polyclonal antibody #3027 at 1:200 or monoclonal #9750 at 1:50 dilution. Scale bar 20 μm. B. A375M cells were untransfected (Nil) or transfected with control or IGF-1R siRNA. Other cell lines were untransfected. Whole cell lysates (50 μg) were analysed by western blot using 1:1000 dilution of #3027 (upper) or #9750 (lower), showing detection of IGF-1R β (98 kDa) and IGF-1R pro-receptor (220 kDa). Membranes were reprobed for β-tubulin as loading control. Dotted line: one lane removed. C. Manual IHC on control TMA using #9750 antibody at 1:50, showing representative appearances of FFPE cell pellets made from parallel cultures to those used in B. Scale bar 20 μm. D. IGF-1R IHC on FFPE sections of MCF7 and SKUT-1 cells using #9750 or #14534 at 1:50 in manual (upper) or automated (lower) IHC. Scale bar 20 μm.

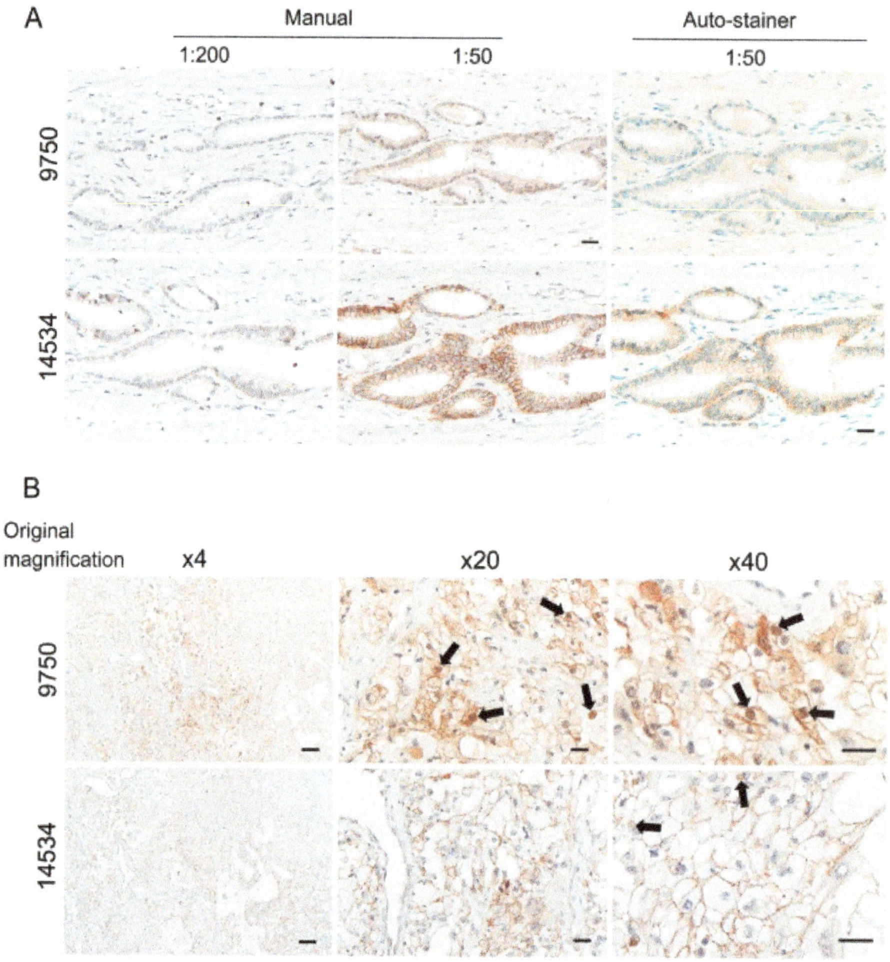

Figure 2: Comparison of manual and automated IGF-1R IHC using monoclonal IGF-1R antibodies in human tumors. A. Adjacent sections of prostate cancer stained using IGF-1R antibodies #9750 or #14534 at 1:200 or 1:50 in manual and automated protocols. Scale bar 20 µm. B. Clear cell renal cancer, fresh sections cut from same tumor block stained in Figure 4B panel H in (Aleksic et al. 2010), manually stained with #9750 or #14534 at 1:50. Scale bar for images taken at X4, 100 µm, and for X20-X40, 20 µm. Black arrows: nuclei positive for IGF-1R.

Having confirmed the specificity of both monoclonal antibodies in control cells of known IGF-1R expression, we performed testing in FFPE samples of human cancer. Staining of prostate cancer using manual and automated IHC showed negligible signal using either antibody at 1:200 dilution, and detectable signal at 1:50 that was more intense in the epithelial than stromal components, as previously noted [5]. The two antibodies showed different staining patterns, with faint membrane and more marked intracellular staining by #9750, and pronounced membrane staining by #14534. In both cases, the staining was much fainter in the auto-stained slides (Figure 2A). Finally, we analysed IGF-1R expression and subcellular localization in clear cell renal cancer, in which we had detected prominent nuclear IGF-1R in our previous study [19]. At low power it was apparent that #9750 gave stronger staining than #14534 (Figure 2B, left). As in prostate cancer (Figure 2A), #14534 showed prominent membrane IGF-1R, while #9750 showed membrane and cytoplasmic signal. In #9750-stained tumor there was clear detection of nuclear IGF-1R that showed cell to cell variation, recapitulating appearances generated by previous lots of #3027 in our prior study (Figure 2B, upper center and right panels; compare Figure 4B panel H in Ref. [19]. In contrast nuclear IGF-1R was only faintly detected by #14534 (Figure 2B lower). Given that nuclear IGF-1R is detectable by a range of methods including subcellular fractionation, immunofluorescence, proximity ligation assay and chromatin immunoprecipitation, and is reported to have prognostic and predictive significance [18-21], we suggest that #9750 is preferable to #14534 when using IHC to study IGF-1R expression and subcellular localization in human tumors.

In conclusion, we developed a specific and sensitive manual IHC protocol using antibody #9750. This is a monoclonal antibody, ensuring consistent antibody supply in future work. Nuclear IGF-1R was only weakly detected by antibody #14534, and auto-staining did not recapitulate appearances of the manual #9750 protocol, likely reflecting differences in antigen retrieval and detection. We provide a detailed protocol for the preferred manual IGF-1R IHC method that we commend for future studies. Adoption of a uniform protocol should reduce inter-study variation and may help to clarify whether responses to anti-IGF drugs associate with IGF-1R expression or subcellular localization.

ACKNOWLEDGEMENTS

This study was supported by funding to TA and VMM from Prostate Cancer UK, National Institute for Health Research (NIHR) Research Capability Funding, NIHR Oxford

Biomedical Research Centre and the Development Fund of the Oxford Cancer Research Centre. We are grateful to Adam Peltan, New England Biolabs UK for technical support.

REFERENCES

1. Baserga R, Hongo A, Rubini M, Prisco M, Valentinis B (1997) The IGF-I receptor in cell growth, transformation and apoptosis. Biochim Biophys Acta 1332: F105-126.
2. Chitnis MM, Yuen JS, Protheroe AS, Pollak M, Macaulay VM (2008) The type 1 insulin-like growth factor receptor pathway. Clin Cancer Res 14: 6364-6370.
3. Tennant MK, Thrasher JB, Twomey PA, Drivdahl RH, Birnbaum RS, et al. (1996) Protein and messenger ribonucleic acid (mRNA) for the type 1 insulin-like growth factor (IGF) receptor is decreased and IGF-II mRNA is increased in human prostate carcinoma compared to benign prostate epithelium. J Endocrinol Metab 81: 3774-82.
4. Chott A, Sun Z, Morganstern D, Pan J, Li T, et al. (1999) Tyrosine kinases expressed in vivo by human prostate cancer bone marrow metastases and loss of the type 1 insulin-like growth factor receptor. Am J Pathol 155: 1271-1279.
5. Hellawell GO, Turner GD, Davies DR, Poulsom R, Brewster SF, et al. (2002) Expression of the type 1 insulin-like growth factor receptor is up-regulated in primary prostate cancer and commonly persists in metastatic disease. Cancer Res 62: 2942-2950.
6. Grzmil M, Hemmerlein B, Thelen P, Schweyer S, Burfeind P (2004) Blockade of the type I IGF receptor expression in human prostate cancer cells inhibits proliferation and invasion, up-regulates IGF binding protein-3, and suppresses MMP-2 expression. J Pathol 202: 50-59.
7. Liao Y, Abel U, Grobholz R, Hermani A, Trojan L, et al. (2005) Up-regulation of insulin-like growth factor axis components in human primary prostate cancer correlates with tumor grade. Hum Pathol 36: 1186-1196.
8. Ryan CJ, Haqq CM, Simko J, Nonaka DF, Chan JM, et al. (2007) Expression of insulin-like growth factor-1 receptor in local and metastatic prostate cancer. Urol Oncol 25: 134-140.
9. Tolcher AW, Sarantopoulos J, Patnaik A, Papadopoulos K, Lin CC, et al. (2009) Phase I, pharmacokinetic, and pharmacodynamic study of AMG 479, a fully human monoclonal antibody to insulin-like growth factor receptor 1. J Clin Oncol 27: 5800-5807.
10. King H, Aleksic T, Haluska P, Macaulay VM (2014) Can we unlock the potential of IGF-1R inhibition in cancer therapy? See comment in PubMed Commons below Cancer Treat Rev 40: 1096-1105.
11. Cao L, Yu Y, Darko I, Currier D, Mayeenuddin LH, et al. (2008) Addiction to elevated insulin-like growth factor I receptor and initial modulation of the AKT pathway define the responsiveness of rhabdomyosarcoma to the targeting antibody. Cancer Res 68: 8039-8048.
12. Zha J, O'Brien C, Savage H, Huw LY, Zhong F, et al. (2009) Molecular predictors of response to a humanized anti-insulin-like growth factor-I receptor monoclonal antibody in breast and colorectal cancer. Mol Cancer Ther 8: 2110-2121.
13. Gong Y, Yao E, Shen R, Goel A, Arcila M, et al. (2009) High expression levels of total IGF-1R and sensitivity of NSCLC cells in vitro to an anti-IGF-1R antibody (R1507). PLoS One 4: e7273.
14. Huang F, Greer A, Hurlburt W, Han X, Hafezi R, et al. (2009) The mechanisms of differential sensitivity to an insulin-like growth factor-1 receptor inhibitor (BMS-536924) and rationale for combining with EGFR/HER2 inhibitors. Cancer Res 69: 161-170.
15. Browne BC, Eustace AJ, Kennedy S, O'Brien NA, Pedersen K, et al. (2012) Evaluation of IGF1R and phosphorylated IGF1R as targets in HER2-positive breast cancer cell lines and tumours.Breast Cancer Res Treat 136: 717-727.
16. Wynes ME, Asuncion S, Dziadziuszko BR, Glisson R, Wisuba BS, et al. (2012) Insulin-like growth factor (IGF-1R) protein expression (PE) and gene copy number (9GCN) for discrimination of response and outcome to figitumumab in NSCLC. J ClinOncol 30: 7597.
17. Schwartz GK, Tap WD, Qin LX, Livingston MB, Undevia SD, et al. (2013) Cixutumumab and temsirolimus for patients with bone and soft-tissue sarcoma: a multicentre, open-label, phase 2 trial. Lancet Oncol 14: 371-382.
18. Sehat B, Tofigh A, Lin Y, Trocmé E, Liljedahl U, et al. (2010) SUMOylation mediates the nuclear translocation and signaling of the IGF-1 receptor.Sci Signal 3: ra10.
19. Aleksic T, Chitnis MM, Perestenko OV, Gao S, Thomas PH, et al. (2010) Type 1 insulin-like growth factor receptor translocates to the nucleus of human tumor cells. Cancer Res 70: 6412-6419.
20. Sarfstein R, Pasmanik-Chor M, Yeheskel A, Edry L, Shomron N, et al. (2012) Insulin-like growth factor-I receptor (IGF-IR) translocates to nucleus and autoregulates IGF-IR gene expression in breast cancer cells. J Biol Chem 287: 2766-2776.
21. Asmane I, Watkin E, Alberti L, Duc A, Marec-Berard P, et al. (2012) Insulin-like growth factor type 1 receptor (IGF-1R) exclusive nuclear staining: a predictive biomarker for IGF-1R monoclonal antibody (Ab) therapy in sarcomas. Eur J Cancer 48: 3027-3035.
22. Chitnis MM, Lodhia KA, Aleksic T, Gao S, Protheroe AS, et al. (2014) IGF-1R inhibition enhances radiosensitivity and delays double-strand break repair by both non-homologous end-joining and homologous recombination. Oncogene 33: 5262-5273.
23. Dale OT, Aleksic T, Shah KA, Han C, Mehanna H, et al. (2015) IGF-1R expression is associated with HPV-negative status and adverse survival in head and neck squamous cell cancer. Carcinogenesis 36: 648-655.
24. Turney BW, Turner GD, Brewster SF, Macaulay VM (2011) Serial analysis of resected prostate cancer suggests up-regulation of type 1 IGF receptor with disease progression. BJU Int 107: 1488-1499.
25. Lodhia KA, Gao S, Aleksic T, Esashi F, Macaulay VM (2015) Suppression of homologous recombination

sensitizes human tumor cells to IGF-1R inhibition. Int J Cancer 136: 2961-2966.

26. Ramcharan R, Aleksic T, Kamdoum WP, Gao S, Pfister SX, et al. (2015) IGF-1R inhibition induces schedule-dependent sensitization of human melanoma to temozolomide. Oncotarget 6: 39877-39890.

CHAPTER 2 | IMMUNOPATHOLOGY

Wilson IB Onuigbo

Keywords: Cancer, Metastasis, Lymph nodes, Necrosis

INTRODUCTION

On account of its position in the human body, lung cancer is without parallel in colonization capability [1,2]. Moreover, the numbers thrown into the circulation are of the order of millions [3]. Surely, these must reach all tissues indiscriminately. And, yet, there are discernible pattern formations in the lymph node system.

LYMPH NODE PATTERNS

Over the years, I have provided some results in this ravaging realm of oncology. This was thanks to the great goodwill of the late Professor Cappell, who reported my earliest work in glowing terms [4]. Little wonder that my grooming ground was the University Department of Pathology at the Glasgow Western Infirmary, an Institution described in the Bulletin of the History of Medicine [5] as being second to none in Britain. There, I introduced, instead of the usual casual display of bodily parts on the Table, the Mono-Block Formalin-Fixation Method [6] (Figure 1).

The accruing developments are worthy of chronological classification as follows:

- 1961. Centrifugal metastasis occurs, the proximal lymph nodes being earlier and more grossly involved [7].
- 1962. Contralateral metastasis may occur in the neck, the line of cross-over to the other side being apparent [8].
- 1962. Triple carcinomata in one lung were reported. The squamous celled growth spread to a contiguous node and another near paraesophageal node. The polygonal-cell carcinoma showed two neighboring invaded nodes. The adenocarcinoma, unlike the others, spread over considerable areas, involving no less than 72 lymph nodes, the growths occurring bilaterally but asymmetrically [9].
- 1963. The situation of the earliest deposits within the retrogradely situated abdominal nodes revealed, as shown in 6 statements, that this was in the convex border, where incoming lymph vessels arrive and not in the concave border, where outgoing lymph vessels emerge [10]. This was necessarily interpreted in terms of the formation of new lymph vessels. This phenomenon is nowadays called "lymphangiogenesis" whose review I have provided elsewhere [11].
- 1964. A general consideration of lymph node metastases in lung cancer was vicariously undertaken. This led to the delineation of what I called "natural laws" as follows [12]:

  Ipsilateral nodes are invaded more grossly than contralateral ones.

  Contiguous nodes are invaded more grossly than distant nodes.

  Contiguous nodes are invaded in a more orderly fashion than distant nodes.

  Particular nodes are invaded while others may be skipped.

  Early metastases are truly discrete while subsequent dispersal may through coalescence simulate direct extension.

Therefore, I concluded with a last phrase, namely, the need "to chart virgin fields of knowledge."

DISCUSSION

In sum, from ancient times, lymph nodes were believed to be "suitable soils" for cancer colonization [13]. Lo and behold!

Citation: Wilson IB (2015) Immunopathology. Immunochem Immunopathol 1: 110. doi:10.4172/2469- 9756.1000110.

Because of the wholesale nourishing function of the blood supply, its contained cancer cells must be reaching all the lymph nodes. Nevertheless comparable colonization does not materialize. Instead, there is an orderly pattern of spread whose topography is not that of blood spread but of lymph spread. Incidentally, in an embryonic paper on lung cancer [14], I had the temerity to recommend that research should be carried out in order to elucidate "a possible difference in immunological potentiality between blood and lymph."

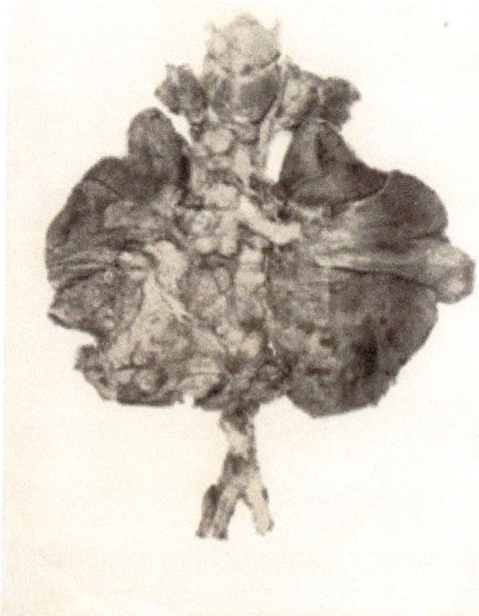

Figure 1: Early stage of axial preservation showing the as yet to be removed lungs. Note the aortic bifurcation and the lymph nodes nearby.

Today, the giant status of immunology is of great concern here as regards cancer, especially lung cancer. It seems to me that immunology should be geared specifically towards decoding the secrets of Nature in lung cancer. In other words, the chequered existence of the bloodborne lung cancer cell requires penetrating and purposive decoding researches [15,16].

Concerning such researches, the importance of the microenvironment is increasingly being realized [17,18]. However, we should go back to 1798 when Sir Astley Cooper, through animal experimentation and necropsy investigation, emphasized that red cells occur in the thoracic duct which is important to the "human economy" [19]. Concerning its duty, my experience revealed the most important evidence of accompanying necrosis itself. As I concluded pertinently, "Necrosis of the cancer cells was apparent in 3 cases, but it was clear that this had occurred in association with large aggregates of the malignant cells and that among such aggregated cells red blood corpuscles abounded." [20].

It is to be noted that this form of necrosis is associated with the phenomenon of metastasis itself, unlike the Necrosis which occurs in situ within the primary tumor itself. The latter has long been attributed to "Tumor Necrosis Factor" [21] which has been as defined thus: "Tumor necrosis was defined when there were necrotic tissues in the tumor mass at low magnification." [22].

The great point is that the thoracic duct necrosis is part and parcel of the metastasis formation, i.e., not merely of tumor formation. This is important because the ductal cancer cells had begun the active process of metastasis by first detaching ably from the primary focus and secondly transporting themselves during the next phase! On this account, I have named the thoracic duct Factor as the "Erythrocyte Associated Necrosis Factor" (EANF) [23]. This Factor is reminiscent of when, long ago, bleeding was a great problem. Thereafter, the Coagulation Factor was discovered and its treatment became assured [24]. It is, therefore, my hypothesis that, if EANF is discovered, the omens will be good!

FUTURE PROSPECTS

Now, developments have attained to such a height that there are

(i) the old cannulation undertaken simply in the thoracic duct [25], and

(ii) the new technique of intravital videomicroscopy [26]. Therefore, since the killer lung cancers superbaound [27], the patients, who give their consent as legally required [28], should be cannulated in order to retrieve the two necessary subsets required in scientific investigation, namely, the living individual cancer cells and the dying massed cancer cells commingled with red corpuscles. In this way, the newly founded, blossoming, well-funded translational laboratories should swing into action [29]. The future owes them the duty to replicate EANF [30].

Incidentally, EANF is likely to be molecular. Indeed, as I like to see it, immunology can and should be guided towards decoding the signals which Nature herself has been sending out in the bodies of patients dying with lung cancer. Elsewhere, I noted that the medical masters of yester years believed that Nature's own ways need to be not only identified but also exploited [31]. Hitherto, I had made this appeal in journals such as Single Cell Biology [32] and International Journal of Surgery [33]. Accordingly, let this Journal, Immunochemistry and Immunopathology, lend a helping hand. Thus, as Jubb's associates reminded all, "The rapid pace of drug discovery and drug development in oncology, immunology and ophthalmology brings new challenges" [34]. Therefore, it is to be hoped that breakthroughs will, sooner than later, emerge and point in the direction of that target therapy which can conduce to cancer cure.

In this context, as I showed historically [35], a major problem has long been the perplexing tissue-specific pattern of metastatic progression in cancer which has been weighed on the scale of "seed" and "soil." With this in mind, Kaplan's group [36] looked into several questions, including genetic regulation and activation of specific chemokines/cytokines and proteases, loss of deletion allows for acquisition of unique and specific properties that connect tumor cells with the metastatic microenvironment. Be that as it may, I am persuaded that the thoracic duct has provided a readily accessible microenvironment for translational research on EANF [32]. Indeed, a fruitful future is to be expected in immunopathology with special reference to the thoracic duct.

REFERENCES

1. Daniels M, Goh F, Wright CM, Sriram KB, Relan V, et al. (2012) Whole genome sequencing for lung cancer. J Thorac Dis 4: 155-163.

2. Spiro SG, Gould MK, Colice GL (2007) Initial evaluation of the patient with lung cancer: symptoms, signs, laboratory tests, and paraneoplastic syndromes: ACCP evidenced-based clinical practice guidelines. 2nd edn. Chest 132: 149S-160S.
3. Peck K, Sher YP, Shih JY, Roffler SR, Wu CW, et al. (1998) Detection and quantitation of circulating cancer cells in the peripheral blood of lung cancer patients. Cancer Res 58: 2761-2765.
4. Robert Muir, Daniel FC (1958) Muir's Text-Book of Pathology. 7th edn. London: Arnoled. p. 505.
5. Jacyna LS (1988) The laboratory and the clinic: the impact of pathology on surgical diagnosis in the Glasgow Western Infirmary, 1875-1910. Bull Hist Med 62: 384-406.
6. Onuigbo WIB (1963) A mono-block formalin-fixation method for investigating cancer metastasis. Z Krebsforsch 65: 209-210.
7. Onuigbo WIB (1961) Centrifugal metastasis in lung cancer. Br J Dis Chest 55: 86-90.
8. Onuigbo WIB (1962) Contralateral cervical node metastases in lung cancer. Thorax 17: 201-204.
9. Onuigbo WIB (1962) Multiple carcinomata of the lung (a case with three primary tumours). Br J Dis Chest 56: 144-146.
10. Onuigbo WIB (1963) A modified theory of retrograde lymphatic metastasis in lung cancer. Br J Dis Chest 57: 120-125.
11. Onuigbo WIB (2014) Lymphangiogenesis in cancer: A Review. Biochem Physiol 3: 138.
12. Onuigbo WIB (1964) Lymph node metastases in lung cancer. Geriatrics 19: 380-388.
13. Onuigbo WIB (1975) Origins of the soil theory of cancer metastasis. Mater Med Pol 7: 254-255.
14. Onuigbo WIB (1957) Some observations on the spread of lung cancer in the body. Br J Cancer 11: 175-180.
15. Onuigbo WIB (1974) The spread of lung cancer to the heart, pericardium and great vessels. Jpn Heart J 15: 234-238.
16. Onuigbo WIB (2000) Ten anomalous patterns of lung cancer spread with a single explanatory hypothesis. Med Hypotheses 55: 227-231.
17. Joyce JA, Pollard JW (2009) Microenvironmental regulation of metastasis. Nat Rev Cancer 9: 239-252.
18. Fidler IJ, Kim SJ, Langley RR (2007) The role of the organ microenvironment in the biology and therapy of cancer metastasis. J Cell Biochem 101: 927-936.
19. Cooper A, Babington W, Haighton J, Smith R, Cheston RB (1798) Medical records and researches. Harvard University, London, T. Cox.
20. Onuigbo WIB (1967) The carriage of cancer cells by the thoracic duct. Br J Cancer 21: 496-500.
21. Sidhu RS, Bollon AP (1993) Tumor necrosis factor activities and cancer therapy--a perspective. Pharmacol Ther 57: 79-128.
22. Park SY, Lee HS, Jang HJ, Lee GK, Chung KY, et al. (2011) Tumor necrosis as a prognostic factor for stage IA non-small cell lung cancer. Ann Thorac Surg 91: 1668-1673.
23. Onuigbo WIB (2013) Nature's necrosis factor when associated with erythrocytes may not only explain the surprises in lung cancer metastases but also suggest target therapy. Med Hypotheses 80: 698-700.
24. Laurence DR, Bennette PN (1987) Clinical Pharmacology. 6th edn. ELBS: Churchill. Livingstone 567-570.
25. Mittleider D, Dykes TA, Cicuto KP, Amberson SM, Leusner CR (2008) Retrograde cannulation of the thoracic duct and embolization of the cisterna chyli in the treatment of chylous ascites. J Vasc Interv Radiol 19: 285-290.
26. Chambers AF, MacDonald IC, Schmidt EE, Koop S, Morris VL, et al. (1995) Steps in tumor metastasis: new concepts from intravital videomicroscopy. Cancer Metastasis Rev 14: 279-301.
27. Zhan P, Song Y (2012) Status quo and prospects of the translational research on lung cancer in China. Transl Lung Cancer Res 1: 91-93.
28. Onuigbo WIB (2014) Historical Origins of Informed Consent in Cancer Surgery. Forensic Res 5: 246-247.
29. Woolf SH (2008) The meaning of translational research and why it matters. JAMA 299: 211-213.
30. Onuigbo WIB (2014) Is there a natural translational system suitable for the target therapy of lung cancer? Trans Med 4: 130.
31. Onuigbo WIB (2015) The visionary views of medical masters of yester years on Nature's norms point to present prospects in the target therapy of cancer. Biol Med 7: 221.
32. Onuigbo WIB (2014) The scientific significance of the role of the thoracic duct in cancer cell carriage: A review. Single Cell Biol 3: 104.
33. Onuigbo WIB (2014) Anomalous lung cancer cell carriage: a historical review with present prospects. Int J Surg 12: 734-736.
34. Jubb AM, Koeppen H, Reis-Filho JS (2014) Pathology in drug discovery and development. J Pathol 232: 99-102.
35. Onuigbo WIB (1963) A history of the cell theory of cancer metastasis. Gesnerus 20: 90-95.
36. Kaplan RN, Rafii S, Lyden D (2006) Preparing the "soil": the premetastatic niche. Cancer Res 66: 11089-11093.

CHAPTER 3 | IMMUNOHISTOCHEMISTRY

Danielle E. Green, Thejus T. Jayakrishnan, Michael Hwang, Sam G. Pappas, T. Clark Gamblin and Kiran K. Turaga

Keywords: Colorectal neoplasms, Appendiceal neoplasms, Peritoneal neoplasms, Microarray analysis, Immunohistochemistry, DNA mutational analysis

INTRODUCTION

Predictive and prognostic biomarkers have been studied in different cancers with the aim of developing personalized medicine for patients (1, 2). The role of immunohistochemistry (IHC)-microarray analysis of pathological specimens in this paradigm is currently being investigated, and preliminary data do suggest potential utility (3, 4). Few studies have examined the value of gene expression and molecular profiling of specimens in the setting of peritoneal metastases (PM) (5–7). However, the role of IHC-microarray analysis of specimens from PM of appendiceal or colorectal origin is not well elucidated.

Gene expression profiling has pointed toward phenotypic clustering with distinct survival outcomes for patients with PM (8). Vascular endothelial growth factor (VEGF) has been suggested as a potential prognostic marker for patients with PM from mucinous adenocarcinoma originating in the appendix or colon (9, 10). In colorectal cancer, there is evidence to support the association of malignant transformation and peritoneal dissemination with BRAF/KRAS mutations (11–14). Genes in the RAF family encode kinases regulated by the Ras pathway and mediate cell responses to growth signals. As such, BRAF is seen as a gene downstream from KRAS. Interestingly, BRAF and KRAS mutations have been observed to be mutually exclusive even though they exert equal effects on tumorigenesis (15).

Also important in colorectal cancer, cyclooxygenase-2 (COX-2) is an enzyme that is upregulated in colorectal cancer (16, 17). COX-2 inhibitors, like aspirin, have a protective effect on the development of colorectal cancer, and have been shown to improve survival in COX-2 overexpressing tumors (18, 19). The therapeutic value of COX-2 inhibition in appendiceal tumors is not clearly defined although studies have demonstrated increased expression (20).

Demonstration of the clinical utility of molecular profiling in guiding successful systemic therapy have resulted in a surge in the use of commercial molecular profiling services (21). The purpose of this study was to assess the feasibility of routine IHC-microarray and mutational analysis of patients with PM of appendiceal and colorectal primaries using a commercially available molecular profiling service. This is important in the context of mucinous contents of these tumors that could impact the sampling and analysis.

MATERIALS AND METHODS

Subjects

A retrospective chart review with Institutional Review Board (IRB) approval was performed to identify all patients that had appendiceal or colorectal primaries with PM that also had tissue biopsies for molecular profiling (Caris Molecular Intelligence™) sent to Caris Life Sciences lab (Phoenix, AZ, USA), which is a central Clinical Laboratory Improvement Amendments-certified laboratory. Additional demographics, histology, surgery, and treatment details were collected from medical records. Resultant biomarker data were then stratified by Peritoneal Carcinomatosis Index (PCI), histology, and treatment characteristics. All patients were treated at the regional cancer therapy program at the Medical College of Wisconsin (MCW) between April 2008 and June 2012. Patients with insufficient tissue for molecular profiling to be performed or having primaries other than the colon or appendix were excluded from the study.

Patient Samples

Our standard practice for patients with high grade appendiceal adenocarcinoma or colorectal carcinomatosis is to evaluate

Citation: Danielle E. Green ,Thejus T. Jayakrishnan , Michael Hwang , Sam G. Pappas ,T. Clark Gamblin and Kiran K. Turaga, Immunohistochemistry, http://dx.doi.org/10.3389/fsurg.2014.00050

the patients with a staging laparoscopy after four to six cycles of systemic chemotherapy. Biopsies for pathological and biochemical analysis were obtained during laparoscopy and shipped to Caris lab using standard protocol aimed to provide theranostic information (21). Sufficiency of the sample for biochemical analysis (Caris Molecular Intelligence™) was determined at the lab. Primary antibodies used for IHC are COX-2 (SP21), ERCC1 (8F1), PTEN (6H2.1), SPARC monoclonal (122511), SPARC polyclonal (polyclonal), TOP2A (3F6), TOPO1 (1D6), TS (TS106/4H4B1), and RRM1 (polyclonal). Avidin-biotin systems and polymer-based, biotin-free systems were used for detection of the antibodies. The chromogenic reporter, 3,3′-diaminobenzidine (DAB), was used to allow for a colorimetric visualization of the antibody yielding a brown stain that can be analyzed with a light microscope. The intensity of the staining was scored as 0, 1+, 2+, or 3+, and the percentage of staining cells was scored as 0–100% by a board-certified pathologist. Thresholds to determine patient benefit to therapeutic agents included the following: negative TS, staining smaller than or equal to 1+, 25%; negative ERCC1, percentage of staining smaller than or equal to 25%; high TOP2A, percentage of staining >10%. DNA microarray was performed on total RNA extracted from tumor tissue and was converted to cDNA. This cDNA sample was then subjected to a whole genome microarray analysis using Illumina cDNA-mediated annealing, selection, extension, and ligation (DASL) process with the HumanHT-12 v4 beadChip (Illumina Inc., San Diego, CA, USA). After direct hybridization and scanning of the bead array, the expression of a subset of 88 transcripts were then compared to tissue-specific normal control pools and the statistical significance of the difference between the patient tumor sample and control is determined. Direct sequence analysis was performed on genomic DNA isolated from a tumor sample using custom primers designed to flank, amplify and sequence codons 12 and 13 in exon 2 and codon 61 in exon 3 of the KRAS gene, and codons 464–469 of exon 11 and codon 600 of exon 15 in the BRAF gene.

Treatment

Following laparoscopic evaluation, patients were classified as extensive disease for exclusion from Cytoreductive Surgery with hyperthermic intra-peritoneal chemoperfusion (CRS + HIPEC) for PCI scores higher than 11 for gastric cancer, and 19 for colorectal and non-gastric primaries. After cytoreduction, HIPEC was performed using the closed technique and dosing of therapy was based on standard published consensus guidelines (22).

Statistical Analysis

Statistical calculations were performed using STATA software version 12.1 (StataCorp, TX, USA). Non-parametric methods of Kruskal Wallis and chi-square tests were employed. Survival outcomes were explored using Cox proportional hazards model. Alpha was fixed at 0.05 for statistical significance.

Results

The baseline characteristics and survival of the subjects are described in Table 1. Of the 16 patients, 11 had colon primaries and 5 had appendix primaries. Biopsies were sufficient in size for IHC to be performed on 16 patient samples vs. 7 for microarray. Patients with colon cancer were twice as likely to undergo neoadjuvant chemotherapy vs. those with appendiceal cancer that were twice as likely to undergo HIPEC upfront.

Table 1: Baseline characteristics and survival of colon and appendix cancer patients included in the study

	All patients ($n = 16$)	Colon ($n = 11$)	Appendix ($n = 5$)	*p*-value
Age (median and range in years)	51 (42–60)	51 (38–72)	51 (40–56)	0.42
Female	11 (69%)	8 (73%)	3 (60%)	1.00
AJCC6 T-stage T4	11 (69%)	8 (73%)	3 (60%)	1.00
Neoadjuvant chemotherapy	11 (69%)	9 (82%)	2 (40%)	0.24
PCI score (median and range)	17 (13–26)	17 (8–27)	17 (12–20)	0.82
CRS + HIPEC	8 (50%)	4 (36%)	4 (80%)	0.28
Median survival (months)	-	30	60	0.50

AJCC, American Joint Committee on Cancer; PCI, Peritoneal Carcinomatosis Index; CRS + HIPEC, cytoreductive surgery with hyperthermic intra-peritoneal chemoperfusion.

Immunohistochemistry (IHC)

Immunohistochemistry results are described in Table 2. Differences in percent staining or staining intensity were not significantly different between the two cancer primaries (p-value = 0.20). Of note, COX-2 was not differently expressed between the two groups with 80% staining in colorectal vs. 100% in appendiceal (p-value = 0.52).

Table 2: Immunohistochemistry (IHC) findings stratified by histological subtype

Biomarker (IHC)	Colon (N = 11)	Appendix (N = 5)	p-value
COX-2	80%	100%	0.52
ERCC1	100%	100%	1.00
PTEN	100%	100%	1.00
SPARC	36%	20%	1.00
TOP2A	100%	80%	0.31
TOPO1	100%	100%	1.00
TS	82%	80%	1.00

COX-2, cyclooxygenase-2; ERCC1, excision repair cross-complementing rodent repair deficiency, complementation group 1; PTEN, phosphatase and tensin homolog; SPARC, secreted protein acidic cysteine-rich; TOP2A, topoisomerase (DNA) 2 alpha; TOPO1, topoisomerase (DNA) 1; TS, thymidylate synthase.

Mutational Analysis

The results of mutational analysis (n = 15) are represented in Figure 1. Patients with appendiceal primary were all BRAF wild type, but were split between KRAS wild type (40%) and KRAS mutant (40%). The analysis was reported as "indeterminate KRAS" for 1 patient (20%). Patients with colon primary had more variation in their mutations with the most common mutation being BRAF mutated with KRAS wild type (40%) vs. 20% with BRAF wild type–KRAS wild type vs. 20% BRAF wild type–KRAS mutant. Of two patients who did not have BRAF mutation analysis performed, one was KRAS mutant.

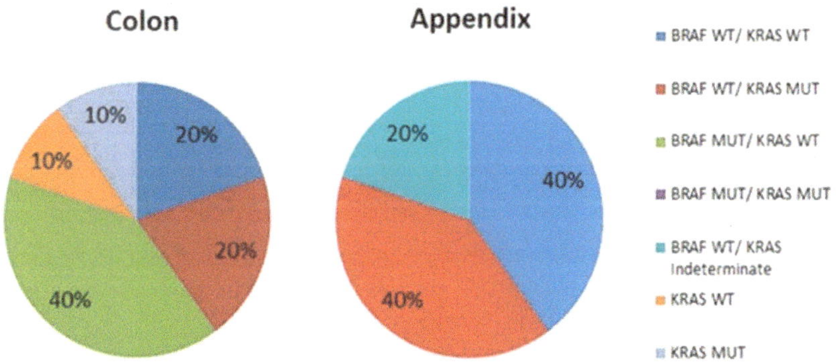

Figure 1: Mutational analysis of peritoneal metastases from colon and appendix primaries. WT, wild type; MUT, mutated.

Survival

The results of survival analysis are described in Table 3. When biomarkers of interest were compared with survival data, COX-2 was the only biomarker that significantly impacted survival (expression associated with a hazards ratio of 0.06, p-value = 0.02). SPARC (Poly) expression also showed trends toward survival benefit (hazards ratio 0.15, p-value = 0.08).

Table 3: Unadjusted survival analysis stratified by biomarkers identified in immunohistochemistry (IHC)

Biomarker	Hazards ratio (95% CI)	p-value
COX-2	0.06 (0.005–0.71)	0.02
RRM1	0.26 (0.04–1.57)	0.14
SPARC (Poly)	0.15 (0.02–1.3)	0.08
TS	1.00	1.00

COX-2, cyclooxygenase-2; RRM1, ribonucleotide reductase M1; SPARC, secreted protein acidic cysteine-rich; TS, thymidylate synthase.

DISCUSSION

Use of a commercial molecular profiling service can yield significant information toward the understanding of biology and treatment response of PM in patients with appendiceal or colorectal primaries. While concerns of mucinous disease interfering with the test exist, we found that majority of the patients were able to successfully undergo IHC evaluation of their samples, although microarray could not be performed in some.

Previous studies have revealed that the phenotypes could be clustered based on the gene expression profile. Levine et al. reported gene expression profiling in 41 samples of patients with PM of appendiceal and colorectal origin and showed that the two groups were genomically different with impact on survival (8). They identified 3 different phenotype clusters with the following results: high risk colorectal cancer group with worst prognosis (0% 5 years OS), high- and low-risk appendiceal subgroups (25 and 70% 10-year OS, respectively) (8).

The important role of BRAF/KRAS mutations in the tumorogenesis pathway has been well elucidated (11, 23). Chan et al. showed higher prevalence of BRAF or KRAS mutations (90%) in serrated polyps with dysplasia compared to polyps without dysplasia (54%), thereby suggesting a role in malignant transformation (23). Some authors failed to show increased prevalence of BRAF mutations in dysplastic specimens compared to non-dysplastic serrated polyps and have argued that these mutations were associated with serrated morphology rather than malignant transformation (11, 24). Mutations in KRAS have been associated with metastatic colorectal cancer including peritoneal dissemination with implications for therapy (12, 25–27). Mutations in BRAF are involved in sporadic colorectal tumorigenesis with proclivity to develop PM, as well as poor survival outcomes compared to those with KRAS mutations (13, 14).

In attempting to understand the profile of these tumors, the high proportion of BRAF mutated tumors in the colorectal primary patients with PM is remarkable. Increasing evidence suggests that the phenotype of BRAF mutated tumors presents with PM, and aggressive biology, which is what we found in this small cohort of patients (13, 14). Distinct in their genetic code, appendiceal tumors did not express BRAF mutations, which confirm a distinct origin from their counterparts, as suggested by other authors as well (28, 29). Our study confirmed the high prevalence of KRAS mutations (40%) in patients with appendiceal primaries, which are similar to previous studies in which one found 45% with KRAS mutations and another 91% with KRAS mutations among those patients with appendiceal primaries with PM (30). We did not encounter patients that exhibited both BRAF and KRAS mutations simultaneously, which is also consistent with previous reports (15).

There is a possible survival benefit for patients with COX-2 expression especially in the setting of PM, which may lend credence to the use of aspirin or other NSAIDs in the management of patients with peritoneal carcinomatosis. Although previous studies have identified the benefit of COX inhibitors in the treatment and prevention of colorectal cancer, these data have not included disease with PM (18, 19). Molecular studies on appendiceal adenocarcinoma also revealed increased expression of COX-2 but failed to identify a prognostic value or therapeutic benefit with targeted therapy (20). In light of this, more data would need to be collected to analyze the effect COX inhibitors on PM with high COX-2 expression.

The purpose of molecular profiling is to guide therapies. Appendiceal cancer is a rare primary and molecular profiling of this histological subtype could be extremely useful when dealing with high grade disease to determine potential molecular targets. We were limited in our analysis due to our small sample size of 16 and also the insufficient sample for more than half of our patients (56%) to have microarray analysis performed. In this study, microarray analysis was limited by the amount of tumor biopsied as well as by the mucinous content of the tumor. While this sample may be too small and therefore underpowered to detect potential targets for intervention, it does demonstrate the feasibility of this novel technique for patients with PM. It is noteworthy to point out that we were able capture variations in the expression of molecular markers and trends in survival benefit despite the small size.

CONCLUSION

Immunohistochemistry and mutational analysis using commercially available molecular profiling testing is feasible for patients undergoing surgery for their PM, although mucin content might interfere with microarray analysis. BRAF mutations and COX-2 expression deserve further investigation in the prognostication and management of patients with colorectal and appendiceal primaries.

Conflict of Interest Statement

Dr. Kiran K. Turaga has received honorarium from Castle Life Sciences. The other authors have no disclosures to make. Dr. Joanne Xiu from CARIS Life Sciences assisted with manuscript review to verify accuracy of the methods of the techniques used for IHC and microarray analysis. There was no financial conflict of interest between the company and the authors of the manuscript.

ACKNOWLEDGMENTS

We would like to acknowledge the role of Dr. Joanne Xiu, PhD from CARIS Life Sciences who assisted with review of the methods of the study to verify accuracy of the technique. Role of Funding Source: This study was supported by the Sebastian Raclaw Abdominal Cancer Fund. The study sponsor had no involvement in the study.

REFERENCES

1. Duffy MJ, Crown J. Precision treatment for cancer: role of prognostic and predictive markers. Crit Rev Clin Lab Sci (2014) 51:30–45. doi:10.3109/10408363.2013.865700

2. Thunnissen E, van der Oord K, den Bakker M. Prognostic and predictive biomarkers in lung cancer. A review. Virchows Arch (2014) 464(3):347–58. doi:10.1007/s00428-014-1535-4

3. Toon CW, Chou A, Clarkson A, DeSilva K, Houang M, Chan JC, et al. Immunohistochemistry for myc predicts

survival in colorectal cancer. PLoS One (2014) 9:e87456. doi:10.1371/journal.pone.0087456

4. Luo RZ, Cai PQ, Li M, Fu J, Zhang ZY, Chen JW, et al. Decreased expression of PTPN12 correlates with tumor recurrence and poor survival of patients with hepatocellular carcinoma. PLoS One (2014) 9:e85592. doi:10.1371/journal. pone.0085592

5. Kleivi K, Lind GE, Diep CB, Meling GI, Brandal LT, Nesland JM, et al. Gene expression profiles of primary colorectal carcinomas, liver metastases, and carcinomatoses. Mol Cancer (2007) 6:2. doi:10.1186/1476-4598-6-2

6. Takeno A, Takemasa I, Seno S, Yamasaki M, Motoori M, Miyata H, et al. Gene expression profile prospectively predicts peritoneal relapse after curative surgery of gastric cancer. Ann Surg Oncol (2010) 17:1033–42. doi:10.1245/s10434-009- 0854-1

7. Takei Y, Takigahira M, Mihara K, Tarumi Y, Yanagihara K. The metastasisassociated microRNA miR-516a-3p is a novel therapeutic target for inhibiting peritoneal dissemination of human scirrhous gastric cancer. Cancer Res (2011) 71:1442–53. doi:10.1158/0008-5472.CAN-10-2530

8. Levine EA, Blazer DG III, Kim MK, Shen P, Stewart JH IV, Guy C, et al. Gene expression profiling of peritoneal metastases from appendiceal and colon cancer demonstrates unique biologic signatures and predicts patient outcomes. J Am Coll Surg (2012) 214:599–606. doi:10.1016/j.jamcollsurg.2011.12.028

9. Logan-Collins JM, Lowy AM, Robinson-Smith TM, Kumar S, Sussman JJ, James LE, et al. VEGF expression predicts survival in patients with peritoneal surface metastases from mucinous adenocarcinoma of the appendix and colon. Ann Surg Oncol (2008) 15:738–44. doi:10.1245/s10434-007-9699-7

10. Jimenez WA, Sardi A, Ledakis P, Nieroda C, Sittig M, Gushchin V. The role of VEGFR-2 expression in outcomes and survival of patients with peritoneal carcinomatosis from appendiceal cancer. Eur J Surg Oncol (2013) 39:1415–22. doi:10.1016/j.ejso.2013.08.032

11. Giehl K. Oncogenic Ras in tumour progression and metastasis. Biol Chem (2005) 386:193–205. doi:10.1515/BC.2005.025

12. Miranda E, Destro A, Malesci A, Balladore E, Bianchi P, Baryshnikova E, et al. Genetic and epigenetic changes in primary metastatic and nonmetastatic colorectal cancer. Br J Cancer (2006) 95:1101–7. doi:10.1038/sj.bjc.6603337

13. Yokota T, Ura T, Shibata N, Takahari D, Shitara K, Nomura M, et al. BRAF mutation is a powerful prognostic factor in advanced and recurrent colorectal cancer. Br J Cancer (2011) 104:856–62. doi:10.1038/bjc.2011.19

14. Domingo E, Niessen RC, Oliveira C, Alhopuro P, Moutinho C, Espín E, et al. BRAF-V600E is not involved in the colorectal tumorigenesis of HNPCC in patients with functional MLH1 and MSH2 genes. Oncogene (2005) 24:3995–8. doi:10.1038/sj.onc.1208569

15. Rajagopalan H, Bardelli A, Lengauer C, Kinzler KW, Vogelstein B, Velculescu VE. Tumorigenesis: RAF/RAS oncogenes and mismatch-repair status. Nature (2002) 418:934. doi:10.1038/418934a

16. Eberhart CE, Coffey RJ, Radhika A, Giardiello FM, Ferrenbach S, DuBois RN. Up-regulation of cyclooxygenase 2 gene expression in human colorectal adenomas and adenocarcinomas. Gastroenterology (1994) 107:1183–8.

17. DuBois RN, Radhika A, Reddy BS, Entingh AJ. Increased cyclooxygenase- 2 levels in carcinogen-induced rat colonic tumors. Gastroenterology (1996) 110:1259–62. doi:10.1053/gast.1996.v110.pm8613017

18. Chan AT, Ogino S, Fuchs CS. Aspirin use and survival after diagnosis of colorectal cancer. JAMA (2009) 302:649–58. doi:10.1001/jama.2009.1825

19. Chan AT, Ogino S, Fuchs CS. Aspirin and the risk of colorectal cancer in relation to the expression of COX-2. N Engl J Med (2007) 356:2131–42. doi:10.1056/NEJMoa067208

20. Raghav KP, Shetty AV, Kazmi SM, Zhang N, Morris J, Taggart M, et al. Impact of molecular alterations and targeted therapy in appendiceal adenocarcinomas. Oncologist (2013) 18:1270–7. doi:10.1634/theoncologist.2013-0186

21. Von Hoff DD, Stephenson JJ Jr., Rosen P, Loesch DM, Borad MJ, Anthony S, et al. Pilot study using molecular profiling of patients' tumors to find potential targets and select treatments for their refractory cancers. J Clin Oncol (2010) 28:4877–83. doi:10.1200/JCO.2009.26.5983

22. Turaga K, Levine E, Barone R, Sticca R, Petrelli N, Lambert L, et al. Consensus guidelines from the American society of peritoneal surface malignancies on standardizing the delivery of hyperthermic intraperitoneal chemotherapy (HIPEC) in colorectal cancer patients in the United States. Ann Surg Oncol (2014) 21(5):1501–5. doi:10.1245/s10434-013-3061-z

23. Chan TL, Zhao W, Leung SY, Yuen ST. Cancer Genome Project. BRAF and KRAS mutations in colorectal hyperplastic polyps and serrated adenomas. Cancer Res (2003) 63(16):4878–81.

24. Yantiss RK, Panczykowski A, Misdraji J, Hahn HP, Odze RD, Rennert H, et al. A comprehensive study of nondysplastic and dysplastic serrated polyps of the vermiform appendix. Am J Surg Pathol (2007) 31(11):1742–53. doi:10.1097/PAS. 0b013e31806bee6d

25. Kumar SS, Price TJ, Mohyieldin O, Borg M, Townsend A, Hardingham JE. KRAS G13D mutation and sensitivity to cetuximab or panitumumab in a colorectal cancer cell line model. Gastrointest Cancer Res (2014) 7:23–6.

26. Lin YL, Liang YH, Tsai JH, Liau JY, Liang JT, Lin BR, et al. Oxaliplatin-based chemotherapy is more beneficial in KRAS mutant than in KRAS wild-type metastatic colorectal cancer patients. PLoS One (2014) 9:e86789. doi:10.1371/ journal.pone.0086789

27. Lee J, Hong YS, Hong JY, Han SW, Kim TW, Kang HJ, et al. Effect of simvastatin plus cetuximab/irinotecan for KRAS mutant colorectal cancer and predictive value of the RAS signature for treatment response to cetuximab.

Invest New Drugs (2014) 32(3):535–41. doi:10.1007/s10637-014-0065-x

28. Pai RK, Hartman DJ, Gonzalo DH, Lai KK, Downs-Kelly E, Goldblum JR, et al. Serrated lesions of the appendix frequently harbor KRAS mutations and not BRAF mutations indicating a distinctly different serrated neoplastic pathway in the appendix. Hum Pathol (2014) 45:227–35. doi:10.1016/j.humpath.2013.10. 021

29. Taggart MW, Galbincea J, Mansfield PF, Fournier KF, Royal RE, Overman MJ, et al. High-level microsatellite instability in appendiceal carcinomas. Am J Surg Pathol (2013) 37:1192–200. doi:10.1097/PAS.0b013e318282649b

30. Lilleberg SL, Foster JM, Sharma P, et al. Use of mutation analysis of pseudomyxoma peritonei and appendiceal adenocarcinomas to identify somatic variants within MAPK, AKT and WNT signaling pathways: potential markers for focused treatment strategies. Gastrointestinal Cancers Symposium. San Francisco, CA: American Society of Clinical Oncology (ASCO) (2009).

CHAPTER 4

IMMUNOHISTOCHEMICAL ANALYSIS

Naoya Maekawa, Satoru Konnai, Tomohiro Okagawa, Asami Nishimori, Ryoyo Ikebuchi, Yusuke Izumi, Satoshi Takagi, Yumiko Kagawa, Chie Nakajima, Yasuhiko Suzuki, Yukinari Kato, Shiro Murata, Kazuhiko Ohashi

INTRODUCTION

Dogs often develop spontaneous cancers, which may cause death [1] or reduce the quality of life of the patients. Among malignant cancers, lymphoma, mast cell tumor (MCT), osteosarcoma (OS), soft tissue sarcoma, and mammary carcinoma are relatively frequent [2,3] and often recognized as fatal diseases in clinical settings. Oral melanoma and hemangiosarcoma (HSA) are also common malignancies in dogs, and patient dogs with these types of cancer usually have poor prognosis [4,5]. The standards of care for each cancer type have been established and successfully improved the prognosis; however, the treatment outcomes are not always satisfying because of the low-to-moderate response rates or limited prolongation of survival times.

Immunotherapies have potential as novel treatment options for cancer. Among those, immune checkpoint inhibitors such as anti-programmed death 1 (PD-1) and anti-PD-ligand 1 (PD-L1) antibodies showed promising effects on several malignancies in humans [6,7]. The immune checkpoint molecule PD-1 is a CD28-family receptor, which suppresses immune responses. PD-1 on T cells negatively regulates T cell receptor signaling and inhibits the induction of cytokines such as interferon gamma (IFN-γ), interleukin 2, and tumor necrosis factor alpha as well as cell proliferation, allowing the maintenance of peripheral tolerance or the persistence of certain pathogens in the host [8]. Two ligands for PD-1 have been reported: PD-ligand 1 (PD-L1) and PD-L2. PD-L2 expression is restricted to certain types of cells or tissues, such as macrophages and dendritic cells, whereas PD-L1 expression can be induced in a wide variety of cell types, including non-hematopoietic cells. PD-L1 expression is not found in most normal tissues; however, its expression is reported in various tumor cells [9,10] and thus is considered as one of the immune evasion mechanisms for cancer. In renal cell carcinoma, gastric cancer, and other cancer patients, PD-L1 expression is known to be associated with poor prognosis [10–12], indicating that PD-L1 could be an important regulator of the immune system when it fights against cancer. Antibody drugs that target this pathway interfere with binding of PD-L1 to PD-1 and can enhance specific immune responses to tumor cells [13,14], subsequently resulting in the regression of cancer [15]. A number of clinical trials have revealed that objective responses can be obtained with anti-PD-1 or anti-PD-L1 antibodies in patients with malignant cancers, including advanced melanoma, non-small cell lung carcinoma, and renal cell carcinoma [6,7], and accumulating evidence demonstrates the potential of immune checkpoint inhibitors in cancer treatment.

However, there are only few reports on the PD-1/PD-L1 axis in dogs, and its association with diseases remains to be elucidated. Previously, we have reported that PD-L1 is expressed in dog melanoma, MCT, and renal cell carcinoma and that PD-L1 blockade by an anti-PD-L1 antibody enhances IFN-γ production by tumor-infiltrating cells [16]. These results suggest that anti-PD-L1 antibodies may have therapeutic effects on cancers in dogs. In this study, to assess which cancer types could be targeted, PD-L1 expression in dog malignant cancers was further investigated. Here, we show that dog oral melanoma, OS, HSA, MCT, mammary adenocarcinoma, and prostate adenocarcinoma express PD-L1, suggesting that the PD-1/PD-L1 axis could be used as an immune evasion mechanism in these cancers. In support of this hypothesis, PD-1 expression was upregulated on tumor-infiltrating lymphocytes obtained from oral melanoma and hepatic tumors. At least, therapeutic potentials of PD-1/PD-L1 blockers in oral melanoma and other PD-L1-positive cancers deserve further investigation.

Citation: Maekawa N, Konnai S, Okagawa T, Nishimori A, Ikebuchi R, Izumi Y, et al. (2016) Immunohistochemical Analysis. PLoS ONE 11(6): e0157176. doi:10.1371/journal. pone.0157176.

MATERIALS AND METHODS

Canine Samples

Animal use throughout this study was approved by the Institutional Animal Care and Use Committee (the serial number of approval was #15–0149), Hokkaido University. No animal was sacrificed for the purpose of this study. Clinical samples of dog tumor tissues were surgically excised at the Veterinary Teaching Hospital, Graduate School of Veterinary Medicine, Hokkaido University and at Veterinary Hospitals in Sapporo city in 2014–2015. Upon the use for this study, informed consent was obtained from all owners of the dogs. Peripheral blood samples of clinically healthy dogs were collected from beagles at the age of 12–15 years kept at the Experimental Animal Facility, Graduate School of Veterinary Medicine, Hokkaido University.

Flow Cytometry

To assess the binding specificity of a recently established anti-PD-L1 monoclonal antibody (mAb) [17], flow cytometric analyses were performed as described previously [16], with some modifications. In brief, canine melanoma cell lines, CMeC and CMM-1, which are PD-L1-negative under normal conditions [16], were transfected with the pEGFP-N2 vector or the pEGFP-N2–cPD-L1 vector [16] using Lipofectamine 2000 (Life Technologies, Carlsbad, CA, USA) according to the manufacturer's instructions. One day after the transfection, the cells were harvested and stained with anti-PD-L1 mAb 6G7-E1 or an isotype-matched control antibody (rat IgM) (BD Biosciences, San Jose, CA, USA) at a final concentration of 10 μg/mL. After washing, the cells were incubated with an allophycocyanin-conjugated anti-rat Ig antibody (Beckman Coulter, Fullerton, CA, USA). Fluorescence was analyzed by a FACSVerse flow cytometer (BD Biosciences) and the FCS Express 4 software (De Novo Software, Glendale, CA, USA). For transfected cells, enhanced green fluorescent protein (EGFP)-positive cells were gated and used for analysis.

To assess whether PD-1 expression is upregulated in the context of canine cancers, flow cytometric analysis was performed with cross-reactive anti-human PD-1 antibody [18]. Peripheral blood mononuclear cells (PBMCs) and TILs from freshly excised dog tumor tissues were obtained as described previously [16]. All single cell suspensions were prepared by the mechanical method. Cells were stained with the optimal concentrations of FITC-conjugated anti-CD4/PE-conjugated anti-CD8 antibody cocktail (AbD Serotec, Oxford, UK) and biotinylated anti-human PD-1 antibody (R&D Systems, Minneapolis, MN, USA) for 30 min at room temperature (RT). After washing, cells were incubated with Streptavidin APC-eFluor 780 (eBioscience, San Diego, CA, USA) for 30 min at RT. Fluorescence of the cells were analyzed by FACS Verse and FACS Express 4 software. Biotinylated normal goat IgG (R&D systems) was used as an isotype-matched control antibody. For the analysis, lymphocytes population was gated by FSC and SSC and within them PD-1 expression on $CD4^+$ cells or $CD8^+$ cells was evaluated.

Specimens

Specimens were randomly selected from formalin-fixed and paraffin-embedded tissues of dog malignant tumors (110 samples in total), which had been submitted for histological diagnosis and kept in a commercial pathology laboratory (North Lab, Hokkaido, Japan). All the melanoma samples (n = 40) used in this study originated from the oral cavity. The MCT samples (n = 5) were all classified into Patnaik grade III [19]. For mammary adenocarcinoma sample (n = 5) analysis, no inflammatory mammary carcinoma samples were included. In addition to the above-mentioned specimens, OS (n = 10), HSA (n = 10), prostate adenocarcinoma (n = 5), skin squamous cell carcinoma (n = 5), diffuse large B-cell lymphoma (n = 5), nasal adenocarcinoma (n = 5), soft tissue sarcoma (n = 5), histiocytic sarcoma (n = 5), transitional cell carcinoma (n = 5), and anal sac gland carcinoma with metastatic disease (n = 5) specimens were studied by immunohistochemistry.

Immunohistochemistry

Immunohistochemical staining was examined by the avidin–biotin peroxidase complex (ABC) procedure. Sections (4 μm) were dewaxed in xylene and hydrated through graded alcohols. To remove endogenous peroxidase, the sections were immersed in a 3% hydrogen peroxide solution at room temperature for 10 min. Following this, the sections were incubated with anti-PD-L1 antibody 6G7-E1 (10 μg/mL). After washing with phosphate-buffered saline, the sections were incubated in a secondary antibody solution (biotin-labeled goat anti-rat IgM) (Jackson ImmnunoResearch Laboratories, West Grove, PA, USA) at room temperature for 30 min. Following the incubation, the sections were reacted using the ABC in the VECTASTAIN Elite ABC Kit (Vector Laboratories, Burlingame, CA, USA) at room temperature for 30 min. Visualization was accomplished using a 0.05% 3,3′-diaminobenzidine solution. Mayer's hematoxylin stain was used as a counterstain. For the negative control, sections were subjected to the same procedures without the primary antibody or with the rat IgM isotype control antibody (Acris Antibodies, Herford, Germany). The specimen was considered positive for PD-L1 if there was histologic evidence of cell staining. No obvious staining was observed in the negative control sections (S1 Fig). To prepare the OS specimens, decalcification was performed using a standard protocol with Plank–Rychlo's solution. Berlin blue staining was performed to distinguish hemosiderin deposits from positive staining in the HSA samples, when required.

Statistical Analysis

In the flow cytometric analysis of PD-1 expression, Mann–Whitney U test was conducted and $p < 0.05$ was considered to be statistically significant.

RESULTS

Anti-PD-L1 antibody 6G7-E1 specifically binds to dog PD-L1

The anti-PD-L1 antibodies that can bind to dog PD-L1 were established previously [16,17]. Among those, 6G7-E1 showed sufficient binding as determined by immunohistochemistry of formalin-fixed and paraffin-embedded dog tumor sections. To test the specificity of 6G7-E1 in detection of dog PD-L1, we first tried Western blotting analysis of canine PD-L1–rabbit IgG Fc fusion protein [16] as a positive control. However, no binding was observed when 6G7-E1 was used as the primary antibody, while an anti-rabbit IgG Fc antibody detected the specific band (data not shown). Because this result suggests that 6G7-E1 recognizes a specific conformation of dog PD-L1, flow cytometric analysis of the canine melanoma cell lines CMeC and CMM-1 was performed. No binding was observed with the non-transfected or mock (EGFP only)-transfected canine melanoma cells, whereas 6G7-E1 was bound to the cells transfected with canine PD-L1–EGFP (Fig 1), indicating specific binding of 6G7-E1 to dog PD-L1.

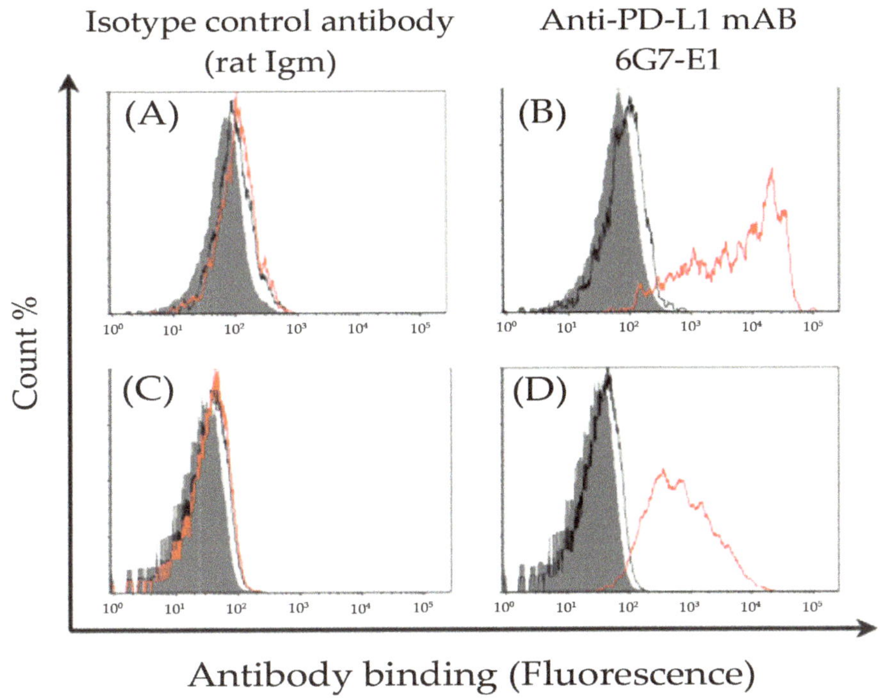

Figure 1: Binding specificity of anti-PD-L1 mAb 6G7-E1.

Canine melanoma cell lines, CMeC and CMM-1, were transfected with the pEGFP-N2 vector (mock) or pEGFP-N2–cPD-L1, and antibody binding was analyzed by a flow cytometer. The shaded area, black line, and red line represent the results for the cells with no treatment, mock-transfected cells, and cPD-L1–EGFP-transfected cells, respectively. (A) Binding of the isotype control antibody to CMeC; (B) binding of 6G7-E1 to CMeC; (C) binding of the isotype control antibody to CMM-1; and (D) binding of 6G7-E1 to CMM-1 are shown in the histograms. No binding of 6G7-E1 was observed in the mock-transfected or untransfected cells, whereas specific binding was observed in the cPD-L1–EGFP-transfected cells.

Canine malignant cancers express PD-L1

Immunohistochemical analysis was performed to detect PD-L1 expression in various malignant cancers. In total, 110 specimens were tested, among which 36 oral melanoma, 7 OS, 6 HSA, 3 grade III MCT, 4 mammary adenocarcinoma, and 3 prostate adenocarcinoma specimens were PD-L1 positive (Figs 2 and 3, and Table 1). Both cytoplasmic staining and cell-surface staining were observed. The rates of PD-L1 expression were 90% (36/40) for oral melanoma, 70% (7/10) for OS, 60% (6/10) for HSA, 60% (3/5) for grade III MCT, 80% (4/5) for mammary adenocarcinoma, and 60% (3/5) for prostate adenocarcinoma (Table 1). The other 7 types of tumors, namely squamous cell carcinoma, diffuse large B-cell lymphoma, nasal adenocarcinoma, soft tissue sarcoma, histiocytic sarcoma, transitional cell carcinoma, and anal sac gland carcinoma did not express PD-L1, although the tested sample size was substantially limited (5 cases for each tumor type).

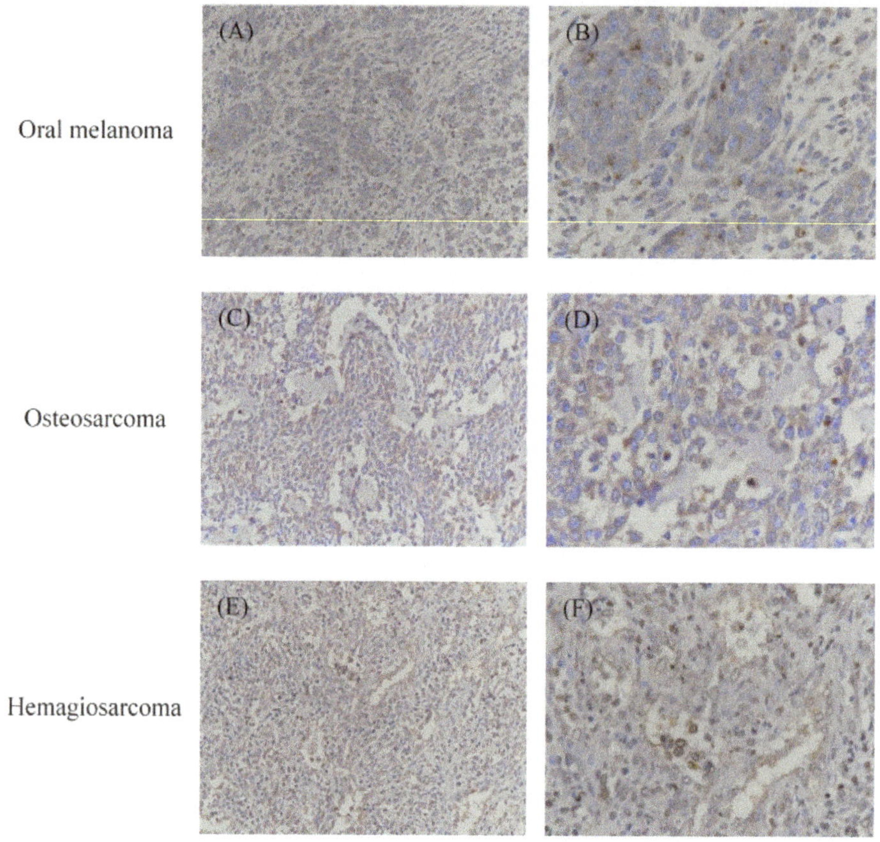

Figure 2: Immunohistochemical analysis of PD-L1 in oral melanoma, osteosarcoma, and hemangiosarcoma.

Formalin-fixed and paraffin-embedded tumor tissues were examined immunohistochemically. The sections were stained with anti-PD-L1 mAb 6G7-E1. Representative positive stainings of (A, B) oral melanoma, (C, D) osteosarcoma, and (E, F) hemangiosarcoma are shown. Original magnification: (A, C, E) 200×; (B, D, F) 400×.

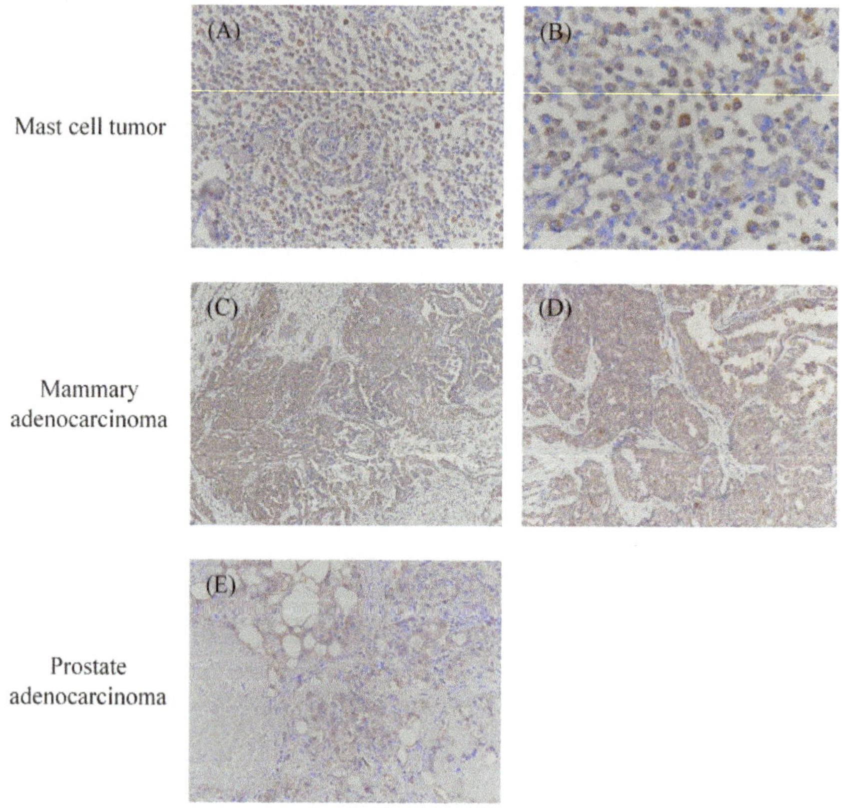

Figure3: Immunohistochemical analysis of PD-L1 in mast cell tumor, mammary adenocarcinoma, and prostate adenocarcinoma.

Formalin-fixed and paraffin-embedded tumor tissues were examined immunohistochemically. The sections were stained with anti-PD-L1 mAb 6G7-E1. Representative positive stainings of (A, B) mast cell tumor, (C, D) mammary adenocarcinoma, and (E, F) prostate adenocarcinoma are shown. Original magnification: (A, D, E) 200×; (B) 400×; (C) 100×.

Table 1: PD-L1 expression in various canine malignant cancers

Pathology	Positive cases/Tested samples
Melanoma (oral)	36/40
Osteosarcoma	7/10
Hemangiosarcoma	6/10
Mast cell tumor (grade III)*	3/5
Mammary adenocarcinoma**	4/5
Prostate adenocarcinoma	3/5
Squamous cell carcinoma (skin)	0/5
Diffuse large B-cell lymphoma	0/5
Nasal adenocarcinoma	0/5
Soft tissue sarcoma	0/5
Histiocytic sarcoma	0/5
Transitional cell carcinoma	0/5
Anal sac gland carcinoma	0/5

The results of immunohistochemical analysis were summarized.

*Grading of mast cell tumor was performed in accordance with the Patnaik grading method [19].

**No inflammatory mammary carcinoma was included in this study.

PD-1 is highly expressed on tumor-infiltrating lymphocytes (TILs) in canine oral melanoma

In order to assess the expression level of PD-1 on tumor-associated lymphocytes, TILs were obtained from surgically excised cancer tissues, and flow cytometric analysis was conducted. Compared to peripheral blood lymphocytes from healthy dogs, PD-1 was highly expressed on both $CD8^+$ and $CD4^+$ TILs from oral melanoma (Fig 4, $p < 0.05$). The positive rate of PD-1 expression on $CD8^+$ or $CD4^+$ TILs was 70.9–96.6% or 80.2–96.8%, respectively (Table 2). In the case of hepatic tumors, more optimal control cells were available; normal tissue-infiltrating lymphocytes (NILs) from the same individuals were used. Both in hepatocellular adenoma and in hepatocellular adenocarcinoma, TILs had higher expression of PD-1 than NILs (S2 Fig), indicating that upregulation of PD-1 expression might be a common phenotype for TILs.

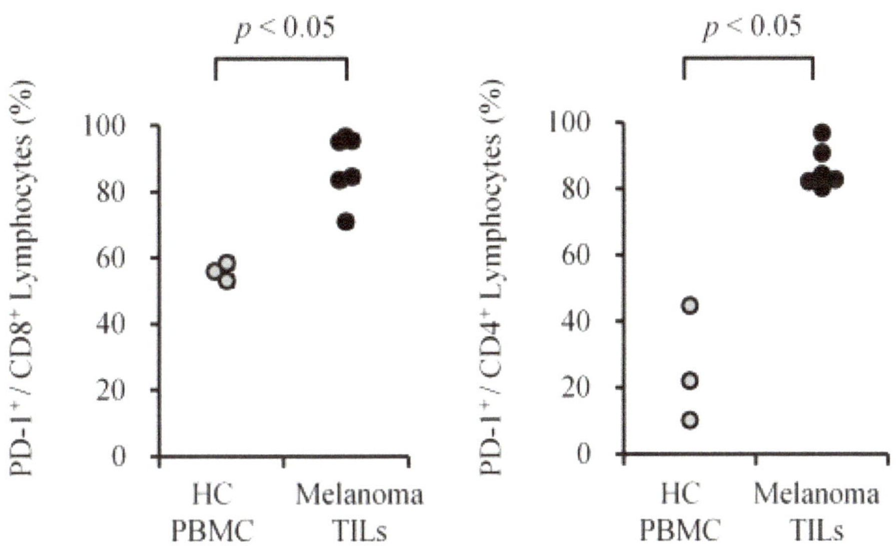

Figure 4: PD-1 expression on tumor-infiltrating lymphocytes (TILs) obtained from oral melanoma. TILs were collected from surgically excised oral melanoma tissues and the expression level of PD-1 was evaluated by flow cytometry. Left panel, PD-1 expression on $CD8^+$lymphocytes. Right panel, PD-1 expression on $CD4^+$ lymphocytes. Peripheral blood mononuclear cells (PBMC) obtained from healthy dogs were used as control (healthy control, HC). $p < 0.05$ was considered statistically significant (Mann–Whitney U test).

Table 2: Oral melanoma samples used in the flow cytometric analysis of PD-1 expression

				PD-1 expression (%)	
Breed	Age	Sex	Site	$CD8^+$	$CD4^+$
American cocker spaniel	12	Male	Maxilla, left	84.4	84.2
Golden retriever	14	Female, spayed	Mandible, left	83.5	82.2
Miniature dachshund	13	Male	Mandible, right	70.9	80.2
Golden retriever	14	Male, castrated	Lip, upper left	95.2	82.7
Chihuahua	13	Female	Maxilla, left	95.1	96.8
Mix	9	Male	Mandible, right	96.6	90.7

Breed of dog, age, sex, tumor site, and positive rate of PD-1 expression (%) on $CD8^+$ or $CD4^+$ lymphocytes were shown in the table.

DISCUSSION

Melanoma is a relatively common type of tumor, which accounts for 7% of all malignant cancers and is the most frequent oral malignancy in dogs [20]. Canine malignant melanoma can occur in the haired skin, oral cavity, nail bed, foot pad, eye, or mucocutaneous junction [20]. Among these forms, oral melanoma is considered a highly malignant cancer because it frequently causes severe local invasion and metastatic disease. Unfortunately, oral melanoma is generally resistant to chemotherapy, making it difficult to treat metastatic lesions, which eventually kill diseased dogs [21]. The absence of effective systemic therapy encourages the development of novel therapeutic modalities, including immunotherapies. In humans, immune checkpoint inhibitors such as anti-PD-1 and anti-PD-L1 antibodies have been used for the treatment of advanced melanoma, showing promising efficacies, with the objective response rates of 28% and 18%, respectively [6,7]. In this study, immunohistochemical analysis demonstrated that as much as 90% (36/40) of dog oral melanoma expressed PD-L1, suggesting that the PD-1/PD-L1 axis is a major mechanism of immune evasion for this form of cancer. This result is well consistent with our previous report, which showed that 100% (8/8) of oral melanoma expressed PD-L1, whereas most melanoma excised from the eye or skin did not express PD-L1 [16]. Moreover, in agreement with these results, PD-1 was highly expressed on both $CD8^+$ and $CD4^+$ TILs obtained from oral melanoma. These TILs seemed functionally exhausted because immunosuppressive motifs, which suppress effector functions of T cells in human and mice, is highly conserved in dog PD-1 [16]. Considering that dog malignant melanoma shares some similarities with human melanoma, inhibitors of the PD-1/PD-L1 axis could also provide therapeutic effects against dog oral melanoma, and dogs could be a good animal model for investigating therapeutic aspects of PD-1/PD-L1 inhibitors against melanoma in clinical studies.

OS is the most common bone cancer in dogs, known for its highly metastatic characteristics. With amputation alone, MST for dogs with OS is only 19 weeks, and approximately 90% of the dogs develop metastatic lesions [22,23]. Therefore, aggressive surgery in combination with systemic chemotherapy has been a standard treatment for canine OS, and new systemic therapies need to be investigated. In humans, anti-PD-L1 antibodies are expected to have therapeutic effects on OS because approximately 75% (12/16) of metastatic OS showed PD-L1 expression. In a mouse model, an anti-PD-L1 antibody improved the function of cytotoxic T lymphocytes and increased the survival of tumor-bearing mice [24]. Because 70% (7/10) of primary OS in dogs were found to express PD-L1, blocking antibodies may also have a therapeutic efficacy against canine OS. However, it may be important to note that, in contrast to its metastatic lesions, no human primary OS expressed PD-L1 [24], whereas dog primary OS expressed PD-L1 at a high rate. The difference in PD-L1 expression should be taken into careful consideration when extrapolating findings from human OS studies to canine OS or vice versa.

Dogs have a relatively high risk for developing HSA [25], which is a malignant cancer originating from vascular endothelial cells. Considering that dog HSA is highly metastatic, adjuvant chemotherapy remains important although it can provide only a modest benefit in survival times [26]. Because angiosarcoma is a rare disease in humans, reports on PD-L1 expression in angiosarcoma have been limited [27,28], and its therapeutic implication has not been well studied. Because PD-L1 expression was found in 60% (6/10) of the dog HSA samples, it is worth investigating the therapeutic potential of PD-1/PD-L1 inhibitors as novel systemic immunotherapies for dog HSA. PD-L1 expression in HSA may share the characteristics of its originating vascular endothelial cells, because vascular endothelial cells express PD-L1 in response to several cytokines such as IFNs [29,30]. It may be reasonable to suggest that HSA utilizes the PD-1/PD-L1 axis as an immune evasion mechanism because PD-L1 on vascular endothelial cells has been reported to negatively regulate $CD8^+$ T-cell responses such as IFN-γ production and cytolytic activity [30].

MCT is the most common cutaneous cancer in dogs, accounting for up to 21% of all canine skin neoplasms [31]. Although the clinical behavior of MCT can vary, histologic grading [19] is widely used and considered to be a reliable prognostic factor for MCT dogs. According to Bostock *et al.*, for high-grade or undifferentiated MCT, MST is only 13 weeks [32] and the metastatic rate is as high as 56 to 96%. In this study, high-grade (Patnaik grade III) MCT was analyzed for PD-L1 expression, and 60% (3/5) of the samples were positively stained. This result is also well consistent with our previous report, in which 66.7% (4/6) of grade III MCTs showed PD-L1 expression [16]. Although some cytotoxic chemotherapy drugs and KIT tyrosine kinase inhibitors such as imatinib and toceranib have been used to treat MCT systemically, immune checkpoint inhibitors targeting the PD-1/PD-L1 axis also have the potential to be included in the treatment of MCT because the emergence of drug resistance is sometimes observed during chemotherapy, including that with KIT inhibitors. Although PD-L1 expression in grade I or II MCT remains to be investigated, PD-L1 expression may be related to the biological behavior of MCT because it drives $CD8^+$ T-cell suppression and facilitates metastasis in mouse cancer models [33]. Further investigations are required to assess whether PD-L1 expression could be used as a prognostic marker for this complicated and heterogeneous cancer.

Mammary gland tumors are the most common neoplasms in sexually intact female dogs, accounting for 70% of all cancer cases in this subpopulation [34]. Among malignant mammary tumors, mammary adenocarcinoma represents a common histopathology, and dogs with mammary adenocarcinoma treated by surgery alone sometimes suffer from a recurrence and/or metastases. Chemotherapy has some benefits for mammary malignancies; however, in many cases it is not curative, and alternative or additional systemic therapies need to be explored. In humans, PD-L1 expression in tumor cells was observed in 34% (15/44) of patients with breast cancer, and its expression was significantly correlated with some important prognostic factors such as the expression of hormone receptors [35]. In dogs, 80% (4/5) of the mammary adenocarcinoma samples expressed PD-L1, although its association with the prognosis remains unclear. A further investigation of the relationship between the expression status of PD-L1 and the prognosis in the case of canine mammary tumors should be conducted, and it is worth to at least evaluate the therapeutic potential of PD-1/PD-L1 inhibitors as novel systemic therapies against this cancer.

Prostate adenocarcinoma is a relatively uncommon disease in male dogs. Although the incidence is low, prostate adenocarcinoma often arises as a clinical problem because local progression and metastases are the common sequelae. At the time of diagnosis, regional and distant metastases can be found in most cases, and MSTs for dogs with no treatment are considered to be less than a month [36]. To date, no consensus for the standard of care has been achieved, and conventional treatments such as surgery, radiation therapy, and chemotherapy are palliative in most dogs. In humans, 50% (8/16) of castration-resistant prostate cancer (CRPC) cases were reported to express PD-L1 [37]; however, none of the CRPC patients who received an anti-PD-1 antibody had an objective response in a clinical trial [6]. No response in the CRPC patients is possibly due to the absence of PD-L1 expression in the tumor tissues, although only a few samples from the enrolled patients were examined and found to be PD-L1-negative [6,38]. In this study, PD-L1 was expressed in 60% (3/5) of the dog prostate adenocarcinoma samples, but its therapeutic implications remain obscure. Further studies of the association of PD-L1 expression with the treatment outcome should be conducted, and dogs could be a powerful animal model for human prostate cancer because dog prostate adenocarcinoma shares some features with human prostate cancer in terms of its spontaneous occurrence, metastatic propensity, and PD-L1 expression.

The other cancers tested in this study did not show any PD-L1 expression. The absence of PD-L1 expression in these tumors may be due to differences in the origin of tumor cells, tumor site, and/or immunologic condition of each cancer. Because the sample size tested in this study was very small, further analysis should be performed before making a conclusion on the expression status of PD-L1 in those cancers. Recently, the regulatory mechanisms of PD-L1 expression in humans have been extensively investigated. One of the mechanism for inducing PD-L1 expression in tumor cells is in response to IFN-γ [9], which is likely produced by immune cells in the tumor microenvironment during antitumor immune responses. Because PD-L1 expression in canine cancer cell lines was induced or enhanced by canine IFN-γ treatment [16], this mechanism is also likely to be involved in the regulation of PD-L1 in dogs. Another mechanism is associated with oncogenic signaling; the loss of the phosphatase and tensin homolog (PTEN) function has been reported to upregulate PD-L1 expression in glioma and triple-negative breast cancer cells [39,40]. In dogs, a mutation and/or loss of PTEN were also reported in melanoma, OS, HSA, and malignant mammary gland tumors [41–44]. This may contribute, at least in part, to the aberrant PD-L1 expression in these cancers in dogs.

To the best of our knowledge, this is the first report of PD-L1 expression in various canine malignant cancers. Expression analysis of PD-L1 has important implications in a clinical application of PD-1/PD-L1 inhibitors in dogs because, in human clinical trials with an anti-PD-1 antibody, PD-L1 expression was reported to be associated with the treatment outcome. The patients with PD-L1-positive tumors had an objective response rate of 36%, while none of the patients with PD-L1-negative tumors had an objective response [6]. Our data provide basic information on the involvement of the PD-1/PD-L1 axis in canine cancer immunology and strongly encourage the development of novel immunotherapies to target the PD-1/PD-L1 pathway in dogs. Because anti-PD-L1 antibodies were shown to have therapeutic potential for canine cancers [16], clinical applications of anti-PD-L1 antibodies deserve further investigation.

Supporting Information

S1 Figure. Representative immunohistochemistry with isotype-matched control antibody. Oral melanoma specimen was stained with rat IgM isotype control antibody. No staining was observed.

Oral melanoma

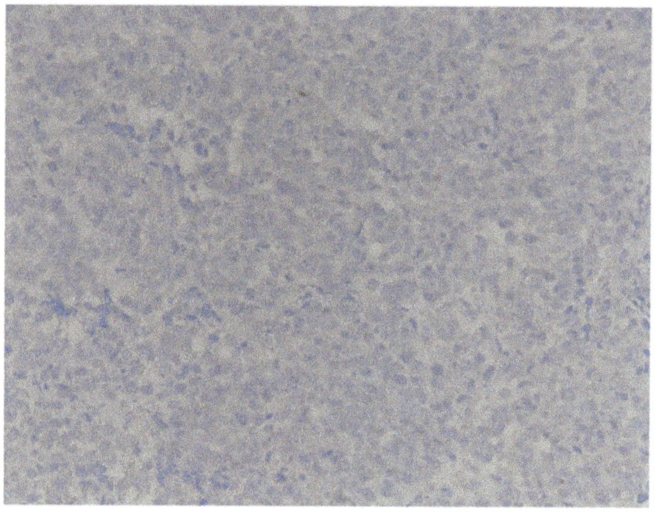

S2 Figure. PD-1 expression on TILs obtained from hepatic tumors. TILs obtained from (A) hepatocellular adenoma and (B) hepatocellular adenocarcinoma were analyzed for PD-1 expression by flow cytometry (red line). Normal tissue-infiltrating lymphocytes (NILs) obtained from adjacent healthy liver tissue of the same individuals (blue line) were used as control. Black line, isotype control for TILs. Shaded area, isotype control for NILs.

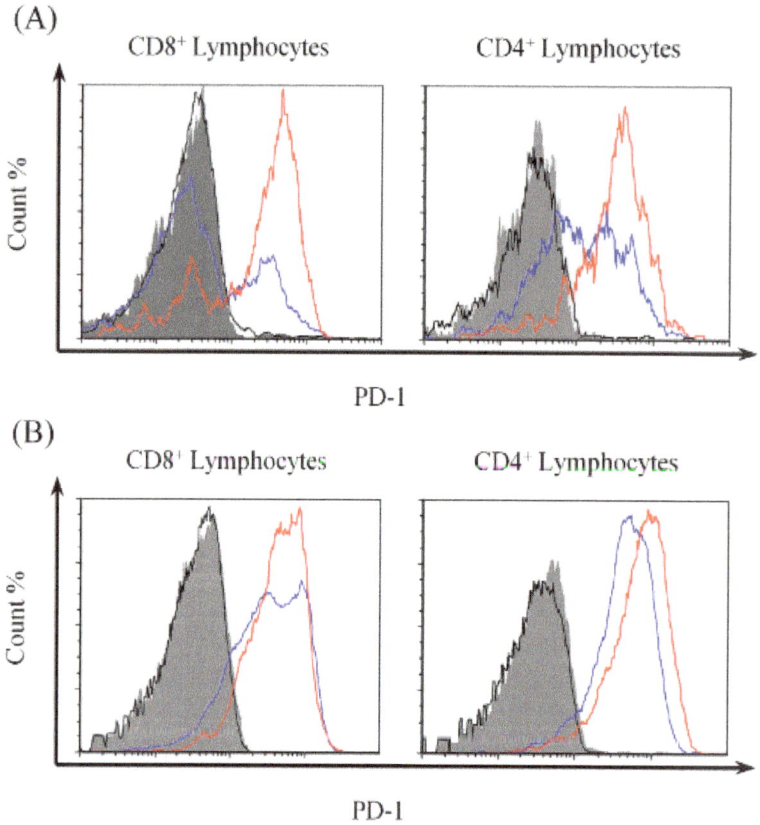

REFERENCES

1. Adams VJ, Evans KM, Sampson J, Wood JLN. Methods and mortality results of a health survey of purebred dogs in the UK. J Small Anim Pract. 2010;51: 512–524. doi: 10.1111/j.1748-5827.2010.00974.x. pmid:21029096
2. Dobson JM, Samuel S, Milstein H, Rogers K, Wood JLN. Canine neoplasia in the UK: estimates of incidence rates from a population of insured dogs. J Small Anim Pract. 2002;43: 240–246. pmid:12074288 doi: 10.1111/j.1748-5827.2002.tb00066.x
3. Bronden LB, Nielsen SS, Toft N, Kristensen AT. Data from the Danish Veterinary Cancer Registry on the occurrence and distribution of neoplasms in dogs in Denmark. Vet Rec. 2010;166: 586–590. doi: 10.1136/vr.b4808. pmid:20453236
4. MacEwen EG, Patnaik AK, Harvey HJ, Hayes AA, Matus R. Canine oral melanoma: comparison of surgery versus surgery plus Corynebacterium parvum. Cancer Invest. 1986;4: 397–402. pmid:3801954 doi: 10.3109/07357908609017520
5. Wood CA, Moore AS, Gliatto JM, Ablin LA, Berg RJ, Rand WM. Prognosis for dogs with stage I or II splenic hemangiosarcoma treated by splenectomy alone: 32 cases (1991–1993). J Am Anim Hosp Assoc. 1998;34: 417–421. pmid:9728473 doi: 10.5326/15473317-34-5-417
6. Topalian SL, Hodi FS, Brahmer JR, Gettinger SN, Smith DC, McDermott DF, et al. Safety, Activity, and Immune Correlates of Anti-PD-1 Antibody in Cancer. N Engl J Med. 2012; 1–12. doi: 10.1056/nejmoa1200690
7. Brahmer JR, Tykodi SS, Chow LQM, Hwu W-J, Topalian SL, Hwu P, et al. Safety and Activity of Anti-PD-L1 Antibody in Patients with Advanced Cancer. N Engl J Med. 2012; 1–11. doi: 10.1056/nejmoa1200694
8. Keir ME, Butte MJ, Freeman GJ, Sharpe AH. PD-1 and Its Ligands in Tolerance and Immunity. Annu Rev Immunol. 2008;26: 677–704. doi: 10.1146/annurev.immunol.26.021607.090331. pmid:18173375
9. Dong H, Strome SE, Salomao DR, Tamura H, Hirano F, Flies DB, et al. Tumor-associated B7-H1 promotes T-cell apoptosis: A potential mechanism of immune evasion. Nat Med. 2002; 793–800. pmid:12091876 doi: 10.1038/nm0902-1039c
10. Sznol M, Chen L. Antagonist Antibodies to PD-1 and B7-H1 (PD-L1) in the Treatment of Advanced Human Cancer. Clin Cancer Res. 2013;19: 1021–1034. doi: 10.1158/1078-0432.CCR-12-2063. pmid:23460533
11. Thompson RH, Kuntz SM, Leibovich BC, Dong H, Lohse CM, Webster WS, et al. Tumor B7-H1 is associated with poor prognosis in renal cell carcinoma patients with long-term follow-up. Cancer Res. 2006;66: 3381–3385. pmid:16585157 doi: 10.1158/0008-5472.can-05-4303
12. Wu C, Zhu Y, Jiang J, Zhao J, Zhang XG, Xu N. Immunohistochemical localization of programmed death-1 ligand-1 (PD-L1) in gastric carcinoma and its clinical significance. Acta Histochem. 2006;108: 19–24. pmid:16530813 doi: 10.1016/j.acthis.2006.01.003
13. Blank C, Kuball J, Voelkl S, Wiendl H, Becker B, Walter B, et al. Blockade of PD-L1 (B7-H1) augments human tumor-specific T cell responses in vitro. Int J Cancer. 2006;119: 317–327. pmid:16482562 doi: 10.1002/ijc.21775
14. Wong RM, Scotland RR, Lau RL, Wang C, Korman AJ, Kast WM, et al. Programmed death-1 blockade enhances expansion and functional capacity of human melanoma antigen-specific CTLs. Int Immunol. 2007;19: 1223–34. pmid:17898045 doi: 10.1093/intimm/dxm091
15. Brahmer JR, Drake CG, Wollner I, Powderly JD, Picus J, Sharfman WH, et al. Phase I study of single-agent anti-programmed death-1 (MDX-1106) in refractory solid tumors: Safety, clinical activity, pharmacodynamics, and immunologic correlates. J Clin Oncol. 2010;28: 3167–3175. doi: 10.1200/JCO.2009.26.7609. pmid:20516446
16. Maekawa N, Konnai S, Ikebuchi R, Okagawa T, Adachi M, Takagi S, et al. Expression of PD-L1 on Canine Tumor Cells and Enhancement of IFN-γ Production from Tumor-Infiltrating Cells by PD-L1 Blockade. PLoS One. 2014;9: e98415. doi: 10.1371/journal.pone.0098415. pmid:24915569
17. Ikebuchi R, Konnai S, Okagawa T, Yokoyama K, Nakajima C, Suzuki Y, et al. Influence of PD-L1 cross-linking on cell death in PD-L1-expressing cell lines and bovine lymphocytes. Immunology. 2014;142: 551–561. doi: 10.1111/imm.12243. pmid:24405267
18. Esch KJ, Juelsgaard R, Martinez PA, Jones DE, Petersen CA. Programmed death 1-mediated T cell exhaustion during visceral leishmaniasis impairs phagocyte function. J Immunol. 2013;191: 5542–5550. doi: 10.4049/jimmunol.1301810. pmid:24154626
19. Patnaik AK, Ehler WJ, MacEwen EG. Canine cutaneous mast cell tumor: morphologic grading and survival time in 83 dogs. Vet Pathol. 1984;21: 469–474. pmid:6435301
20. Smith SH, Goldschmidt MH, McManus PM. A comparative review of melanocytic neoplasms. Vet Pathol. 2002;39: 651–678. pmid:12450197 doi: 10.1354/vp.39-6-651
21. Murphy S, Hayes AM, Blackwood L, Maglennon G, Pattinson H, Sparkes AH. Oral malignant melanoma—the effect of coarse fractionation radiotherapy alone or with adjuvant carboplatin therapy. Vet Comp Oncol. 2005;3: 222–229. doi: 10.1111/j.1476-5810.2005.00082.x. pmid:19754777
22. Spodnick GJ, Berg J, Rand WM, Schelling SH, Couto G, Harvey HJ, et al. Prognosis for dogs with appendicular osteosarcoma treated by amputation alone: 162 cases (1978–1988). J Am Vet Med Assoc. 1992;200: 995–9. pmid:1577656
23. Szewczyk M, Lechowski R, Zabielska K. What do we know about canine osteosarcoma treatment?–review. Vet Res Commun. 2015;39: 61–67. doi: 10.1007/s11259-014-9623-0. pmid:25422073
24. Lussier DM, O'Neill L, Nieves LM, McAfee MS, Holechek SA, Collins AW, et al. Enhanced T-cell immunity to osteosarcoma through antibody blockade of PD-1/PD-L1 interactions. J Immunother. 2015;38: 96–106. doi: 10.1097/CJI.0000000000000065. pmid:25751499

25. MacVean DW, Monlux AW, Anderson PS, Silberg SL, Roszel JF. Frequency of Canine and Feline Tumors in a Defined Population. Vet Pathol. 1978;15: 700–715. pmid:220774 doi: 10.1177/030098587801500602

26. Ogilvie GK, Powers BE, Mallinckrodt CH, Withrow SJ. Surgery and doxorubicin in dogs with hemangiosarcoma. J Vet Intern Med. 1996;10: 379–384. pmid:8947871 doi: 10.1111/j.1939-1676.1996.tb02085.x

27. Kim JR, Moon YJ, Kwon KS, Bae JS, Wagle S, Kim KM, et al. Tumor Infiltrating PD1-Positive Lymphocytes and the Expression of PD-L1 Predict Poor Prognosis of Soft Tissue Sarcomas. PLoS One. 2013;8: e82870. doi: 10.1371/journal.pone.0082870. pmid:24349382

28. D'Angelo SP, Shoushtari AN, Agaram NP, Kuk D, Qin L-X, Carvajal RD, et al. Prevalence of tumor-infiltrating lymphocytes and PD-L1 expression in the soft tissue sarcoma microenvironment. Hum Pathol. Elsevier Inc.; 2015;46: 357–65. doi: 10.1016/j.humpath.2014.11.001. pmid:25540867

29. Eppihimer MJ, Gunn J, Freeman GJ, Greenfield EA, Chernova T, Erickson J, et al. Expression and regulation of the PD-L1 immunoinhibitory molecule on microvascular endothelial cells. Microcirculation. 2002;9: 133–45. pmid:11932780 doi: 10.1038/sj.mn.7800123

30. Rodig N, Ryan T, Allen JA, Pang H, Grabie N, Chernova T, et al. Endothelial expression of PD-L1 and PD-L2 down-regulates CD8+ T cell activation and cytolysis. Eur J Immunol. 2003;33: 3117–26. pmid:14579280 doi: 10.1002/eji.200324270

31. Welle MM, Bley CR, Howard J, Rüfenacht S. Canine mast cell tumours: A review of the pathogenesis, clinical features, pathology and treatment. Vet Dermatol. 2008;19: 321–339. doi: 10.1111/j.1365-3164.2008.00694.x. pmid:18980632

32. Bostock DE, Crocker J, Harris K, Smith P. Nucleolar organiser regions as indicators of post-surgical prognosis in canine spontaneous mast cell tumours. Br J Cancer. 1989;59: 915–8. pmid:2500145 doi: 10.1038/bjc.1989.193

33. Chen L, Gibbons DL, Goswami S, Cortez MA, Ahn Y-H, Byers LA, et al. Metastasis is regulated via microRNA-200/ZEB1 axis control of tumour cell PD-L1 expression and intratumoral immunosuppression. Nat Commun. 2014;5: 5241. doi: 10.1038/ncomms6241. pmid:25348003

34. Merlo DF, Rossi L, Pellegrino C, Ceppi M, Cardellino U, Capurro C, et al. Cancer incidence in pet dogs: findings of the Animal Tumor Registry of Genoa, Italy. J Vet Intern Med. 2008;22: 976–84. doi: 10.1111/j.1939-1676.2008.0133.x. pmid:18564221

35. Ghebeh H, Mohammed S, Al-Omair A, Qattan A, Lehe C, Al-Qudaihi G, et al. The B7-H1 (PD-L1) T lymphocyte-inhibitory molecule is expressed in breast cancer patients with infiltrating ductal carcinoma: correlation with important high-risk prognostic factors. Neoplasia. 2006;8: 190–8. pmid:16611412 doi: 10.1593/neo.05733

36. Sorenmo KU, Goldschmidt MH, Shofer FS, Goldkamp C, Ferracone J. Evaluation of cyclooxygenase-1 and cyclooxygenase-2 expression and the effect of cyclooxygenase inhibitors in canine prostatic carcinoma. Vet Comp Oncol. 2004;2: 13–23. doi: 10.1111/j.1476-5810.2004.00035.x. pmid:19379307

37. Massari F, Ciccaresc C, Caliò A, Munari E, Cima L, Porcaro AB, et al. Magnitude of PD-1, PD-L1 and T Lymphocyte Expression on Tissue from Castration-Resistant Prostate Adenocarcinoma: An Exploratory Analysis. Target Oncol. 2015;[Epub ahead of print]. doi: 10.1007/s11523-015-0396-3

38. Taube JM, Klein AP, Brahmer JR, Xu H, Pan X, Kim JH, et al. Association of PD-1, PD-1 ligands, and other features of the tumor immune microenvironment with response to anti-PD-1 therapy. Clin Cancer Res. 2014;1: 5064–5075. doi: 10.1158/1078-0432.ccr-13-3271

39. Parsa AT, Waldron JS, Panner A, Crane CA, Parney IF, Barry JJ, et al. Loss of tumor suppressor PTEN function increases B7-H1 expression and immunoresistance in glioma. Nat Med. 2007;13: 84–8. pmid:17159987 doi: 10.1038/nm1517

40. Mittendorf EA, Philips AV, Meric-Bernstam F, Qiao N, Wu Y, Harrington S, et al. PD-L1 expression in triple-negative breast cancer. Cancer Immunol Res. 2014;2: 361–70. doi: 10.1158/2326-6066.CIR-13-0127. pmid:24764583

41. Koenig A, Bianco SR, Fosmire S, Wojcieszyn J, Modiano JF. Expression and significance of p53, rb, p21/waf-1, p16/ink-4a, and PTEN tumor suppressors in canine melanoma. Vet Pathol. 2002;39: 458–72. pmid:12126149 doi: 10.1354/vp.39-4-458

42. Levine RA, Forest T, Smith C. Tumor suppressor PTEN is mutated in canine osteosarcoma cell lines and tumors. Vet Pathol. 2002;39: 372–378. pmid:12014501 doi: 10.1354/vp.39-3-372

43. Dickerson EB, Thomas R, Fosmire SP, Lamerato-Kozicki AR, Bianco SR, Wojcieszyn JW, et al. Mutations of phosphatase and tensin homolog deleted from chromosome 10 in canine hemangiosarcoma. Vet Pathol. 2005;42: 618–632. pmid:16145208 doi: 10.1354/vp.42-5-618

44. Kanae Y, Endoh D, Yokota H, Taniyama H, Hayashi M. Tumor Suppressor Gene in Malignant Mammary Gland Tumors of Dogs. Am J Vet Res. 2006;67: 127–133. pmid:16426222 doi: 10.2460/ajvr.67.1.127

CHAPTER 5

"IMMUNOCYTOCHEMISTRY AND FUNCTIONAL FINDINGS IN AN ANIMAL MODEL OF RETINAL DEGENERATION"

Nicolás Cuenca, Laura Fernández-Sánchez, Yves Sauvé, Francisco J. Segura, Gema Martínez-Navarrete, José Manuel Tamarit, Lorena Fuentes-Broto, Ana Sanchez-Cano and Isabel Pinilla

Keywords: Retinal degeneration, retinitis pigmentosa, P23H rat, visual acuity, electroretinogram, optical coherence tomography, autofluorescence, immunohistochemistry

INTRODUCTION

Mutations in the rhodopsin gene are a common cause of retinitis pigmentosa (RP),[1] with P23H being one of the most common autosomal mutations of this gene (Dryja et al., 1990), and accounting for approximately one third of RP cases in the USA (Dryja et al., 2000). The effects of this dominant mutation have been examined, at both anatomical and electrophysiological level (Machida et al., 2000; Cuenca et al., 2004; Pinilla et al., 2005), using the P23H transgenic rat (Lewin et al., 1998). However, these studies have relied on animals bred with an albino background, which is likely to increase the complexity of the retinal degenerative process. The use of pigmented heterozygous P23H animals provides a more precise model to study RP-related retinal degeneration. Furthermore, its slower degeneration rate is more suitable for the development and evaluation of preventive therapeutic approaches. The pigmented background also makes it easier to use functional evaluation tests for visual features such as visual acuity and contrast sensitivity.

The introduction of new optical imaging techniques such as Optical coherence tomography (OCT), a non-invasive method used to examine the retina *in vivo*, changed not only clinical practice, but also research. The fast speed acquiring images of Spectral-Domain OCT (SD-OCT) avoids artifacts and reveals retinal structures with high definition, and 3D visualization in a non-invasive manner. Some animal models had been previously examined with time-domain OCT, but resolution problems were encountered with the use of this technique (Horio et al., 2001; Li et al., 2001). However, SD-OCT has been successfully used to distinguish the retinal layers, with a good correlation with retinal histology in some animal models of retinal degeneration (Fischer et al., 2009; Huber et al., 2009). Clinical devices such as Spectralis OCT (Heidelberg Engineering, Germany), with minor modifications in their acquisition software, have been successfully used to evaluate rodent retinas (Fischer et al., 2009; Huber et al., 2009). The possibility of tracking retinal changes allows retinal degeneration to be monitored over time and therapeutic interventions to be evaluated *in vivo* in the same animal, thus reducing the number of animals required. The system can also be used to evaluate fundus autofluorescence (FAF), a method commonly used in clinical practice to diagnose retinal degeneration, and for angiographic imaging of retinal and choroidal vessels using fluorescein or indocyanine green.

In this study, we used functional and structural tests to study an animal model of RP, the P23H pigmented rat, paying special attention to the usefulness of SD-OCT for the detection of retinal changes in thickness and other features. Furthermore, these results were compared with those provided by immunocytochemistry.

Citation: Cuenca N, Fernández-Sánchez L, Sauvé Y, Segura FJ, Martínez-Navarrete G, Tamarit JM, Fuentes-Broto L, Sanchez-Cano A and Pinilla I (2014) immunocytochemistry and functional findings in an animal model of retinal degeneration. Front. Neuroanat. 8:151. doi: 10.3389/fnana.2014.00151.

MATERIAL AND METHODS

Animals

Male pigmented transgenic rats, heterozygous for the P23H rhodopsin mutation, were bred from a cross between transgenic homozygous P23H Line 1 and normal pigmented Long Evans (LE) rats. The visual performance of the animals was monitored by means of an optomotor test given on a monthly basis ($n = 8$) and full field ERG recordings at P18, P21, P29, P58, P90 and P180 ($n = 4$). SD-OCT was performed at P130. Four normal LE rats crossed with Sprague-Dawley (SD) were used as wild-type controls at age P29. Transgenic rats were obtained from Dr. M. LaVail (UCSF), and bred in a colony at the University of Utah and at the University of Zaragoza, Spain, and maintained under a 12-hour light/dark cycle (light cycle illumination varied from 7 to 30 lux, depending on the front-to-back position within the respective cages). SD rats were obtained from Harlan Laboratories (Barcelona, Spain) and LE rats from Charles River Laboratories (Barcelona, Spain). They were housed and handled with the authorization and supervision of the Institutional Animal Care and Use Committees at both Universities. All procedures were performed in accordance with the ARVO Statement for the Use of Animals in Ophthalmic and Vision Research.

Visual Acuity and Contrast Sensitivity Evaluation

To assess visual parameters, 8 rats were measured at P30, P60, P90, P120, P150 and P180, whereas control wild-type rats were evaluated at P30. The evaluation was carried out using an OptoMotry© system (CerebralMechanics, Lethbridge, Alberta, Canada) (Prusky et al., 2004; Douglas et al., 2005). The device consists of four screens positioned around a square testing chamber. An unrestrained rat is placed on a platform in the center of the square. A virtual cylinder consisting of a sine wave grating is drawn in 3D coordinate space and rotates around the animal, while it is recorded with a video camera. The spatial frequency of the grating is maintained at the viewing position by recentering the cylinder on the rat head. The cylinder is rotated at a constant speed (12°/sec). If the grating is seen by the animal, it tracks the stimulus with reflexive head and neck movements. Spatial frequency thresholds can be measured by systematically increasing the spatial frequency of the grating at 100% contrast until animals no longer track it. This threshold is considered to be maximum visual acuity. A contrast sensitivity curve was generated by identifying the minimum contrast that generates tracking, over a range of spatial frequencies.

Correlation between visual acuity and age was assessed using Pearson's coefficient. Differences in contrast sensitivity between ages were evaluated using a Mann Whitney U test.

Electroretinogram Recordings

Full field ERGs were recorded at P18, P21, P29, P58, P90 and P180, with four animals being studied at each time point. Four normal LE rats crossed with SD were used as wild-type controls at age P29. Following overnight dark adaptation, animals were prepared for recording under dim red light. After being anesthetized with a mixture of ketamine (150 mg/kg i.p.) and xylazine (10 mg/kg i.p.), the animals' head was secured with a stereotaxic head holder and their body temperature was monitored with a rectal thermometer and maintained homoeothermic at 38°C. Pupils were dilated using equal parts of topical phenylephrine (2.5%) and tropicamide (1%). Topical anesthesia with 0.75% bupivacaine was used to prevent any corneal reflexes, and a drop of 0.9% saline was applied regularly to the cornea to prevent dehydration and to allow electrical contact with the recording electrode (gold wire loop). A 25-gauge platinum needle inserted under the scalp between the eyes served as the reference electrode. Amplification (at 1–1000 Hz bandpass, without notch filtering), stimulus presentation and data acquisition were provided by a UTAS-3000 system from LKC Technologies (Gaithersburg, MD).

Mixed b-wave

For quantification of standard dark-adapted b-waves (showing aggregate rod and cone pathway contributions), the stimulus consisted of 3–5 single flash presentations (standard 10-μs duration). For intensity responses, stimuli were presented at sixteen increasing intensities, varying from −3.7 to 2.86 log cds/m^2 in luminance. The effects of rod bleaching, which reduces the b-wave amplitude upon successive flashes, was minimized by increasing inter-stimuli-intervals (ISI), as the stimulus luminance was increased, from 10 s at the lowest stimulus intensity (−3.6 log cds/m^2) up to 2 min at the highest stimulus intensity (1.4 log cds/m^2). The maximum b-wave amplitude was that obtained during the flash intensity series, regardless of the specific stimulus intensity. Criterion amplitudes were established at 20 μV for a- and b-waves. The amplitude of the b-wave was measured from the a-wave negative peak up to the b-wave positive apex, rather than to the peak of oscillations, which can exceed the b-wave apex (Nusinowitz et al., 2001).

Isolation of Cone Response Using a Double Flash Protocol

The double flash protocol was similar to that employed in previous studies (Pinilla et al., 2004). A conditioning flash was followed 1 s later by a probe flash. The role of the conditioning flash in this paradigm is to transiently saturate rods so that they are rendered unresponsive to the probe flash. The intensity of the conditioning flash for complete rod bleaching was set at 1.4 log cds/m^2 for all tests. The response to a probe flash (1.4 log cds/m^2) preceded by the conditioning flash was understood to reflect cone-driven activity. The rod-driven b-wave was obtained by subtracting the trace of the response elicited by the probe from that elicited by the conditioning flash alone. An average of 3–5 traces (set 2 min apart to assure full recovery of rod responsiveness) were usually sufficient to obtain clear responses.

Additional Characterization of Cone Responses Using Photopic Adaptation

After testing as described above, rats were light adapted for 20 min, with a background illumination of 30 cds/m^2 to reach a stable photopic response level. Photopic intensity-responses ranged from −1.6 to 2.9 log cds/m^2 (−1.6, −0.6, 0.4, 1.4, 2.4 and 2.9 log cds/m^2). Flicker responses to white strobe flash presentations with an intensity of 1.36 log cds/m^2 were recorded. Stimuli were presented at 3 Hz, and were then increased in 5

Hz increments from 5 Hz to 50 Hz. When flicker fusion was achieved (3 μV criterion amplitude), the lower frequencies were studied and 60 responses were averaged.

Fundus Imaging System

For comparison with histopathological findings, six eyes from three P23H pigmented rats at P130 and four control rats were studied using a Spectralis HRA-OCT device. Rats were anesthetized by i.p. injection of a mixture of xylazine (10 mg/kg) and ketamine (90 mg/kg), and their pupils were dilated with tropicamide (Tropicamida®, Alcon labs, Barcelona, Spain). In order to improve the image acquisition quality, the rats wore a PMMA afocal contact lens, purchased from Cantoor Nissel (Market Place Brackley, Northamptonshire, UK). Tear substitutive drops were continuously added to improve transparence (Systane®, Alcon Labs, Barcelona, Spain). For examination, the animal was anesthetized using the same anesthetic mixture used for ERG recording, and placed on a platform mounted in the chin rest of the imaging device, with the eye in front of the system, so that the optic nerve could be easily visualized. A heat mat was used to keep the animals warm during the acquisition process.

Combined confocal scanning laser ophthalmoscopy (cSLO) and SD-OCT imaging was performed using a commercially available device (Spectralis HRA OCT system, Spectralis Eye Explorer 5.6b, Heidelberg Engineering, Heidelberg Germany). To adapt the system to the rat eye, a commercially available +25D lens was fit to the system (Heidelberg lens, HE 50744), and the length of the reference pathway was manually adapted according to the manufacturer's instructions. The cSLO system used was an HRA2, using solid source for 488 and 514 nm and an infrared diode laser for 785 and 815 wavelengths. The protocol was always centered on the optic nerve. To evaluate the different thicknesses, one researcher (IP) manually changed the segmentation lines after acquisition. Values were obtained for total retinal thickness, Outer Nuclear Layer (ONL) + Retinal Pigment Epithelium (RPE) thickness, ONL thickness and Inner Plexiform Layer (IPL) thickness. Peripheral areas were used to assess intraindividual differences between superior and inferior retina thickness and temporal and nasal values. The mean values of all square areas, except those surrounding the optic nerve, were compared to evaluate differences between groups using a t test. These mean values were provided by the protocol used for the examination (Spectralis posterior pole protocol) using the optic nerve as the fixation position.

From each animal, a total of 5 single thickness profiles of the posterior map analysis were separately measured: crossing the optic nerve (section 31/61), middle upper (section 45/61) and upper (section 61/61), and middle lower (section 15/61) and lower (section 1/61). Thickness in each profile was measured at positions every 0.5 mm and compared between groups.

To acquire FAF images, fluorescence was excited using laser diodes at 488 nm and recorded between 500 and 700 nm. Fluorescein angiography was performed injecting 0.1 ml of 10% sodium fluorescein intraperitoneally.

Immunostaining

Animals were euthanized with CO_2 at P21, P40, P58, P90, P120 and P180, and their eyes were then enucleated. The eyecups were fixed in 4% paraformaldehyde in 0.1 M PBS at pH 7.4 for 1 h, and then washed in 0.1 M PBS before being cryoprotected in 10% sucrose for 1 h, 20% sucrose for 1 h and 30% sucrose overnight at 4°C. The next day, they were embedded in OCT medium and 10-μm thick retinal sections were cut on a cryostat in a horizontal plane and mounted on glass slides. Sections were treated for immunostaining as previously described (Cuenca et al., 2004), using the primary antibodies shown in Table 1. Slides were then mounted in watermount (Vector Labs) and coverslipped for viewing by means of confocal microscopy (Leica TCS SP2 Confocal System). Pinholes measured 77 μm and the widths of optical sections were 0.9 μm. Final images were obtained from the projections of 4–7 single frames. To control for non-specific staining, some sections were stained omitting the primary antibody.

Table 1: Primary antibodies

Molecular marker (Initials)	Antibody	Source and catalog number	Working dilution
Bassoon	Mouse monoclonal	Stressgen (VAM-PS003)	1:1000
Calbindin D-28K (CB)	Rabbit polyclonal	Swant (CB-38a)	1:500
Protein kinase C, α isoform (PKCα)	Rabbit polyclonal	Santa Cruz Biotechnology (sc-10800)	1:100
Rhodopsin (Rho)	Rabbit polyclonal	Chemicon-Millipore, #AB9279 (Temecula, CA, USA)	1:200
Transducin, Gαc subunit (Gt)	Rabbit polyclonal	Cytosignal (PAB-00801-G)	1:200
Recoverin	Mouse monoclonal	J. F. McGinnis, University of Oklahoma (Oklahoma City, OK, USA	1 :1000

Relationship between OCT and Immunochemistry Measurements

For comparing the OCT and immunochemistry findings, four control and six P23H rat sections were measured at P120 to correlate the thickness of the different layers. The measurements for the histology sections were taken in the central area, close to the optic nerve in 8 retinal sections. The OCT measurements were made in the central retina with the values obtained previously described. ImageJ software (National Institutes of Health, Bethesda, MD, USA) was used for the morphometric analysis of confocal images. Results were analyzed by GraphPad Prism (GraphPad Software, Inc. La Jolla, CA 92037 USA). After checking for normal distribution using the Kolmogorov Smirnov test, a two-tailed Student's *t*-test was performed to compare the OCT with immunohistochemistry measurements. *P* values equal to or less than 0.01 were considered to be statistically significant.

RESULTS

Visual Acuity and Contrast Sensitivity Evaluation

Visual acuity for control rats was 0.54 cyc/deg. A progressive visual acuity loss with age was observed in P23H (Figure 1A), with values of 0.500 cyc/deg at P30, 0.459 cyc/deg at P60, 0.382 cyc/deg at P90, 0.285 cyc/deg at P120, 0.253 cyc/deg at P150 and 0.182 cyc/deg at P180. This decline in visual acuity was well fit by a linear regression model, with a Pearson R^2 value of 0.9903. The same trend was observed for the contrast sensitivity curve (Figure 1B). Peaks of 54.56 (P30), 50.30 (P60), 35.82 (P90), 22.04 (P120), 10.69 (P150) and 2.98 (P180) were obtained for a spatial frequency of 0.089 cycles/deg. The control rat value for this spatial frequency was 56.15.

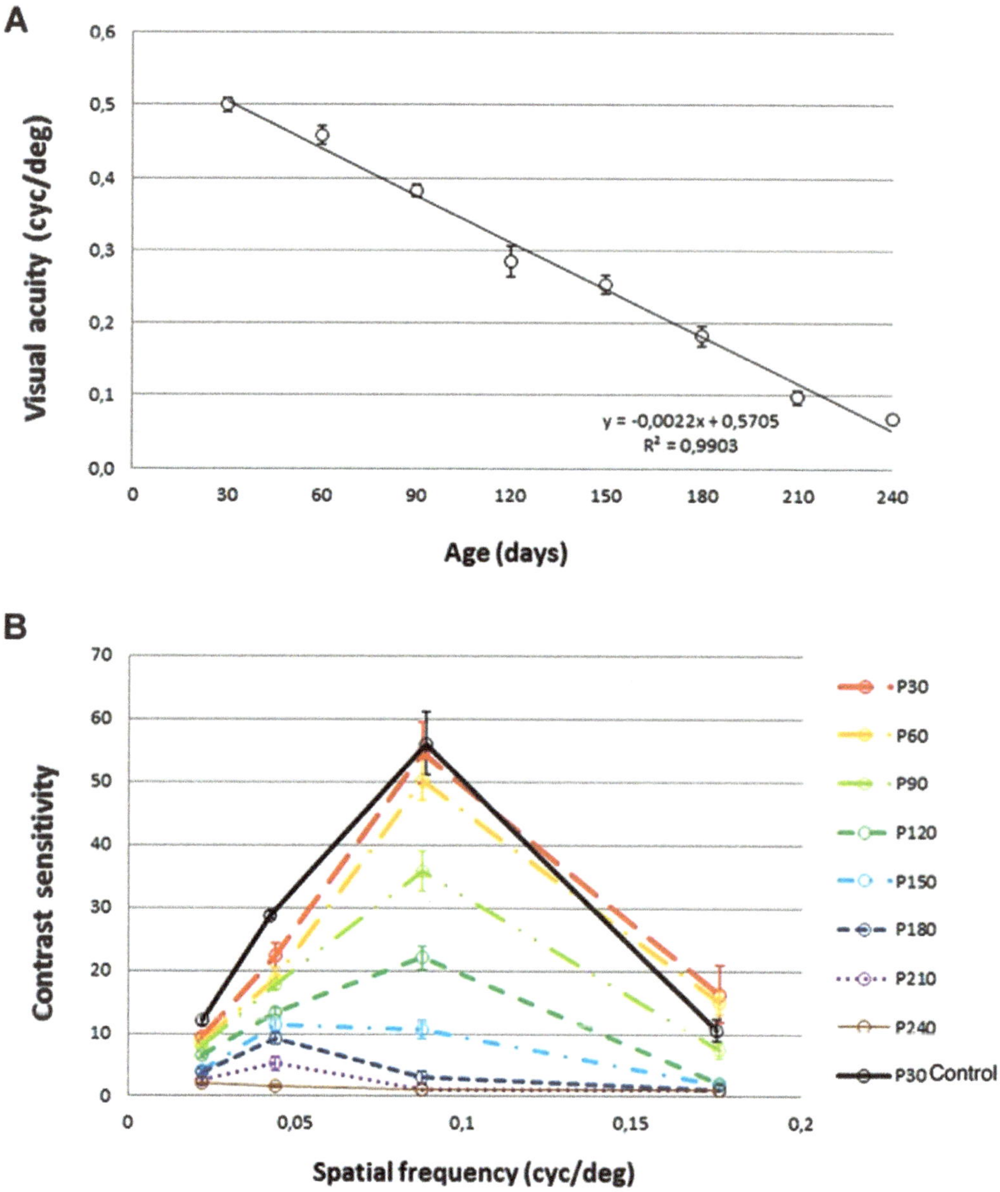

Figure 1: Visual acuity (A) and contrast sensitivity (B) from rats aged 30 days to 240 days. Values are compared to those of normal LExSD rats. Each point represents the mean value of 8 rats. Euthanization for histology limited the data at 150, 180, 210 and 240 days to 7 rats. Vertical bars represent the SEM. **(A)** Linear fit: Visual acuity = −0.0022 × age + 0.5705, R^2 = 0.9903.

Both the visual acuity and contrast sensitivity parameters began to decline at 30 days of age, and continued this trend throughout all the time points studied until the end of the experiment, when some degree of visual acuity still remained.

ERG Results

Scotopic a-waves were already reduced in amplitude at P18, achieving maximal values of 223 ± 27 µV (Figure 2A). Instead of increasing from P18 to P29, as would be expected (Dembinska et al., 2002) a-wave amplitudes reached a maximum of 206 ± 11 µV at age P29. This value amounted to only 34% of the corresponding value in wild-type LExSD rats aged P29 (604 ± 45 µV). Despite being affected at early time points, a-waves from pigmented P23H rats could still be elicited up to P180, the latest time points studied (Figure 2A).

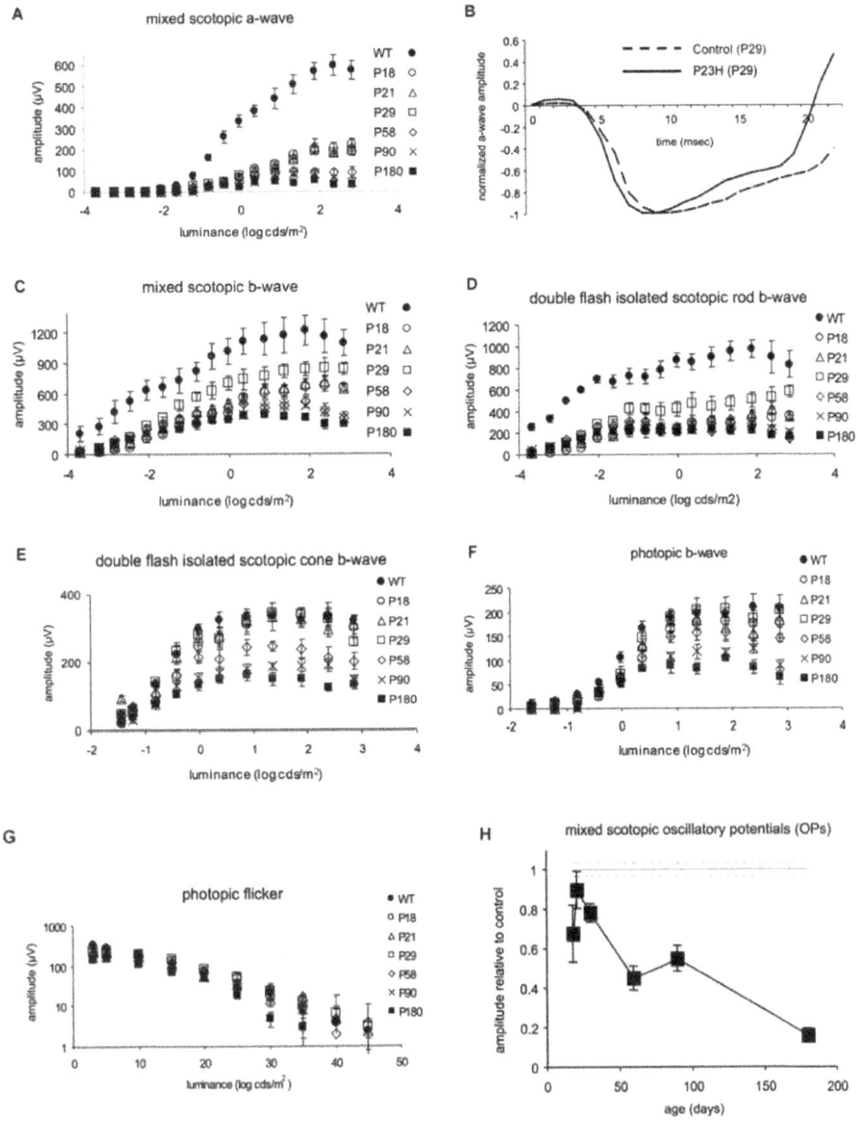

Figure 2: Functional comparison by ERG between pigmented P23H L-1 and control rats. **(A)** ERG amplitude *vs.* flash intensity (V-log I) series of mixed scotopic a-waves from LExSD and P23H rats. **(B)** Example of a-waves recorded at age P29 in normal (dotted line) and P23H (continuous line) rats. Amplitude values are normalized with respect to the maximal amplitudes; absolute amplitudes were 540 µV and 159 µV in normal rats and P23H rats, respectively. Stimulus luminance: 0.38 log cds/m^2. **(C, D)** ERG amplitude vs. flash intensity (V-log I) series of mixed scotopic b-waves (panel **C**) and double flash isolated scotopic rod b-waves (panel **D**) Amplitudes increased from P18 to P29 in P23H rats and subsequently decreased in P23H rats with increasing age. **(E, F)** ERG amplitude vs. flash intensity (V-log I) series of cone b-waves recorded under scotopic (panel **E**) and photopic (panel **F**) adaptation. In P23H rats, amplitudes reached LExSD values from P18 to P29, and then progressively declined. **(G)** Amplitude of the flicker ERG response as a function of stimulus frequency for LExSD rats and P23H rats. Flicker amplitudes and fusions reached LE values at P29, and then dropped very slowly until P180 **(H)** Mixed scotopic OPs Values are expressed as percentage of P23H OP amplitude values relative to the average values in LExSD rats. The percentage increased from P18 to P29 and then gradually decreased until P180, when OPs were still clearly recordable. Error bars represent the standard error of the mean.

In addition to being reduced in amplitude, the mixed scotopic a-waves in P23H rats had faster leading edges than in wild-type LExSD rats, indicating greater sensitivity. Figure 2B shows an example at 29 days of age, when the a-wave amplitude in P23H rats was only 29% of that in wild-type rats. Here, a-wave traces have been normalized against their respective maximal a-wave amplitude. As such, the resulting b-wave in P23H rats appears relatively higher than in wild-type rats because in the former the b-wave amplitude is relatively better preserved than the a-wave (see the trend of the respective ascending b-wave traces on the far right of Figure 2B).

At all ages, b-waves were less affected by the P23H rhodopsin transgene than were a-waves. While maximal b-wave amplitudes in both rod- and cone-driven ERG responses increased from P18 to P29, only cone-driven b-wave responses reached developmental maturity in pigmented P23H rats (Figures 2C–F). Although double flash-isolated rod-driven responses were already affected at P29, with a- and b-waves peaking at 203 and 564 μV vs. 610 and 998 μV in wild-type rats, these responses were still elicited at P180 (a- and b-wave maximal amplitudes of 60 and 211 μV). The rod-driven contribution to mixed scotopic b-waves was slightly lower in P23H (70%) as compared to LExSD (79%) rats, but remained steady at 58% by P180 (Figure 2D). Double-flash isolated scotopic cone b-waves (Figure 2E) and photopic single flash b-waves (Figure 2F) were comparable to those recorded in wild-type LExSD rats at P29. After P29, cone-driven single flash responses underwent slow, protracted deterioration (Figure 2F). By P180, maximal photopic b-waves still reached half of the amplitudes recorded in wild-type rats. Flicker ERGs (Figure 2G) confirmed the findings obtained with single flash cone-driven responses. Flicker amplitudes were comparable between P23H and wild-type rats at P29 (271 ± 30 μV *vs.* 306 ± 22 μV, respectively). Flicker fusions were also comparable at this age (42 ± 6 Hz and 42 ± 3 Hz in P23H and wild-type LExSD rats, respectively). By P180, flicker fusions in P23H rats were reduced in a statistically significant manner (31 ± 4 Hz compared to 42 ± 3 Hz in wild-type rats), as were maximal amplitude values (147 ± 19 μV in P23H rats *vs.* 306 ± 22 μV in control rats).

An indication of inner retina activity can be obtained by measuring the amplitude of oscillatory potentials (OP; Figure 2H). As with cone-driven b-waves, OP amplitudes increased from P18 until P29, at which point these values were comparable to those in age-matched wild-type rats. After P29, OP amplitudes decreased gradually to 16 ± 4% of the OP amplitudes in wild-type rats.

In summary, in P23H rats, only cone-driven b-waves (and mixed scotopic OPs) reached similar maximum amplitude values as in wild-type rats (Figure 2H). While mixed scotopic a-waves were the most severely affected ERG component, all components underwent a similar rapid reduction in maximal amplitude from P29 to P58, followed by a mild protracted drop from P90 to P180.

OCT Findings

In all animals, a basic examination using en face cSLO imaging was performed to identify any retinal abnormalities. The examination included red-free (513 nm), infrared (830 nm) and FAF (492 nm) imaging. Fluorescence angiography was used to analyze retinal vessels (Figure 3).

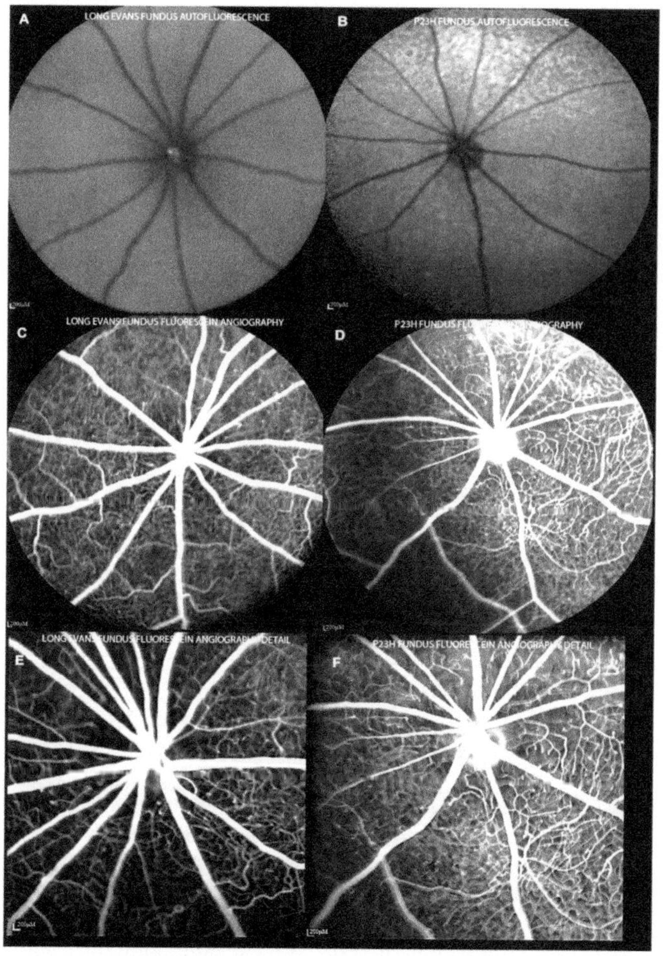

Figure 3: Autofluorescence and angiography images of control and P23H pigmented rats at P130. Autofluorescence images show a normal pattern in control rats **(A)** and hyperfluorescent spots in degenerative rats **(B)**. Angiograms of control **(C,E)** and P23H rats **(D,F)**, showing a normal radial pattern and capillary network at this age.

Almost all the rats analyzed showed features of the Bergmeister papilla, a remnant of the developmental vascular vitreous. No other abnormalities were seen in the red-free and infrared examination (Figures 4A,B).

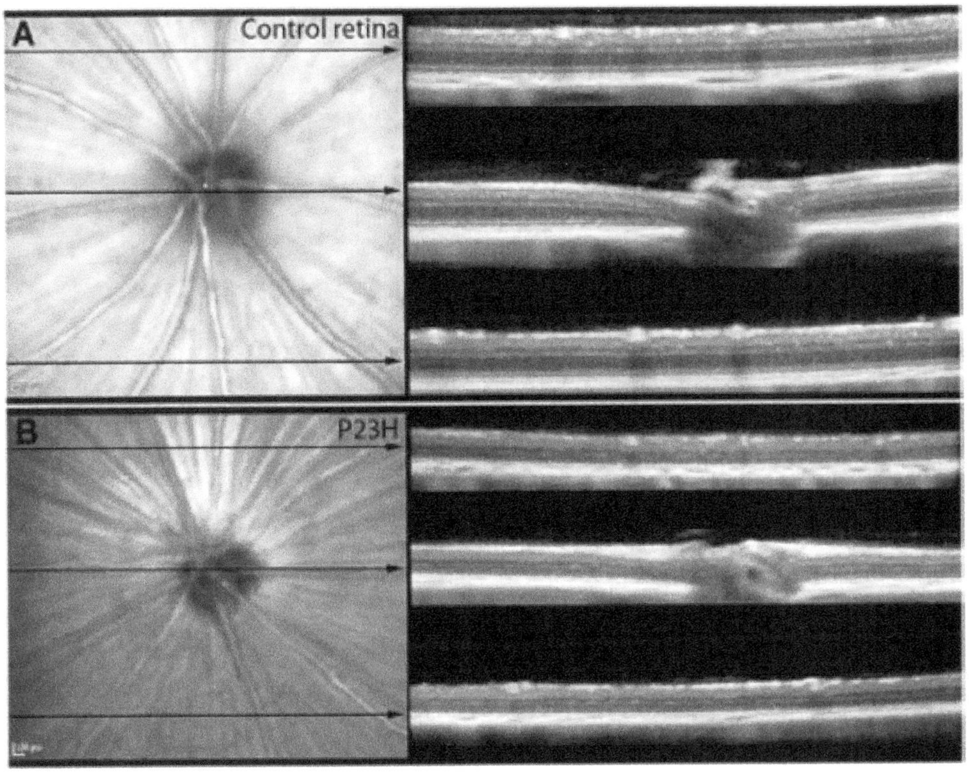

Figure 4: Red-free images and OCT sections of control and P23H pigmented L1. Red-free images and OCT sections of control rats **(A)** and P23H pigmented line 1 at P130 **(B)**. Red-free image showed the optic nerve and the major retinal vessels. The three sections showed the decreased thickness in the P23H rats, with a clear reduction of the ONL layer and changes in the hyperreflective layer. Note that the IPL is well preserved in the RP model.

Control rats showed no autofluorescence in their fundus (Figure 3A). Change in FAF in the P23H rats was noted as sparse autofluorescent dots (Figure 3B). No relevant changes were observed in the angiography pattern (Figures 3C–F). Major retinal vessels emerged from the optic nerve in a radial fashion, and retinal vessels ramified and narrowed into a sparse capillary network. Both great vessels and the capillary network in P23H pigmented rat showed no permeability changes and no lost areas of capillary circuitry at this age.

Structurally, the sections showed changes between control and P23H rats. Control rats exhibited a normal OCT profile, with hyporeflectivity at the nuclear layers and hyperreflectivity in the plexiform layers and external retina, including outer segments, RPE and choroid. In normal rats, ganglion cells and their fibers are distributed together at the internal retina, limited by the internal limiting membrane (ILM); vessels were shown transversally cut with high reflectivity in their walls, distributed between the ganglion cells and the retinal nerve fiber layer. A hyperreflective IPL was followed by a hyporeflective INL, a high reflectivity OPL and a low reflectivity ONL. The four hyperreflectivity layers could be clearly observed at the external retina (Figures 4A, 5A; Spaide and Curcio, 2011). In transgenic rats, the ONL appeared clearly diminished in all the retinal profiles (Figures 4B, 5C). The RPE was disrupted and also diminished in thickness. Although the OPL was easy to find, the ELM showed gaps in its continuity and was more difficult to recognize (Figures 4B, 5C). The hyperreflective lines of the external retina were less evident in the P23H pigmented rat. The thickness of the IPL appeared almost normal. Figure 5 shows the retinal profiles obtained by OCT in control (Figure 5A) and P23H (Figure 5C) rats and its comparison with immunohistochemistry staining (Figures 5B,D). We applied both techniques in order to compare the data acquired in P23H and control rats at P120 (Figure 5E). The usefulness of OCT measurements for evaluating the progression of retinal disease is clear, albeit the data comparing their values with histology measurements are limited. Figure 6 shows an example of thickness maps of control and P23H rats. Mean peripheral areas were statistically higher in control vs. P23H rats. No differences were found between superior and inferior areas and nasal and temporal thicknesses in rats from the same group with any of the techniques.

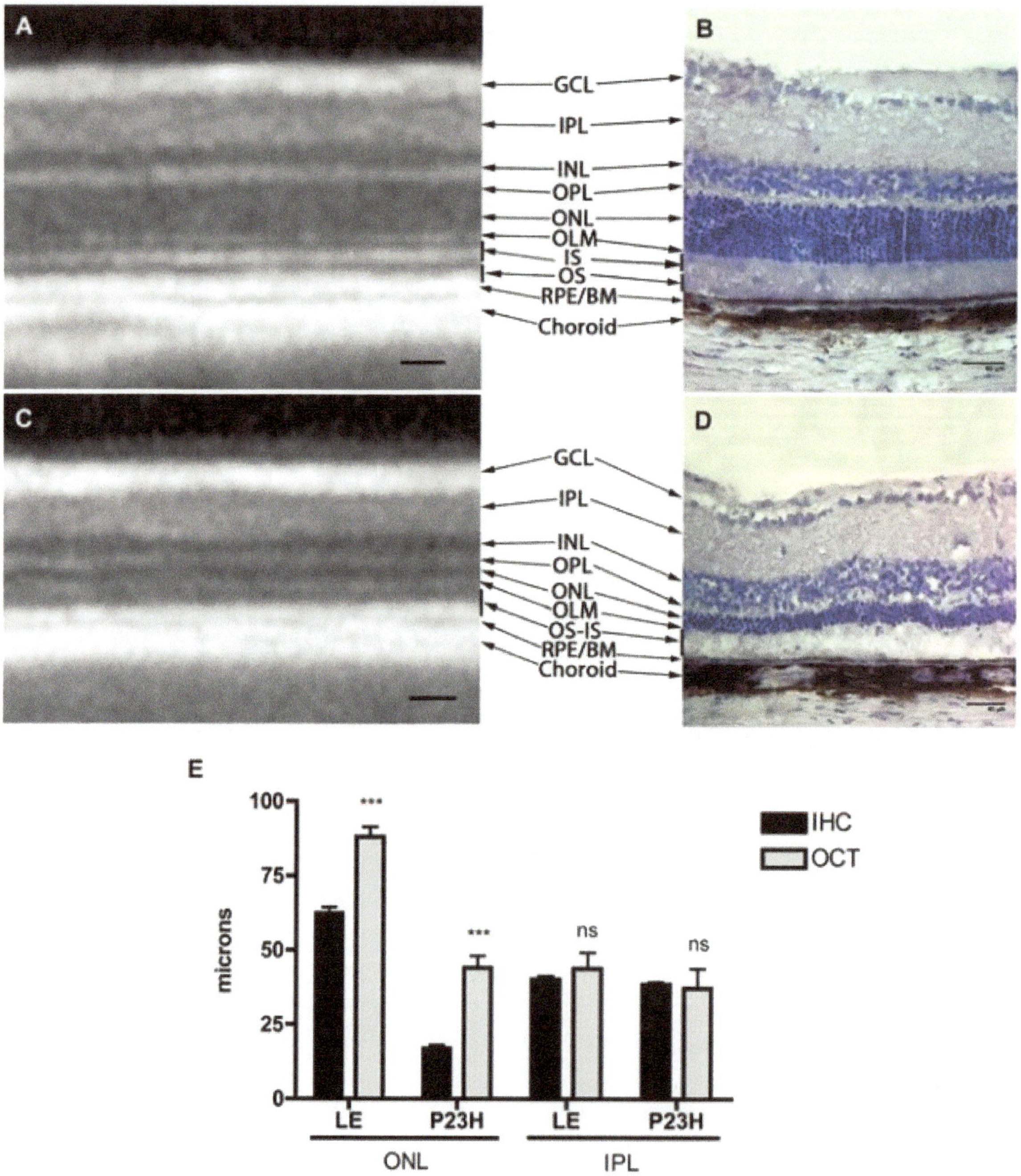

Figure 5: Comparison between OCT and immunohistochemistry. Figure shows an OCT section of a normal **(A)** and P23H rat retina **(C)** with hyper and hyporeflective layers and their correlation with normal **(B)**and RP **(D)** histology.

The lower graph **(E)** shows retinal thickness values in healthy and diseased animals quantified by OCT and immunohistochemistry techniques. Mean values ± SD of different retinal layers measured by immunohistochemistry and OCT profiles. (***) $p < 0.001$. GCL: ganglion cell layer; IPL: inner plexiform layer; INL: inner nuclear layer; OPL: outer plexiform layer; ONL: outer nuclear layer; OLM: outer limiting membrane; IS: inner segments, OS: outer segments; RPE: retinal pigmented epithelium; BM: Bruch membrane. Scale bar: 40 μm.

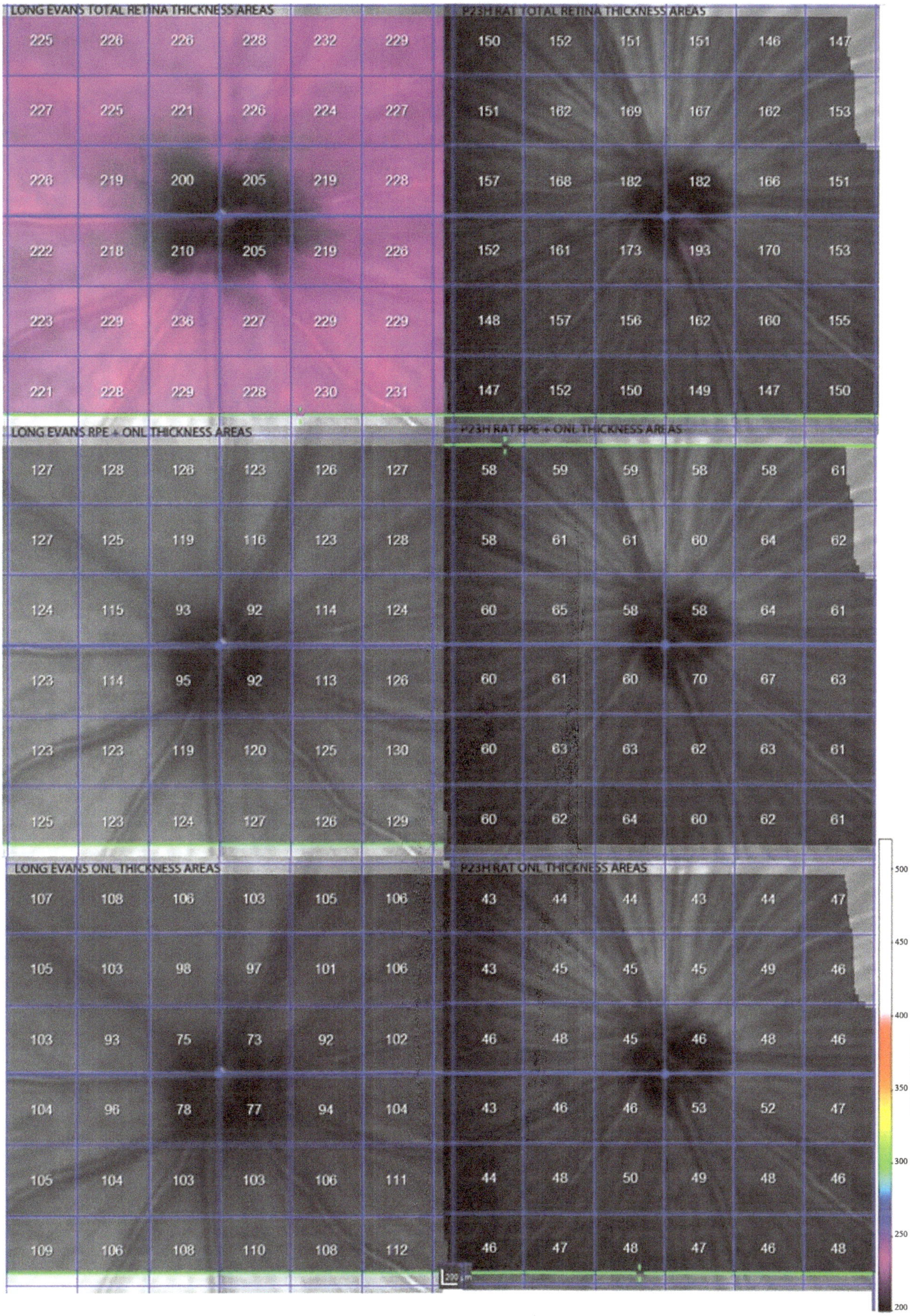

Figure 6: Example of retinal maps of control and P23H pigmented line 1 rats at P130. Mean retinal thickness value in microns is shown inside each square. Maps correspond to total retinal maps, RPE + ONL thickness and ONL thickness. All values were statistically lower in P23H rats.

All the values obtained in the retinal thickness profiles and maps of transgenic rats were significantly lower than those of control rats, with the exception of IPL thickness (Figure 5E). Total thickness retinal values were diminished in transgenic rats and the reduction was evident in the segmented layers (total retina thickness, ONL + RPE, and ONL). The main decrease was observed for ONL measurements. In addition, we found no differences between the data obtained with OCT and immunohistochemistry in the inner retina, while the outer retina showed differences between both techniques, with higher OCT ($p < 0.001$) than immunochemistry measurement values (Figure 5E).

Anatomical Findings

Anatomical studies were performed to compare them with the visual acuity, ERG and OCT image findings. For correlation with functional findings, we focused on cells involved in the generation of a- and b-waves, such as photoreceptors and their corresponding bipolar cells, respectively, and in the plexiform layers to check the synaptic relationship between the retinal cells.

Photoreceptors

Recoverin was used to identify all photoreceptor cells, while cone photoreceptors were specifically stained using gamma-transducin (Figure 7). In wild-type rats, photoreceptor cell bodies were aligned in rows of up to 14–15 cells in thickness (Figure 7A). These cells displayed well-developed outer segments and axon terminals. Cone cell bodies were located in the external third of the ONL (Figures 7A,B).

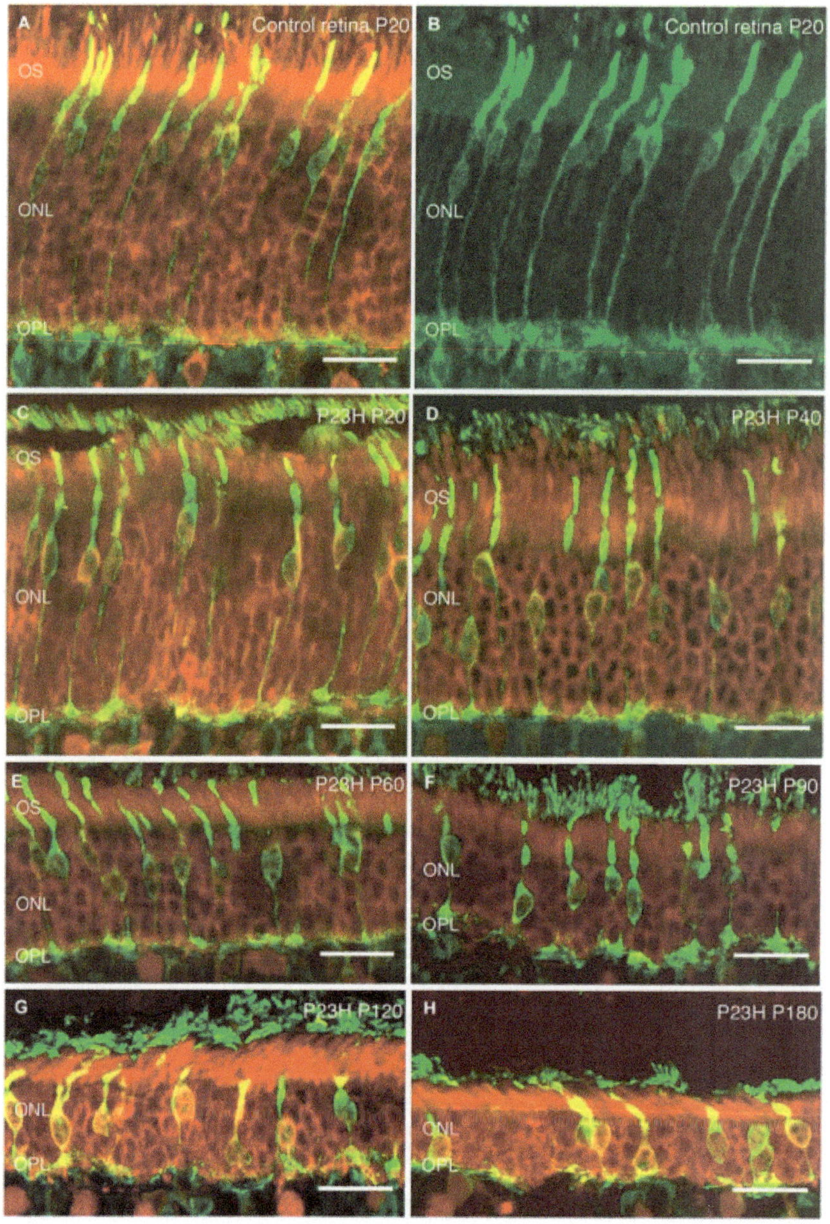

Figure 7: Photoreceptor changes in P23H pigmented L1 compared to control rats. Cryostat sections of a control (P20) and a P23H rat retina immunostained with antibodies against a specific marker for photoreceptor cells, recoverin (red); and a specific marker for cone and cone bipolar subtypes, γ-transducin (green). Photoreceptor cells in control rat retina stained with recoverin **(A)** and cone-photoreceptor cells stained with transducin **(A,B)**. P23H-L1 shows a decrease in photoreceptor rows and morphology changes from P20 to P180 **(C–H)**. OS: Outer segments; ONL: outer nuclear layer; OPL: Outer plexiform layer. Scale bar: 20 μm.

At P20, the retinas of heterozygous P23H pigmented rats exhibited a similar number of photoreceptor rows as in wild-type rats. At this age, subtle changes in cone morphology were apparent: cell bodies were not merely confined to the external part of the ONL, rather they could also be found in the center of the ONL (Figure 7C).

At P40, the photoreceptor layer was reduced to 6–7 rows in thickness (Figure 7D). Cone cell bodies were distributed throughout almost the entire ONL. Cone outer and inner segments and axon terminals presented normal morphology, although the length of cone axon terminals looked shorter compared with control animals (Figure 7D).

These changes in length became clearer at P60, when the ONL was reduced to 4–5 cells in thickness and the outer segments showed the first signs of being truncated (Figure 7E).

The number of ONL cells was progressively reduced to 4–5 cells at P90 (Figure 7F) and 2–3 cell rows at P120 (Figure 7G). At both ages (P90, P120) (Figures 7F,G), the outer segments were clearly more truncated than at P60 (Figure 7E).

At the oldest age studied (P180), only 2 layers of photoreceptors remained in P23H retinas (Figure 7H). The proportion of cones *vs.* rods was increased, and the cones showed rounded cell bodies and increased immunoreactivity to transducin (Figure 7H). The overall cell length was severely reduced, most of the cones lost their outer segments and there was an obvious lack of axon and pedicles.

Rhodopsin is an essential protein involved in rod phototransduction, located specifically in the rod outer segment. Using antibodies against rhodopsin, the rods in LE rat retina (P21) showed a specific stain in their outer segments, with a well-organized and parallel distribution (Figure 8A).

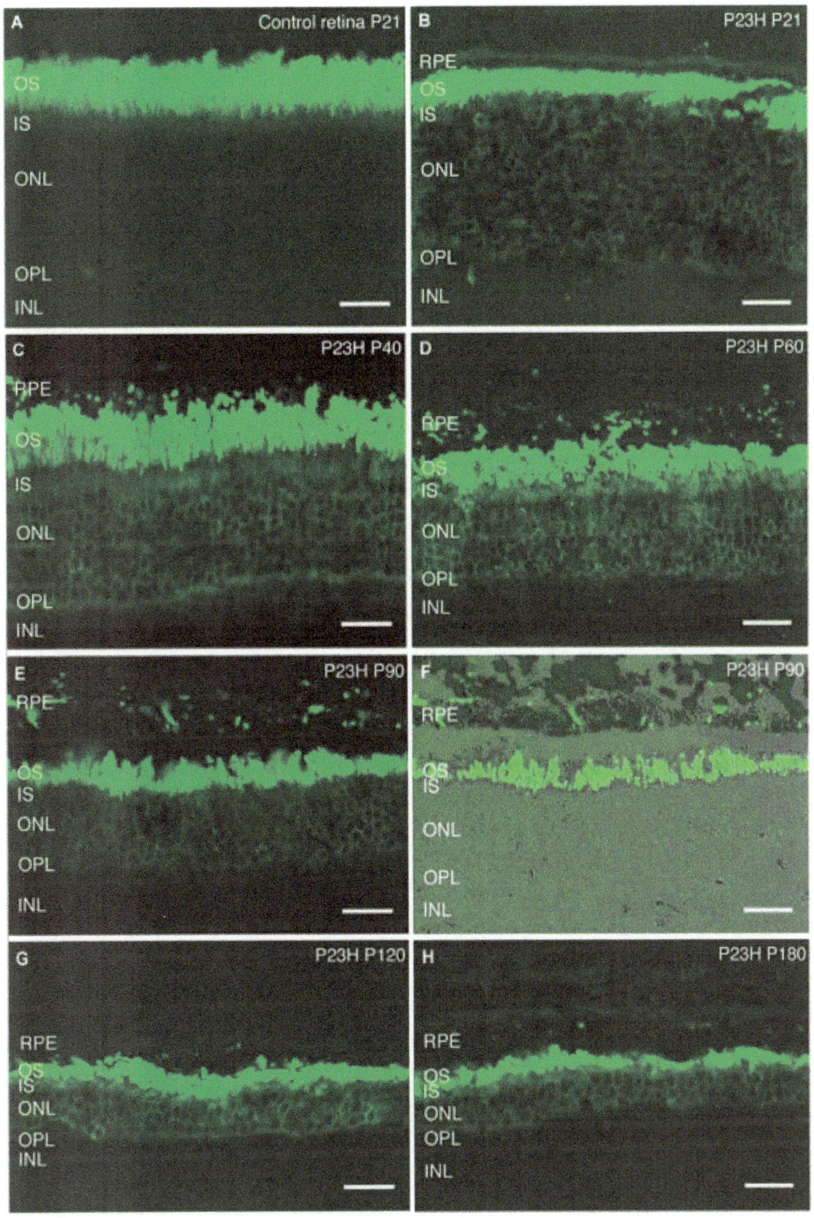

Figure 8: Rhodopsin changes with the degeneration of P23H pigmented L1 rats. Retinal sections stained with an antibody against rhodopsin showing rod outer segments in the control rat retina **(A)** compared to the P23H retina at the same age **(B)**. Ongoing retinal degeneration in P23H-L1 albino rats with aging **(C–H)** includes a progressive loss of photoreceptor rows, shortening of photoreceptor outer segments and mis-localization of rhodopsin along the cell. RPE: retinal pigment epithelium; OS: outer segments; IS: inner segments; ONL: outer nuclear layer; OPL: outer plexiform layer; INL: inner nuclear layer. Scale bar: 20 μm.

Although the number of photoreceptors did not significantly decrease, rhodopsin staining in P23H pigmented rat retinas at P20 was no longer only localized in the outer segments (Figure 8B). Rhodopsin immunostaining could also be seen in the inner segments, the surface of rod cell bodies and their axons as a sign of rod degeneration at this age (Figure 8B). The mislocated rhodopsin staining of the rod inner segments and cell bodies was observed at all ages from P20 to P180 (Figures 8B–H). At P40, rod outer segments maintained their well aligned distribution (Figure 8C). However, at P60, they were shorter, truncated and had lost their parallel distribution (Figure 8D). An increase in rod outer segments phagosomes inside the RPE was observed at this age (Figure 8D). Figures 8E,F show phagosomes of rod outer segments inside the RPE at P90. The progressive impairment and shortening of rod outer segments could be observed at P120 and P180 (Figures 8G,F).

Synaptic Connectivity Changes in the OPL

The OPL is the layer in which synaptic contacts between photoreceptors and bipolar and horizontal cells take place (Kolb et al., 2001). We studied the morphological changes during the progression of photoreceptor degeneration at the OPL in the pigmented P23H rat. For this purpose, we used antibodies against calbindin to identify horizontal cells, PKC-α for visualizing ON-rod bipolar cells and bassoon to stain the synaptic ribbon on the axon terminals of cones and rods.

There is only one type of horizontal cell in the rat retina (Peichl and González-Soriano, 1994). It is a B-type horizontal cell with dendrites postsynaptic to cone pedicles and its axon making synaptic contacts with rod spherules. Figure 9 shows horizontal cell bodies and their axons immunostained with antibodies against calbindin (green). The synaptic ribbons of photoreceptors, identified with antibodies against bassoon (red), are located on top of horizontal tip terminals (Figures 9A,B red spots). As a result of rod photoreceptor degeneration in P23H retinas, the calbindin positive horizontal cells also showed degenerative changes (Figures 9C–H). At P20 and P40, the morphology and distribution of horizontal cells in P23H retinas were comparable to those of the control LE rat (Figures 9C,D), but bassoon immunoreactive spots were decreased, indicating a loss of contacts between rod and horizontal cells. By P60 and P90, there was a progressive disorganization of horizontal cell bodies, dendrites and axon terminals (Figures 9E,F, green processes). The cell bodies appeared to be in poor condition and were inverted, with atrophied dendrites condensing into blobs of stain. By 3 months of age, the horizontal cells in P23H retinas had sprouted abnormal processes from both dendrites and axon terminals trying to reach the remaining patches of photoreceptor synaptic terminals (Figure 9F). At P120 and P180, the horizontal cell processes appeared hypertrophic and beaded, and the number of process fibers were reduced and discontinuously distributed (Figures 9G,H). A loss of contacts with photoreceptor axon terminals was evidenced by the reduced number of bassoon immunoreactive spots (Figures 9G,H).

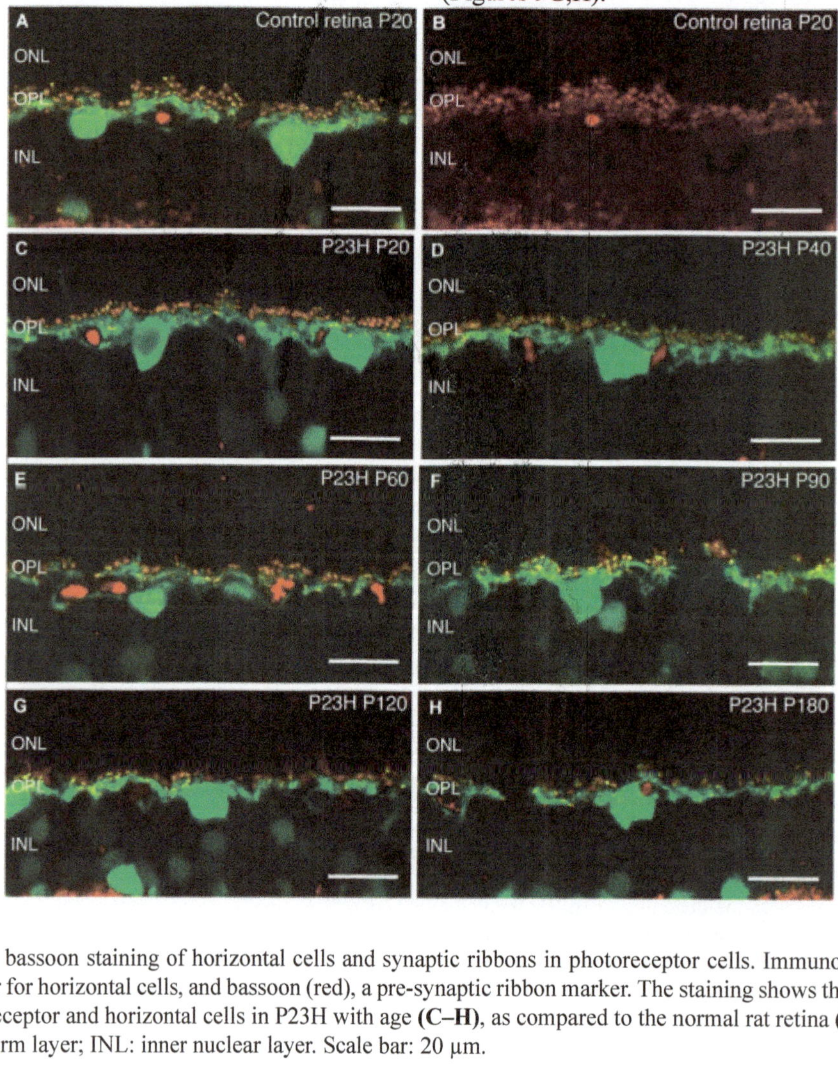

Figure 9: Calbindin and bassoon staining of horizontal cells and synaptic ribbons in photoreceptor cells. Immunostaining against calbindin (green), a specific marker for horizontal cells, and bassoon (red), a pre-synaptic ribbon marker. The staining shows the degeneration of synaptic contacts between photoreceptor and horizontal cells in P23H with age **(C–H)**, as compared to the normal rat retina **(A,B)**. ONL: outer nuclear layer; OPL: outer plexiform layer; INL: inner nuclear layer. Scale bar: 20 μm.

Rod bipolar cells are the only output cells of rod photoreceptors in the OPL. It is therefore important to see whether rod bipolar cells are particularly vulnerable during the course of rod photoreceptor degeneration. Rod bipolar cells can be labeled by antibodies against PKCα (Greferath et al., 1990). In control retinas, bipolar cells had a tuft of dendrites extending into the OPL, and double labeling with bassoon showed contacts with their presynaptic elements (Figures 10A,B). At P20 and P40, the morphology of rod bipolar cell dendrites in P23H rats was similar to that of the LE controls (Figure 10B, green), however a decrease of bassoon immunoreactive spots was evident (Figures 10C,D). At P60 and P90, the dendrites of rod bipolar cells in the OPL were thinner and shorter, and the OPL plexus was discontinuous and wavy, while a loss of contacts was also obvious Figures 10E,F. As degeneration proceeded, further changes became evident. Many of the cells lost their dendrites by P120 (Figure 10G, green) and a few bassoon immunoreactive spots could be observed (Figure 10G). By P180, a reduction of bipolar cells bodies took place. No dendritic plexus in the OPL was visible, and scarce bassoon spots were located directly on top of the cell bodies (Figures 10G,H), suggesting that the output of the remaining photoreceptors was dramatically impaired.

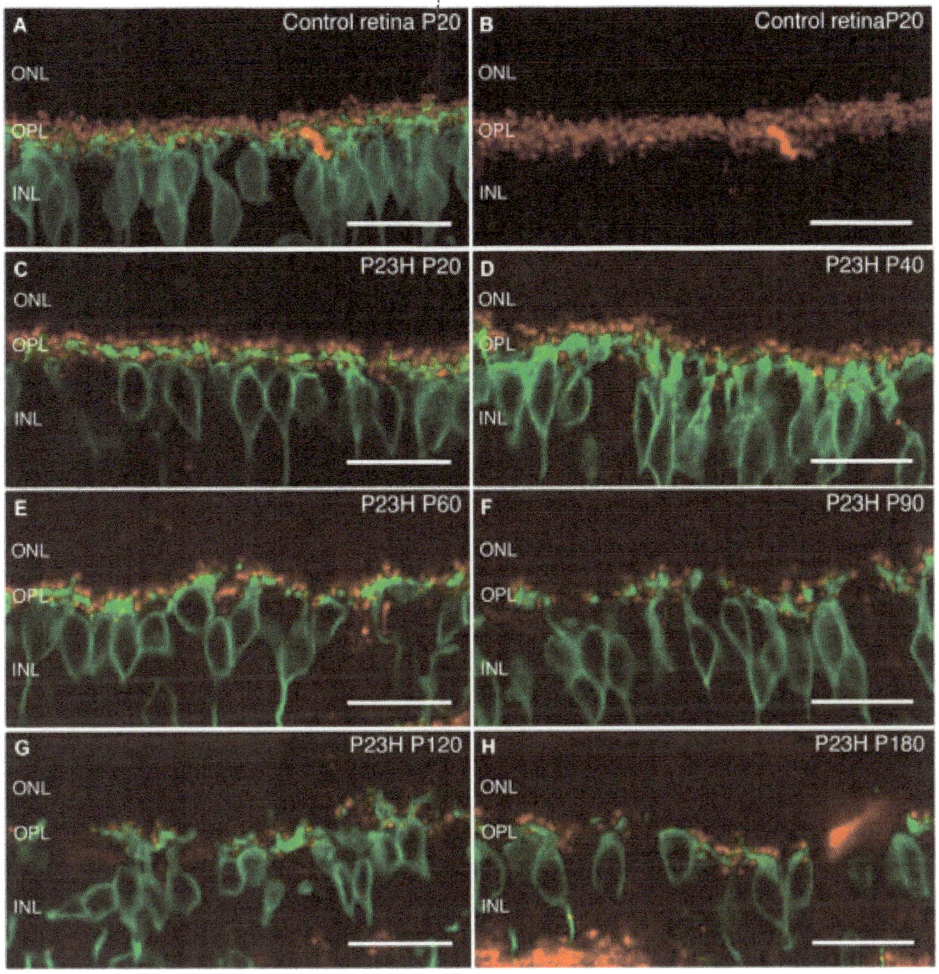

Figure 10: Rod bipolar cells and ribbon synapses changes during retinal degeneration of P23H pigmented L1 rats. Vertical sections stain with antibodies against protein kinase α (PKCα) in green to visualize rod bipolar cells, and against bassoon to visualize ribbon synapses in red. Control retinas show a dense plexus of synaptic contacts between bipolar and photoreceptor cells at the OPL level **(A,B)**. At P20, the P23H retina **(C)** already shows a small decrease as compared to control retinas. During aging **(C–H)**, there is a continuous reduction in the number of the synaptic contacts. ONL: outer nuclear layer; OPL: outer plexiform layer; INL: inner nuclear layer. Scale bar: 20 μm.

Synaptic Connectivity Changes at the IPL

To determine whether morphological changes took place in the IPL during photoreceptor degeneration, we studied two types of bipolar cells and the IPL bands stained with bassoon.

PKCα antibodies labeled ON-rod bipolar cells, and although some amacrine cells were also labeled, they can be easily distinguished by the characteristic distribution of their processes within the IPL.

Rod bipolar cells. In normal retinas, rod bipolar cell bodies were localized in the outer part of the INL (Figure 11A). These had a tuft of dendrites extending into the OPL and a single axon that extended through the IPL (with a few small side branches) and ended at stratum S5 of the IPL with end-bulbs and lateral terminal varicosities (Figure 11A).

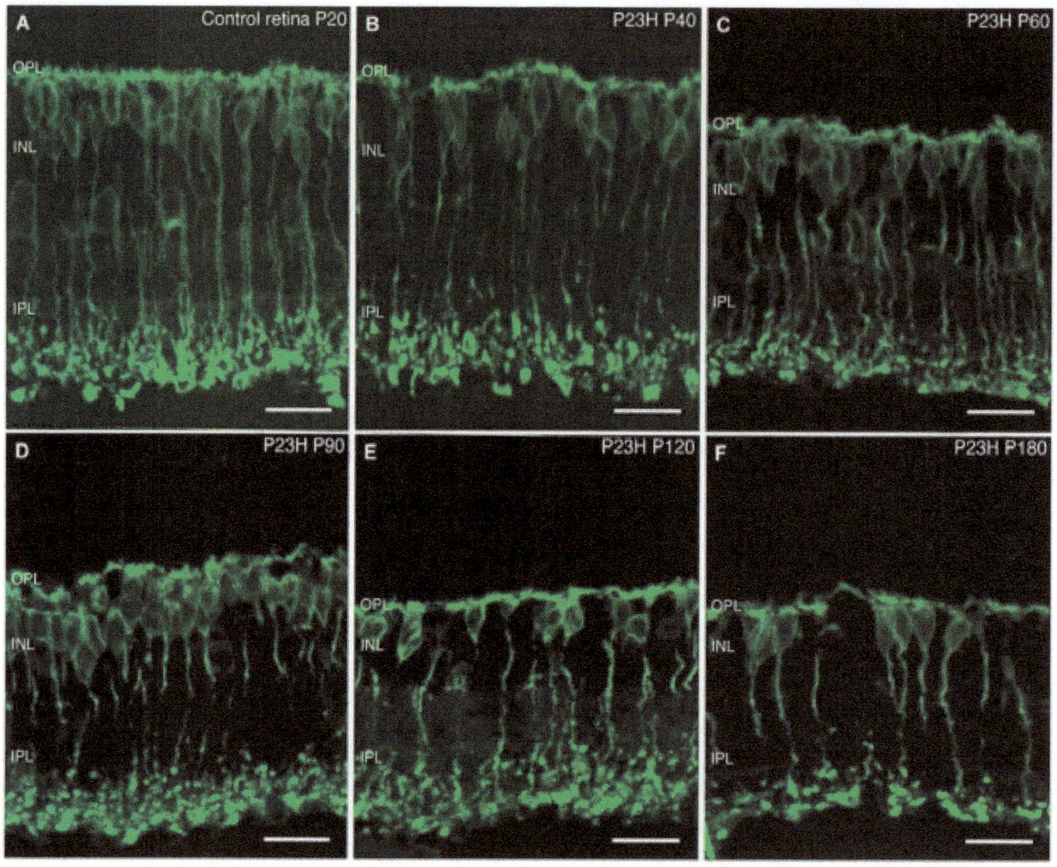

Figure 11: Rod bipolar cell changes during retinal degeneration of P23H pigmented L1 rat. Sections stained against PKCα for identifying rod bipolar cells in control retinas **(A)** and during P23H rat retinal degeneration **(B–F)**. Evident signs of rod bipolar cells degeneration started at P60; from this age and onward, there is a shortening of rod bipolar dendrites, a decrease in their immunoreactivity and loss of bipolar axon terminals. OPL: outer plexiform layer; INL: inner nuclear layer; IPL: inner plexiform layer. Scale bar: 20 μm.

ON-rod bipolar cells exhibited morphological changes during photoreceptor degeneration. From a normal morphology observed at P40 (Figure 11B), rod bipolar cells began to exhibit signs of degenerative changes at P60, with a reduction of their dendritic branches. Also, the cell bodies and axons lost their normal alignment and become shorter than in the control retinas (Figure 11C). Moreover, their axon terminal varicosities were smaller, and their axon terminal end clubs were particularly diminished. As the degeneration progressed from P60 to 180, rod bipolar cells experienced a reduction in number, had even fewer dendrites, and their axon terminal end-bulbs were also markedly less numerous (Figures 11C–F). Their axons became beaded and their terminal varicosities reduced. With further aging, the rod bipolar cell morphology became more disorganized, with cell bodies no longer displaying a regular laminar structure in the INL, and it was clear that the axon terminals were scarcely present at all (Figure 11F).

Cone bipolar cells. In addition to photoreceptors, recoverin antibodies also label two types of cone bipolar cells in the rat retina (McGinnis et al., 1999; Cuenca et al., 2004). At P20, these two types of cone bipolar cells remained unchanged as compared to the control retinas. Type 8 ON-cone bipolar cells had a diffuse plexus of axons, terminating in the inner IPL, in strata S4-S5. Their cell body, located near the OPL, was weakly immunoreactive to recoverin (Figure 12A arrows). The second, Type 2, was an OFF-cone bipolar cell (Figure 12A, arrowheads), with strong immunoreactivity in the cell body, located near the middle of the INL, and an axon making a dense continuous plexus in strata S1 and S2 of the IPL. By P40 and P60, the general morphology of these cone bipolar cells was not drastically modified, and the only apparent change was a decrease in cell body density (Figures 12B,C).

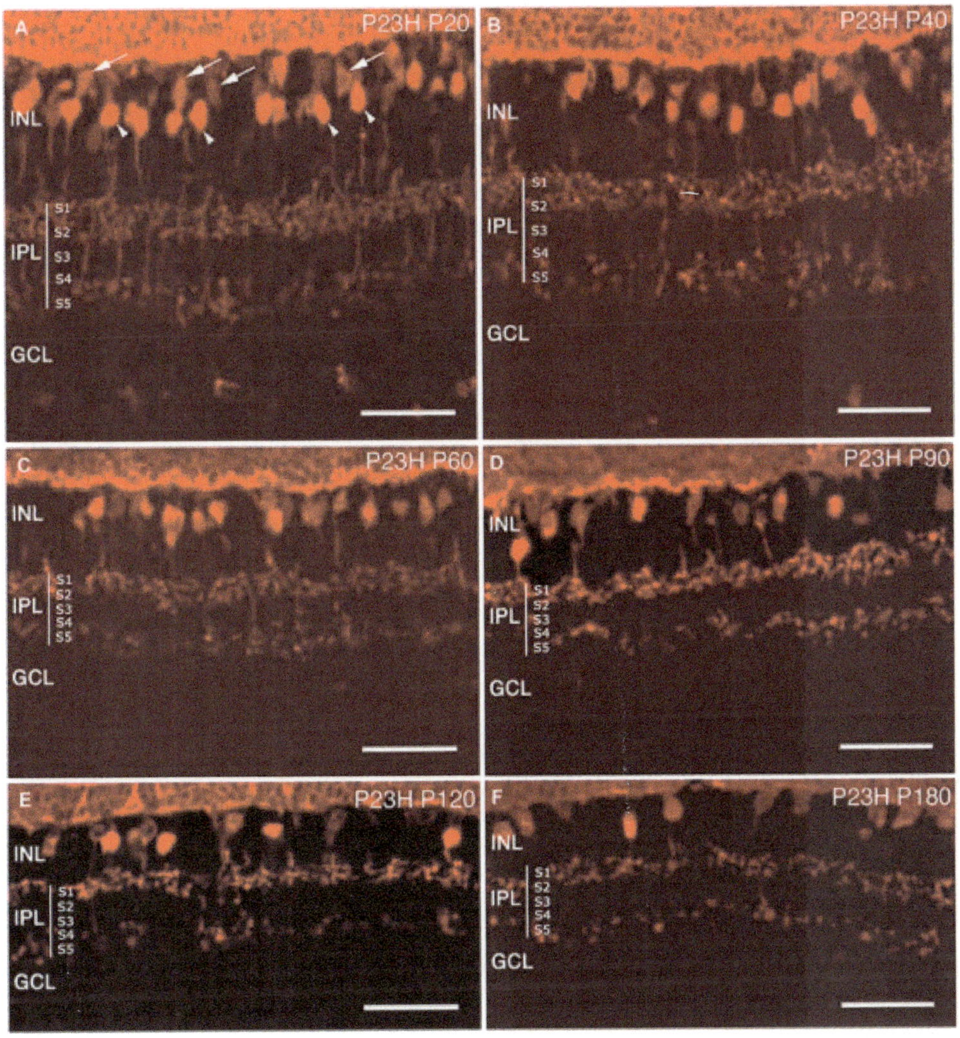

Figure 12: Cone bipolar cell modifications during retinal degeneration of P23H pigmented L1 rats. Retinal sections stained with antibodies against recoverin in order to visualize the degenerative process of cone bipolar cells in P23H **(B–F)** rat retina, compared to the control **(A)**. Along the degenerative process, cone bipolar cells show changes from P60 onwards, with profuse axonal loss at the IPL level. INL: inner nuclear layer; IPL: inner plexiform layer; S1: Stratum 1; S2: Stratum 2; S3: Stratum 3; S4: Stratum 4; S5: Stratum 5; GCL: ganglion cell layer. Scale bar: 40 μm.

At P90 and P120 (Figures 12D,E), the cell bodies of these two types of cone bipolar cells appeared smaller as compared to previous ages. The plexus in strata S1 and S2 was discontinuous, with gaps created by the disappearance of OFF-bipolar axon terminals. ON-bipolar cells were still present, but the terminals in stratum S5 appeared to be more sparsely distributed. At P180, the decrease of cone bipolar cells was evident and the axons of both cone bipolar cells were shorter, less complex and discontinuous, and their terminals exhibited a beaded morphology, indicating a loss of axon terminals (Figure 12F).

Bassoon at the IPL. In the IPL, bassoon is concentrated at the conventional GABAergic amacrine synapses, but is absent from the bipolar cell ribbon synapses (Brandstätter et al., 1999). Staining of vertical retinal sections of LE rats showed immunoreactivity in both synaptic layers of the retina (Figure 13A). Spots of bassoon immunoreactivity were found covering the entire IPL, with decreasing intensity from strata S1 to S5. There were distinct bands of strong immunoreactivity in strata S1, S2 and S3, with less intense staining at the S3/S4 border of the IPL (Figure 13A). At P20 (Figure 13B), bassoon immunoreactivity in the IPL remained unchanged in P23H rats as compared to LE rats. Bassoon staining was clearly diminished at P60, an age at which bassoon immunoreactive bands in the IPL were difficult to distinguish (Figure 13C). From P60 to P180, immunoreactivity decreased in synapses within the IPL over time, and the bands had become less distinct, in some cases disappearing altogether (Figures 13D–F).

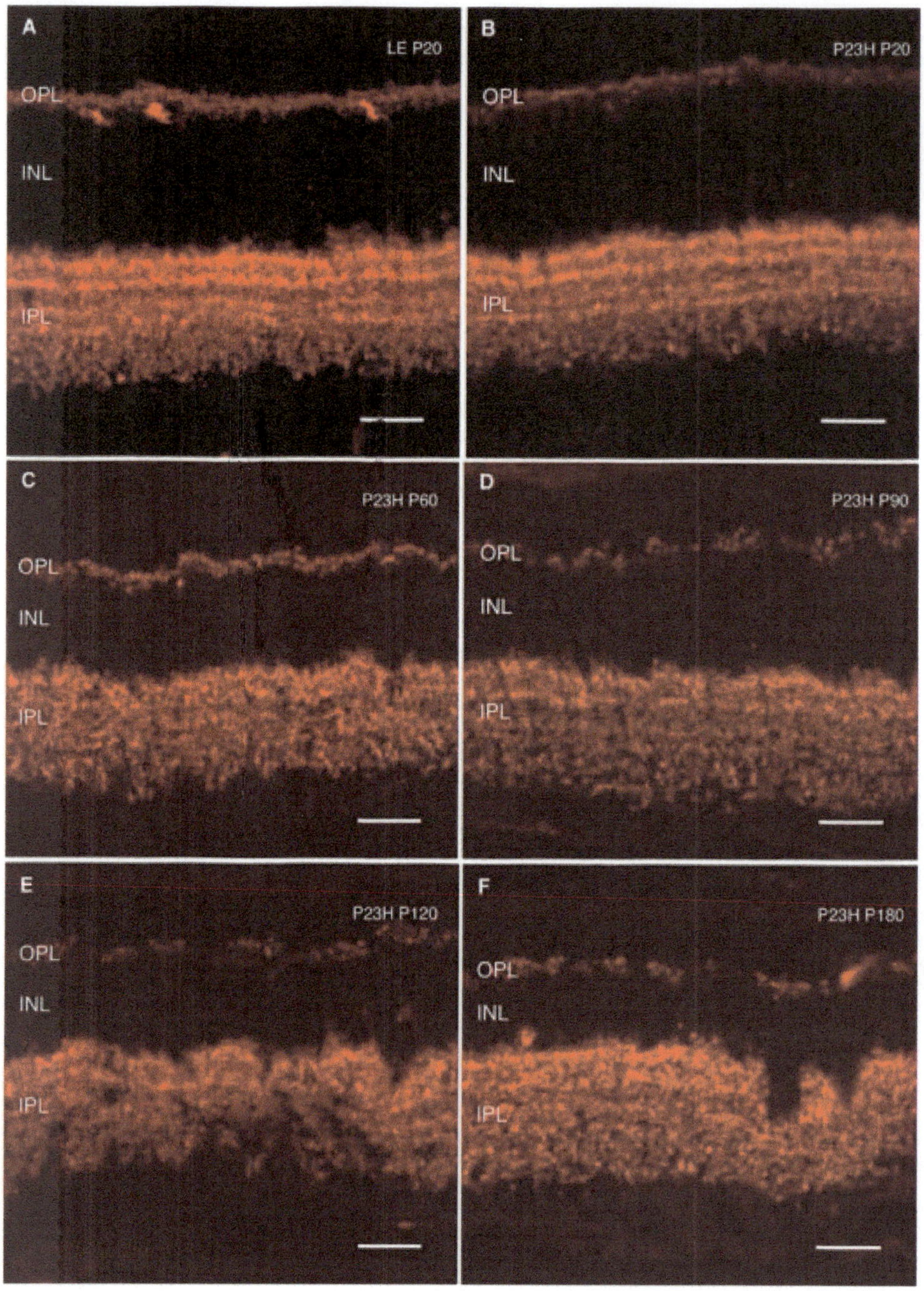

Figure 13: Synaptic connectivity. Cryostat sections stained against Bassoon (red) to visualize pre-synaptic ribbons. Bassoon immunostaining in P23H rat retinas was decreased **(B–F)**, as compared to control retinas **(A)**. A loss of connectivity was seen at the OPL, as well as increased disorganization at the IPL layer. ONL: outer nuclear layer; OPL: outer plexiform layer; INL: inner nuclear layer; IPL: inner plexiform layer. Scale bar: 20 μm.

DISCUSSION

The P23H rat is a dominant autosomal model of RP, used extensively for therapeutic approaches. The P23H albino rat model shows a faster retinal degeneration due to albinism, which make it quite different from the human disease. In contrast P23H pigmented rats present slowest degeneration being closer to P23H human condition. The retinas of genetically inbred albino rodents have been shown to be particularly susceptible to photic injury induced by moderate and high levels of light exposure (LaVail et al., 1987a,b; Naash et al., 1989). It is important to use a pigmented background, closer to the human retina, and to guarantee that pigmentation will not interfere with the retinal degenerative process. Pigmented rats are easier to use for visual acuity evaluation with the optomotor system and to define the lines of the OCT exploration. Their visual acuity resolution is higher than that of albino rats, which helps to distinguish the effect of the degeneration from the result of any therapeutic approach that we use on them. Not all rhodopsin mutations seem to have the same susceptibility to light damage. Some rodent models with faster retinal degeneration are more resistant to light exposure. For instance, retinal degeneration in the S334ter transgenic rat is not exacerbated by light exposure (Lowe et al., 2005). Other genetic factors have also been reported to be involved in the light sensitivity of different rodent strains (LaVail et al., 1987a,b,c). The heterozygous transgenic P23H albino rat has been found to be highly susceptible to retinal damage from exposure to intense light (Bicknell et al., 2002; Vaughan et al., 2003; Lowe et al., 2005). These studies point to the role of light damage in exacerbating RP-related degeneration in P23H mutant rats.

SD-OCT as a Non-Invasive Imaging Technique to Evaluate Retinal Degeneration

OCT is an important tool for retinal evaluation in all kinds of ophthalmological diseases. The fast acquisition and the high number of scans have made SD-OCT a valuable tool in ophthalmic research. The resolution of cross sectional images obtained by third generation OCT has been described as being similar to low power micrographs obtained from light microscopy (Huber et al., 2009). In our study, retinal thicknesses presented a good correlation with histological findings, and OCT proved able to assess the loss of retinal thickness with degeneration, as it showed a clear reduction in the ONL layer, as would be expected in a rod-loss disease. Other authors have shown a good correlation between retinal thickness measured by SD-OCT (Spectralis OCT) in wild-type mice and transgenic animals (rd1, Rho−/−, RPE65−/−) and histological findings (Huber et al., 2009; Jiao et al., 2013; Berger et al., 2014). Their results improved depending on the fixation protocol; thicknesses showed a better correlation when they used a direct embedding method as opposed to overnight fixation. Our previously described protocol used fixation and cryoprotection overnight, with increasing sucrose concentration. Using our standard protocol, the values obtained by immunohistochemistry are significantly lower than those measured *in vivo* during OCT exploration. However, the decreasing trend at the ONL level was clear with both techniques, and both methods exhibited an almost perfect correlation between them in terms of these measures. These findings were not supported by the IPL measurements, despite the fact that the IPL was the best preserved layer with both methods. The main reason for this finding is probably the difficulty in establishing a good limit for the layer, not only with OCT, but also histochemistry. The IPL is the latest layer to be affected, and its measurements remain close in value to those obtained in normal rats. In the immunohistochemistry examination, the S5 stratus was sometimes difficult to establish; OCT limits are clear at these ages, but it may be difficult to establish them in older rats (data not shown), due to cellular and vascular changes during retinal remodeling.

FAF findings are consistent with other retinal degenerative diseases, where photoreceptor debris and the accumulation of lipid degradation products are shown as hyperfluorescent dots. The findings resembled those found in RPE65−/− mice, but not so much as our own results for albino P23H rats (data not shown). Albino rodents are more susceptible to light-induced damage and show faster accumulation of lipid degradation products. P23H albino homozygous rats have an appearance resembling that of pigmented heterozygous rats at 2 months of age, with no changes at P21 (unpublished data). Albino wild-type mice BALB/c showed hyperfluorescent dots at early ages (Huber et al., 2009). Changes in FAF related to A2E accumulation has been described in other animal models of retinal degeneration (Charbel Issa et al., 2013).

Although is well known that retinal vessels change with degeneration (Villegas-Pérez et al., 1998; Fernández-Sánchez et al., 2012), Fluorescence angiography failed to show these changes at the age studied (4 months of age). All retinal vessels conserved their morphology, with no changes in their walls or any other signs or staining.

Functional Assessment using an Optomotor Test

The visual function of retinal degenerative animal models has been measured in previous studies using an OptoMotry system (Umino et al., 2006; McGill et al., 2007; Zhou et al., 2009; Lu et al., 2010). However, this study is the first to describe the spatial frequency and contrast sensitivity thresholds in the P23H-1 rat. Our results in control pigmented rats are similar to those reported by other studies (Douglas et al., 2005). Visual acuity reached 0.540 cyc/deg. The contrast sensitivity curve displayed a typical inverted-U shape. Both visual acuity and contrast sensitivity decreased with age in P23H-1 rats. At P30, visual performance was close to that found in control rats, and the results were consistent with those observed with ERG. As in control rats, the cone driven a-wave had reached maturity, but by this age, the rod driven b-wave was already reduced. Both functional tests demonstrate a gradual decrease in visual acuity, contrast sensitivity and ERG responses from the P30 age point to early in the P240 interval, showing a progressive photoreceptor deterioration that affects first the rods and then the cones. This agrees with the progressive loss of photoreceptors, which first affects the rods, and then both the rods and cones.

Effect of Albino Vs. Pigmented Background in Heterozygous P23H Line 1 Rats

The comparison of the present ERG results with previously published results from similar tests applied to heterozygous P23H line 1 rats, bred on an albino background (Machida et al., 2000), supports the hypothesis that albinism exacerbates the P23H-related retinal degeneration. While mixed scotopic maximal a-wave and b-wave amplitudes were initially better preserved in pigmented animals (at ages P29 and P28 in pigmented and albino rats, respectively), they underwent a similar decline up to the last time points tested (P180 and P203 in pigmented and albino rats, respectively). However, maximal photopic b-wave amplitudes did have higher proportions as compared to the respective wild types at early and late time points. These comparative findings support the suggestion that cone function might be more affected than rod function over time by the lack of pigmentation. Finally, the findings that the a-wave leading edge is faster in pigmented P23H than in wild types, as reported in albino P23H rats (Machida et al., 2000), suggests that pigmentation has no effect on rod phototransduction.

At the anatomical level, heterozygous P23H line 1 rats bred on an albino background showed a progressive loss of rod photoreceptors over several months. By P28, the ONL had lost approximately 40% of its cells (Machida et al., 2000). At this age, we observed rhodopsin mislocated along the remaining rod photoreceptor cells, which is a regular trait in RP diseases (Cuenca et al., 2004, 2005; Barhoum et al., 2008; Martinez-Navarrete et al., 2011). By P180, the ONL had fewer than two rows of cells remaining, and they were essentially cones. Our results indicate that pigmented P23H rats at age P21 had a similar number of photoreceptor rows as wild-type LE rats, while around 12 rows of cells remained at P40. This number then fell to 6 rows at P58, with a further progressive decline until P180, when only 2 layers of photoreceptors were left, consisting mainly of cone photoreceptor cells. As in other RP models reported by different group (Cuenca et al., 2014), the loss of rod photoreceptors leads to morphological changes in other retinal cells. Cone photoreceptor cells undergo changes affecting their length, the position of their cell bodies in the ONL, as well as changes in their outer segments, which become shorter and swollen than in control retinas.

The loss of photoreceptor cells is reflected as a reduction of synaptic contacts between photoreceptors and their postsynaptic bipolar and horizontal cells. Changes in bipolar cells were slower and more subtle than those reported in albino P23H rats (Cuenca et al., 2004): they became apparent only around P60, while this set of changes in bipolar cells appeared around P40 in the albino rat. The degenerative trends observed in the horizontal cell distribution and organization in P23H-L1 pigmented rats at P90 is almost achieved at P40 in the albino rat (Cuenca et al., 2004). All these observations confirm that the degenerative process that took place in the inner retina is closely related to the rod degeneration rate in each line, and should be considered in the design of RP therapies.

Relevance to the Development of Preventive Therapeutic Approaches

The good correlation shown between OCT and histology results is the important key to our work. The possibility of evaluating the retina using non-invasive techniques reduces the number of animals that need to be sacrificed and still provides good data about the progression of the disease and the integrity of the retinal layers. Retinal thickness is not the only variable to provide valuable results; the autofluorescent findings also contribute information about the integrity of the RPE layer.

Pigmented RP rodent models have clear benefits over the albino ones. As in other models, albinism itself exacerbates the retinal degenerative processes. The changes seen in the inner retina are slower that those reported for the albino background in terms of the rate of decline in ERG responsiveness. Preservation of the retinal circuitry is an important factor in the effectiveness of potential preventive treatments. In addition, pigmented rats perform better on behavioral tests aimed at assessing vision. For these reasons, a pigmented background might be optimal when relying on P23H transgenic rats to develop and study experimental therapies, such as cell-based therapy.

The finding that cone function is unaffected by P29 provides us with the opportunity to study approaches aimed at the full functional prevention of blindness, using therapeutic approaches in the pigmented heterozygous P23H line 1 rat, providing that it is bred on a pigmented background. It should be noted that in our study, we were unable to detect a functional correlate of the subtle changes in cone cell body distribution at P21. Whether this morphological change has any impact on retinal function remains to be clarified.

Acknowledgments

The authors would like to thank Dr. James F. McGinnis (University of Oklahoma) for providing the anti-recoverin antibodies. Dr. Pinilla and Dr. Cuenca were supported by grants from the Spanish Ministry of Economy and Competitiveness-FEDER (BFU2012-36845), Instituto de Salud Carlos III (FIS PI13/01124, PS0901854, PI042399 and RETICS RD12/0034/0010), Fundación Gangoiti, ONCE (Organización Nacional de Ciegos Españoles) and FUNDALUCE. Dr. Yves Sauvé is a recipient of the Barbara Tuck/MacPhee Family Vision Research Award in Macular Degeneration.

REFERENCES

1. Barhoum, R., Martínez-Navarrete, G., Corrochano, S., Germain, F., Fernandez-Sanchez, L., de la Rosa, E. J., et al. (2008). Functional and structural modifications during retinal degeneration in the rd10 mouse. Neuroscience 155, 698–713. doi: 10.1016/j.neuroscience.2008.06.042
2. Berger, A., Cavallero, S., Dominguez, E., Barbe, P., Simonutti, M., Sahel, J. A., et al. (2014). Spectral-domain optical coherence tomography of the rodent eye: highlighting layers of the outer retina using signal averaging and comparison with histology. PLoS One 9:e96494. doi: 10.1371/journal.pone.0096494
3. Bicknell, I. R., Darrow, R., Barsalou, L., Fliesler, S. J., and Organisciak, D. T. (2002). Alterations in retinal rod outer segment fatty acids and light-damage susceptibility in P23H rats. Mol. Vis. 8, 333–340.
4. Brandstätter, J. H., Fletcher, E. L., Garner, C. C., Gundelfinger, E. D., and Wässle, H. (1999). Differential expression of the presynaptic cytomatrix protein bassoon among ribbon synapses in the mammalian retina. Eur. J. Neurosci. 11, 3683–3693. doi: 10.1046/j.1460-9568.1999.00793.x
5. Charbel Issa, P., Barnard, A. R., Singh, M. S., Carter, E., Jiang, Z., Radu, R. A., et al. (2013). Fundus autofluorescence in the Abca4(−/−) mouse model of Stargardt disease–correlation with accumulation of A2E, retinal function and histology. Invest. Ophthalmol. Vis. Sci. 54, 5602–5612. doi: 10.1167/iovs.13-11688
6. Cuenca, N., Fernández-Sánchez, L., Campello, L., Maneu, V., De la Villa, P., Lax, P., et al. (2014). Cellular responses following retinal injuries and therapeutic approaches for neurodegenerative diseases. Prog. Retin. Eye Res. 43C, 17–75. doi: 10.1016/j.preteyeres.2014.07.001
7. Cuenca, N., Pinilla, I., Sauvé, Y., Lu, B., Wang, S., and Lund, R. D. (2004). Regressive and reactive changes in the connectivity patterns of rod and cone pathways of P23H transgenic rat retina. Neuroscience 127, 301–317. doi: 10.1016/j.neuroscience.2004.04.042
8. Cuenca, N., Pinilla, I., Sauvé, Y., and Lund, R. (2005). Early changes in synaptic connectivity following progressive photoreceptor degeneration in RCS rats. Eur. J. Neurosci. 22, 1057–1072. doi: 10.1111/j.1460-9568.2005.04300.x
9. Dembinska, O., Rojas, L. M., Chemtob, S., and Lachapelle, P. (2002). Evidence for a brief period of enhanced oxygen susceptibility in the rat model of oxygen-induced retinopathy. Invest. Ophthalmol. Vis. Sci. 43, 2481–2490.
10. Douglas, R. M., Alam, N. M., Silver, B. D., Mcgill, T. J.,

Tschetter, W. W., and Prusky, G. T. (2005). Independent visual threshold measurements in the two eyes of freely moving rats and mice using a virtual-reality optokinetic system. Vis. Neurosci. 22, 677–684. doi: 10.1017/s0952523805225166

11. Dryja, T. P., McEvoy, J. A., McGee, T. L., and Berson, E. L. (2000). Novel rhodopsin mutations Gly114Val and Gln184Pro in dominant retinitis pigmentosa. Invest. Ophthalmol. Vis. Sci. 41, 3124–3127.
12. Dryja, T. P., McGee, T. L., Reichel, E., Hahn, L. B., Cowley, G. S., Yandell, D. W., et al. (1990). A point mutation of the rhodopsin gene in one form of retinitis pigmentosa. Nature 343, 364–366. doi: 10.1038/343364a0
13. Fernández-Sánchez, L., Lax, P., Esquiva, G., Martín-Nieto, J., Pinilla, I., and Cuenca, N. (2012). Safranal, a saffron constituent, attenuates retinal degeneration in P23H rats. PLoS One 7:e43074. doi: 10.1371/journal.pone.0043074
14. Fischer, M. D., Huber, G., Beck, S. C., Tanimoto, N., Muehlfriedel, R., Fahl, E., et al. (2009). Noninvasive, in vivo assessment of mouse retinal structure using optical coherence tomography. PLoS One 4:e7507. doi: 10.1371/journal.pone.0007507
15. Greferath, U., Grunert, U., and Wassle, H. (1990). Rod bipolar cells in the mammalian retina show protein kinase C-like immunoreactivity. J. Comp. Neurol. 301, 433–442. doi: 10.1002/cne.903010308
16. Horio, N., Kachi, S., Hori, K., Okamoto, Y., Yamamoto, E., Terasaki, H., et al. (2001). Progressive change of optical coherence tomography scans in retinal degeneration slow mice. Arch. Ophthalmol. 119, 1329–1332. doi: 10.1001/archopht.119.9.1329
17. Huber, G., Beck, S. C., Grimm, C., Sahaboglu-Tekgoz, A., Paquet-Durand, F., Wenzel, A., et al. (2009). Spectral domain optical coherence tomography in mouse models of retinal degeneration. Invest. Ophthalmol. Vis. Sci. 50, 5888–5895. doi: 10.1167/iovs.09-3724
18. Jiao, J., Mo, B., Wei, H., and Jiang, Y. R. (2013). Comparative study of laser-induced choroidal neovascularization in rats by paraffin sections, frozen sections and high-resolution optical coherence tomography. Graefes Arch. Clin. Exp. Ophthalmol. 251, 301–307. doi: 10.1007/s00417-012-2204-4
19. Kolb, H., Nelson, R., Ahnelt, P., and Cuenca, N. (2001). Cellular organization of the vertebrate retina. Prog. Brain Res. 131, 3–26.
20. LaVail, M. M., Gorrin, G. M., and Repaci, M. A. (1987a). Strain differences in sensitivity to light-induced photoreceptor degeneration in albino mice. Curr. Eye Res. 6, 825–834. doi: 10.3109/02713688709034850
21. LaVail, M. M., Gorrin, G. M., Repaci, M. A., Thomas, L. A., and Ginsberg, H. M. (1987b). Genetic regulation of light damage to photoreceptors. Invest. Ophthalmol. Vis. Sci. 28, 1043–1048.
22. LaVail, M. M., Gorrin, G. M., Repaci, M. A., and Yasumura, D. (1987c). Light-induced retinal degeneration in albino mice and rats: strain and species differences. Prog. Clin. Biol. Res. 247, 439–454.
23. Lewin, A. S., Drenser, K. A., Hauswirth, W. W., Nishikawa, S., Yasumura, D., Flannery, J. G., et al. (1998). Ribozyme rescue of photoreceptor cells in a transgenic rat model of autosomal dominant retinitis pigmentosa. Nat. Med. 4, 967–971. doi: 10.1038/2077
24. Li, Q., Timmers, A. M., Hunter, K., Gonzalez-Pola, C., Lewin, A. S., Reitze, D. H., et al. (2001). Noninvasive imaging by optical coherence tomography to monitor retinal degeneration in the mouse. Invest. Ophthalmol. Vis. Sci. 42, 2981–2989.
25. Lowe, R. J., Duncan, J. L., Yang, H., Donohue-Rolfe, K. M., Matthes, M. T., Yasumura, D., et al. (2005). Retinal degeneration is slowed by eye pigmentation in P23H but not in S334ter mutant rhodopsin transgenic rats. Invest. Ophthalmol. Vis. Sci. 46, E-abstract 2300.
26. Lu, B., Wang, S., Francis, P. J., Li, T., Gamm, D. M., Capowski, E. E., et al. (2010). Cell transplantation to arrest early changes in an ush2a animal model. Invest. Ophthalmol. Vis. Sci. 51, 2269–2276. doi: 10.1167/iovs.09-4526
27. Machida, S., Kondo, M., Jamison, J. A., Khan, N. W., Kononen, L. T., Sugawara, T., et al. (2000). P23H rhodopsin transgenic rat: correlation of retinal function with histopathology. Invest. Ophthalmol. Vis. Sci. 41, 3200–3209.
28. Martinez-Navarrete, G., Seiler, M. J., Aramant, R. B., Fernandez-Sanchez, L., Pinilla, I., and Cuenca, N. (2011). Retinal degeneration in two lines of transgenic S334ter rats. Exp. Eye Res. 92, 227–237. doi: 10.1016/j.exer.2010.12.001
29. McGill, T. J., Lund, R. D., Douglas, R. M., Wang, S., Lu, B., Silver, B. D., et al. (2007). Syngeneic schwann cell transplantation preserves vision in RCS rat without immunosuppression. Invest. Ophthalmol. Vis. Sci. 48, 1906–1912. doi: 10.1167/iovs.06-1117
30. McGinnis, J. F., Stepanik, P. L., Chen, W., Elias, R., Cao, W., and Lerious, V. (1999). Unique retina cell phenotypes revealed by immunological analysis of recoverin expression in rat retina cells. J. Neurosci. Res. 55, 252–260. doi: 10.1002/(sici)1097-4547(19990115)55:2<252::aid-jnr13>3.0.co;2-n
31. Naash, M. I., LaVail, M. M., and Anderson, R. E. (1989). Factors affecting the susceptibility of the retina to light damage. Prog. Clin. Biol. Res. 314, 513–522.
32.
33. Nusinowitz, S., Ridder, W., and Heckenlively, J. R. (2001). "Electrodiagnostic techniques for visual function testing in mice," in Systematic Evaluation of the Mouse Eye: Anatomy, Pathology and Biomethods, eds R. Smith, S. W. M. John, P. M. Nishina and J. P. Sundberg (New York: CRC Press), 320–344.
34. Peichl, L., and González-Soriano, J. (1994). Morphological types of horizontal cell in rodent retinae: a comparison of rat, mouse, gerbil and guinea pig. Vis. Neurosci. 11, 501–517. doi: 10.1017/s095252380000242x
35. Pinilla, I., Lund, R. D., and Sauvé, Y. (2004). Contribution of rod and cone pathways to the dark-adapted electroretinogram (ERG) b-wave following

retinal degeneration in RCS rats. Vision Res. 44, 2467–2474. doi: 10.1016/j.visres.2004.05.020

36. Pinilla, I., Lund, R. D., and Sauvé, Y. (2005). Enhanced cone dysfunction in rats homozygous for the P23H rhodopsin mutation. Neurosci. Lett. 382, 16–21. doi: 10.1016/j.neulet.2005.02.055

37. Prusky, G. T., Alam, N. M., Beekman, S., and Douglas, R. M. (2004). Rapid quantification of adult and developing mouse spatial vision using a virtual optomotor system. Invest. Ophthalmol. Vis. Sci. 45, 4611–4616. doi: 10.1167/iovs.04-0541

38. Spaide, R. F., and Curcio, C. A. (2011). Anatomical correlates to the bands seen in the outer retina by optical coherence tomography: literature review and model. Retina 31, 1609–1619. doi: 10.1097/iae.0b013e3182247535

39. Umino, Y., Everhart, D., Solessio, E., Cusato, K., Pan, J. C., Nguyen, T. H., et al. (2006). Hypoglycemia leads to age-related loss of vision. Proc. Natl. Acad. Sci. U S A 103, 19541–19545. doi: 10.1073/pnas.0604478104

40. Vaughan, D. K., Coulibaly, S. F., Darrow, R. M., and Organisciak, D. T. (2003). A morphometric study of light-induced damage in transgenic rat models of retinitis pigmentosa. Invest. Ophthalmol. Vis. Sci. 44, 848–855. doi: 10.1167/iovs.02-0709

41. Villegas-Pérez, M. P., Lawrence, J. M., Vidal-Sanz, M., Lavail, M. M., and Lund, R. D. (1998). Ganglion cell loss in RCS rat retina: a result of compression of axons by contracting intraretinal vessels linked to the pigment epithelium. J. Comp. Neurol. 392, 58–77. doi: 10.1002/(sici)1096-9861(19980302)392:1<58::aid-cne5>3.3.co;2-e

42. Zhou, X., Li, F., Kong, L., Chodosh, J., and Cao, W. (2009). Anti-inflammatory effect of pigment epithelium-derived factor in DBA/2J mice. Mol. Vis. 15, 438–450.

CHAPTER 6 CALCIUM-BINDING PROTEIN IMMUNOCYTOCHEMISTRY

Priscilla Logerot, Nils O. E. Kru¨tzfeldt, J. Martin Wild, M. Fabiana Kubke

INTRODUCTION

The nucleus mesencephalicus lateralis pars dorsalis (MLd) has been extensively studied both anatomically and electrophysiologically in several avian species, e.g., chicken [1]–[5], guinea fowl [6], mallard [7], barn owl [8]–[15] and pigeon [16]–[18]. Fewer data are available for the MLd of songbirds, which comprise roughly half the number of avian species. In birds generally the nucleus is a major relay in the ascending auditory pathway to the forebrain but in songbirds it also has the special function of mediating auditory feedback for the learning and maintained production of song. We have previously reported on the ascending projections to MLd [19], [20]; in the present paper we describe the regional organization of MLd in zebra finches based on the different staining patterns resulting from the application of antibodies to three calcium binding proteins.

Most of our knowledge of the anatomical organization of MLd in songbirds derives from histochemical and immunohistochemical studies in zebra finches [21]–[24], and from studies that have examined auditory and somatosensory connections of MLd and adjacent structures in various finches [19], [20], [25], [26]. Here we define MLd as the midbrain region receiving ascending projections from the auditory brainstem, as previously described [19], [20]. In the midbrain of the zebra finch, as in other avian species, MLd is located within the intercollicular complex (ICo). Its boundaries can be defined on the basis of its cytoarchitecture, although its ventral and ventrolateral borders can prove difficult to differentiate from the adjacent ICo. MLd was originally shown by Karten [27] (see also [28]) in pigeons to project to the thalamic nucleus ovoidalis (Ov), a finding substantiated in ring doves [29], barn owls [30] and zebra finches [19].

We chose to describe the internal structure of MLd using antibodies against calbindin (CB), calretinin (CR) and parvalbumin (PV), three calcium-binding proteins (CaBPs) that are expressed in different neuronal subpopulations in both the peripheral and central nervous systems, with only a partial overlap [31], [32]. They belong to the EF-hand family of CaBPs [33] and generally bind to calcium ions (Ca^{2+}) [34]. The expression of these three proteins has been used for many years to describe anatomically various sensory pathways and nuclei (for review see [31]), including the auditory torus of amphibians [35], [36], reptiles [37]–[40], birds [3], [5], [11], [12], [14], [21], [22] and mammals [41]–[57]. CaBP immunocytochemistry has been used previously to describe MLd in zebra finches [21], [22], although these studies mainly examined the patterns of expression in male birds (both adults and juveniles) and were performed in the absence of knowledge of the pattern of ascending inputs to MLd in this species. Here we extend these studies to describe the patterns of expression in adult male and female zebra finches, in the context of our knowledge of the ascending inputs to MLd [19], [20] and the electrophysiological in vivo data now available [58]–[62].

Citation: Logerot P, Kru¨tzfeldt NOE, Wild JM, Kubke MF (2011) Calcium-Binding Protein Immunocytochemistry. PLoS ONE 6(6): e20686. doi:10.1371/journal.pone.0020686.

MATERIALS AND METHODS

Animals

The experimental procedures were carried out according to the guidelines of, and were approved by, the Animal Ethics Committee of the University of Auckland (approval #R689). Birds were obtained from a local breeder, housed in a large flight aviary, provided with food and water *ad lib*, and maintained under a constant light/night cycle in the University of Auckland animal facility.

Immunocytochemistry

Each of the 7 birds was deeply anaesthetized with an intramuscular injection of ketamine (Parnell Laboratories, Auckland, New Zealand; 100 mg/kg) and xylazine (Rompun Bayer; 20 mg/kg) and transcardially perfused with 0.9% saline followed by 4% paraformaldehyde in phosphate buffer (PB 0.1 M, pH 7.4) as per University of Auckland Animal Ethics Committee permits. The brains were post-fixed in 4% paraformaldehyde (PFA) before being cryoprotected in 30% sucrose in phosphate buffered saline (PBS 0.01 M, pH 7.4). They were then cut coronally on a freezing microtome and serial, free-floating 35 μm thick sections were collected in PBS in four columns. Sections in one column were mounted on subbed slides and stained with cresyl violet for the identification of cytoarchitecture. Sections in the three other columns were immediately processed for immunocytochemistry. After three 10 minutes rinses (all rinses in this protocol lasted 10 min) in PBS, endogenous peroxidase activity was blocked using 50% methanol and 1% hydrogen peroxide in distilled water for 10 min at room temperature. Sections were then rinsed 3 times in PBS before being incubated in a primary antibody against PV, CB or CR (monoclonal mouse anti-parvalbumin antibody: SWANT clone 235, Basel, Switzerland; monoclonal mouse anti-calbindin D28k: SWANT clone 300, Basel, Switzerland; polyclonal rabbit anti-calretinin antibody: SWANT 7699/4, Basel, Switzerland for 3 males and 3 females; monoclonal mouse anti-calretinin antibody: SWANT 6B3, Basel, Switzerland for one male) at a final dilution of 1:5000 in PBS with 0.4% Triton X-100 (PBS-T) and 2% Normal Horse Serum (NHS) overnight at room temperature. After 3 rinses in PBS, sections were transferred to a biotinylated donkey anti-mouse or anti-rabbit secondary antibody (711-065-150 and 711-065-152, Jackson Immunoresearch Laboratories, Inc., West Grove, PA) in PBS-T with 2% NHS at a dilution of 1:300 for 90 minutes at room temperature and rinsed 6 times in PBS before being incubated in avidin-biotin peroxidase complex (PIE 31001, Global Science and Technology Ltd, Auckland, New Zealand) at 1:1000 in PBS-T for 1 h at room temperature. Following 6 rinses in PBS, sections were finally incubated in a chromagen-solution consisting of 0.025% 3,3′-diamino-benzidine (DAB), 0.005% H_2O_2 and 0.015% $CoCl_2$ in PBS. The reaction was stopped by several washes in PBS. Sections were subsequently mounted on subbed slides, dehydrated in successive ethanol baths, cleared in xylene, and coverslipped using DePeX (Serva, Heidelberg, Germany).

Analysis

All of the material was examined using light microscopy. Comparisons between different staining patterns were performed on adjacent sections, and the overall staining patterns and their boundaries were mapped onto a single, serially cut, cresyl violet-stained zebra finch brain for inter-individual comparisons. Outlines of the nucleus and visible subdivisions, were drawn using a camera lucida and then scanned into a personal computer for digital representation. Sections were also digitally photographed using a Nikon 80i light microscope (5 megapixel camera). Levels were then adjusted using Adobe Photoshop CS4 (Adobe Systems, San Jose, CA).

RESULTS

In the transverse plane MLd has an ovoid shape and is oriented obliquely along a ventrolateral to dorsomedial axis. At its caudal and rostral poles MLd is confined to a position laterally adjacent to the medial edge of ICo, but at intermediate rostrocaudal levels, where it reaches its maximum size, it expands laterally from this edge towards the tectal ventricle, from which it is separated only by a thin periventricular lamina [3]. At caudal levels MLd presents a dorsomedial extension called CM [caudomedial, 3], which has been identified in greenfinches [25], pigeons [18] and chickens [3]. At more rostral levels the dorsomedial border of MLd is straight-edged, where it abuts a core nucleus of the intercollicular complex [3], commonly known as the dorsomedial nucleus (DM). Unlike in pigeons [63] or chickens [64], MLd in zebra finches lacks a clear hilar region on its medial aspect [63], [64], so that its afferents from auditory brainstem nuclei enter the nucleus over a wide dorsoventral extent [19], [20].

Parvalbumin-LI

The general parvalbumin staining pattern in MLd described by us [19] was shown to overlap closely the area in receipt of ascending brainstem auditory afferents, thereby defining the boundaries of MLd (Figure 1). Here we describe regional differences in the pattern of staining in more detail. Two regions within MLd were defined by the PV-LI: inner (MLd.I) and outer (MLd.O) (Figure 2, A–D). MLd.O was characterized by a PV-LI positive neuropil and by the presence of stained fibers and stained and unstained somata (Figure 2, F). (For descriptive purposes, we differentiate between staining of fibers within the neuropil and the rest of the neuropil.) The neuropil in this region showed a dense punctate staining pattern, whereas many of its neurons presented stained processes and those along the lateral edge of MLd exhibited elongated somata concentric with the overlying ventricle (not shown). At the level of DM, a small region on the dorsomedial aspect of MLd that can be identified in Nissl stained sections (Figure 2, B-asterisk, G, H-asterisk) exhibited a staining pattern distinct from that of the MLd.O. This small region had a darker PV-LI positive neuropil, stained fibers and stained somata and processes, but was characterized by an absence of punctate staining.

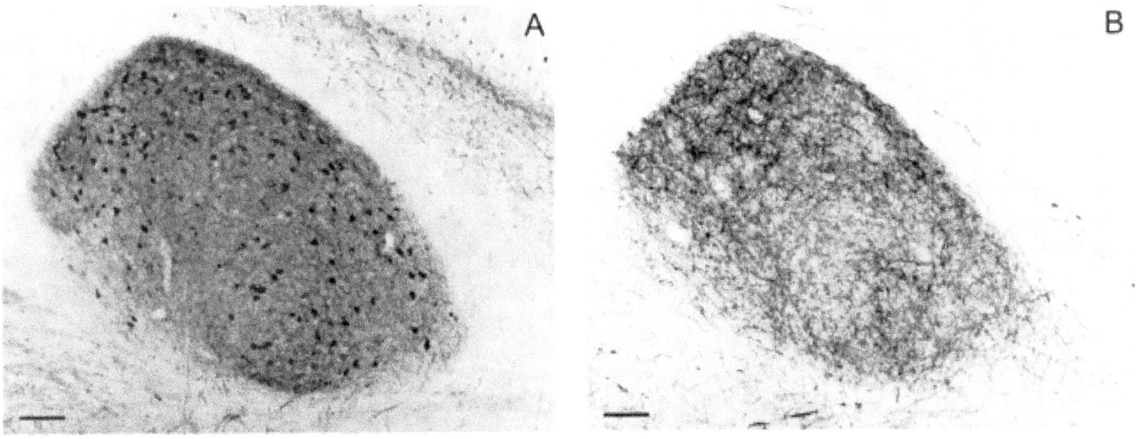

Figure 1: Pattern of parvalbumin-like immunoreactivity (PV-LI) and auditory terminal fields in MLd.

Coronal sections through MLd in two different birds showing the correspondence between the PV-LI (A) and the ascending auditory terminal field obtained from injections to LLV (B). [Image in B was part of 20]. Scale bars=100 μm.

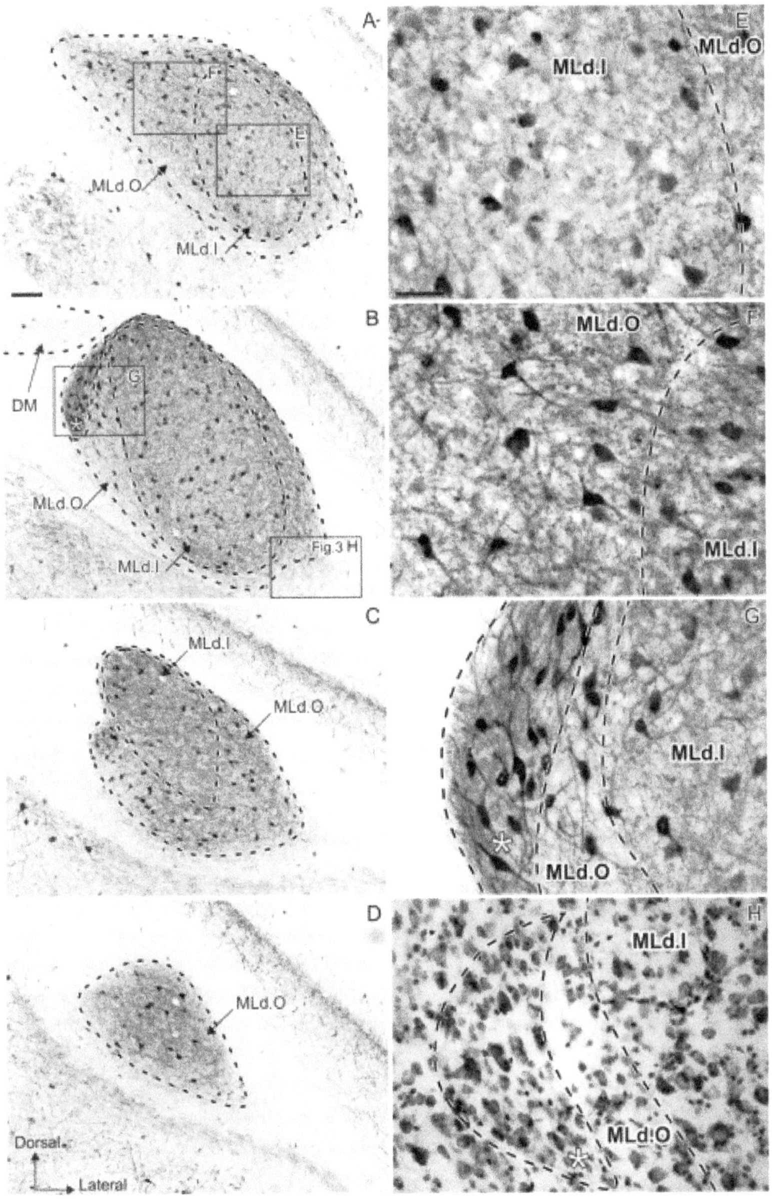

Figure 2: Patterns of parvalbumin-like immunoreactivity (PV-LI).

A–D: caudal (top) to rostral (bottom) coronal sections showing PV-LI through the right MLd of a female zebra finch delineating two regions within the nucleus: MLd.O and MLd.I. The asterisk in **B** indicates the small nucleus within MLd.O that shows a different staining pattern. (DM is outlined for comparison with Figure 6.). **E–G:** high magnifications views of areas boxed in **A** and **B**. **E:** Photomicrograph of MLd.I (inset **E**in panel **A**) showing the specific neuropil staining and low punctuate density of this region. **F:** Photomicrograph of MLd.O (inset **F** in panel **A**) depicting the neuropil staining, high punctuate density and somata with visible processes specific to this region. **G:**high magnification view of the region marked by an asterisk in **B**. Note the darker neuropil staining than that of MLd.O and the absence of punctuate staining. **H:**Photomicrograph of a Nissl stained section also shown in Figure 5B, showing the dorsomedial MLd subnucleus marked with an asterisk in **B**. Scale bar: A–D=100 µm; E–G=50 µm.

The inner region (MLd.I) could be distinguished by an apparent lower density of stained puncta (Figure 2, E; cf Figure 2, F). Like MLd.O, MLd.I also showed an immunopositive neuropil, stained and unstained somata, and some punctate staining. The processes of the stained neurons were, however, not visible in most cases. Incoming fibers - presumably mostly afferents from lower auditory nuclei - were seen mainly through the caudal half MLd. Caudally they were found widely dispersed along the ventromedial edge of the nucleus, while rostrally these were found more restricted to the most ventral edge (data not shown, but see [19], [20]).

Calretinin-LI

Brains of 3 males and 3 females were immunostained using a polyclonal anti-calretinin antibody and 1 other brain from a male was immunostained using a monoclonal anti-calretinin antibody. The staining patterns resulting from use of the monoclonal antibody were better delineated than those from use of the polyclonal, but were otherwise identical and are thus described together. Incubation with antibodies raised against calretinin resulted in a pattern of staining that, as in the case of parvalbumin, revealed two distinct regions within MLd: inner (MLd.O) and outer (MLd.I) (Figure 3, A–D). Caudally, MLd.O occupied a ventral position within the ICo, expanding towards the tectal ventricle at intermediate rostrocaudal levels (Figure 3, A). MLd.O lay on ventrolateral to dorsomedial axis, finally to be located in a dorsal position, underlain by the ICo at more rostral levels. The outer region presented a relatively unstained neuropil, within which some stained somata as well as numerous fibers were observed (Figure 3, E, H). Within this region, the same small, dorsomedial part found to be PV-positive (see above and Figure 2B, G) was either devoid of staining or presented a very light neuropil staining. (Figure 3, B-asterisk, F-asterisk).

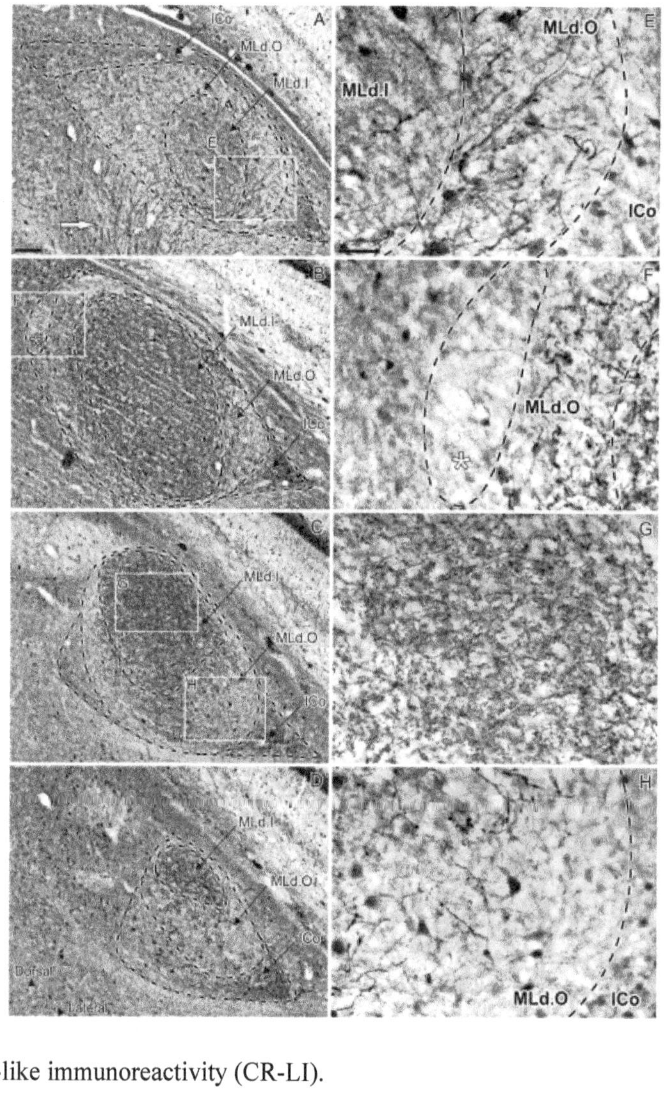

Figure 3: Patterns of calretinin-like immunoreactivity (CR-LI).

A–D: caudal (top) to rostral (bottom) coronal sections showing CR-LI through the right MLd of a male zebra finch delineating MLd.I and MLd.O regions within the nucleus and the ICo as well as the trajectory of presumptive ascending auditory fibers (white arrow in A). The asterisk in **B** indicates the small nucleus within the MLd.O that shows a different staining pattern. **E–G:** high magnifications views of areas boxed in **A**, **B** and **C**. **E:** Photomicrograph of the MLd.I and MLd.O (inset **E** in panel **A**) showing the specific neuropil staining of these regions. **F:** high magnification view of the region marked by an asterisk in **B**. Note the lighter neuropil staining. **G:** Photomicrograph of MLd.I (inset **G** in panel **C**) showing the intense CR-LI staining of the neuropil. **H:** Photomicrograph of the MLd.O (inset **H** in panel **C**) showing the absence of neuropil staining and the presence of a few stained somata and fibers. Scale bar: A–D=100 µm; E–G=50 µm.

MLd.I was readily distinguished from MLd.O by its darkly-stained neuropil (Figure 3, E, G). Some stained somata, as well as perikaryal 'ghosts' and terminal boutons, were observed. MLd.I occupied a central position caudally (Figure 3, A), extended along a ventrolateral to dorsomedial axis at intermediate levels where MLd is at its largest (Figure 3, B and C), and occupied a dorsal position rostrally (Figure 3, D). CR-LI fibers were seen running along the external surface of MLd.I, and some CR-LI fibers were also seen traversing it (Figure 3, E). The trajectory of presumptive ascending afferent fibers was seen mainly through the caudal half of the nucleus. As with the fibers showing PV-LI, CR-LI fibers entered MLd caudally from its internal edge over a wide extent (Figure 3, A), while rostrally they were restricted more ventrally.

The outer and inner regions defined by CR-LI correspond to the outer and inner regions defined by PV-LI. Outside but immediately adjacent to MLd, an external CR-LI positive region was identified (Figure 3, A–D), characterized by an immunopositive neuropil, within which numerous small stained somata were observed; a few of these also showed stained processes. Caudally and rostrally, this region surrounded MLd (Figure 3 A, C and D) and at intermediate levels it was restricted to a ventrolateral position (Figure 3 B). Since this region does not receive ascending auditory inputs [19], [20] it is considered part of ICo [19], [20].

Calbindin-LI

Calbindin-LI was also different in the inner (MLd.I) and outer (MLd.O) regions of MLd (Figure 4, A–D). At its most caudal and rostral levels, MLd showed a CB-LI positive neuropil and stained somata, some of which had immunostained processes and terminal boutons in both MLd.I and MLd.O (Figure 4, C and D). At intermediate levels, MLd.O showed light or no staining of neuropil, with some stained somata. The lateral and dorsal parts of MLd.O had a lightly stained neuropil, while its medial aspect appeared devoid of it (Figure 4, B). Also, the whole region presented some stained somata as well as a low density of terminal boutons. The subnucleus at the dorsomedial corner of MLd that shows distinct PV-LI and CR-LI and is also visible in Nissl stained-sections (Figure 4B asterisk), showed a light neuropil staining and some small stained somata with stained processes. In contrast to calretinin and parvalbumin staining, CB-LI did not stain presumptive afferent fibers to MLd. MLd.I did not present a homogeneous staining throughout the whole nucleus; at intermediate levels it was devoid of neuropil staining but was filled with a considerable number of terminal boutons and a few CB-LI positive large somata, which were less frequently observed than in MLd.O (Figure 4, A, B and E). Caudally and rostrally, however, the neuropil of MLd.I was stained and had greater density of somata (Figure 4, C, D and F). As in the CR-LI stained material, CB-LI was observed surrounding MLd caudally and rostrally, while occupying a ventrolateral position at intermediate levels (Figure 4, A–D). It was characterized by a CB-LI positive dark neuropil, some stained fibers and terminal boutons, and numerous small stained somata, some with stained proximal processes (Figure 4, G). This region is not the recipient of ascending auditory inputs and is therefore considered part of ICo rather than of MLd.

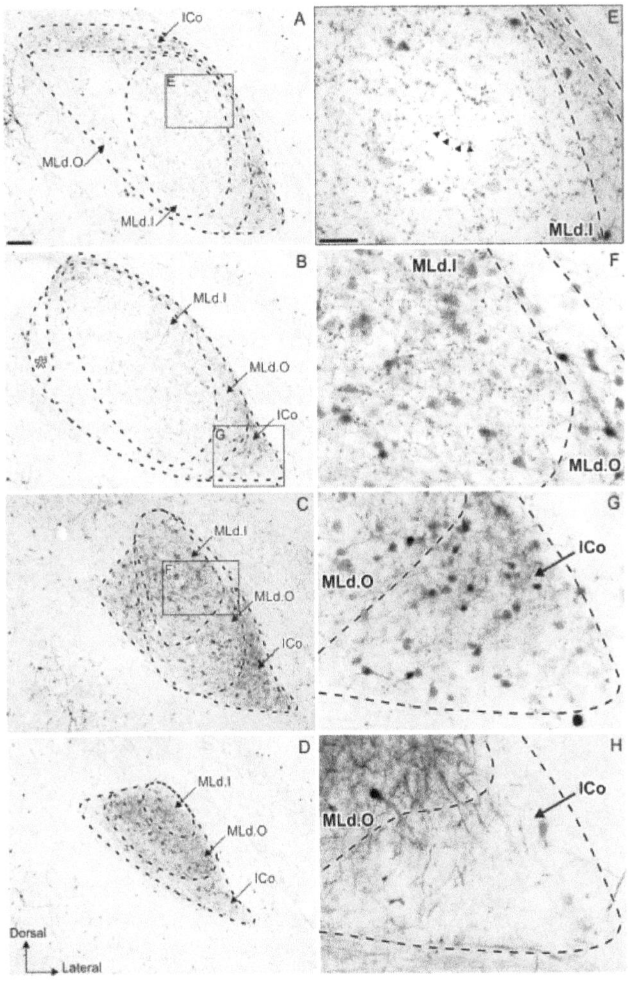

Figure 4: Patterns of calbindin-like immunoreactivity (CB-LI).

A–D: caudal (top) to rostral (bottom) coronal sections showing CB-LI through the right MLd of a female zebra finch delineating MLd.I and MLd.O within the nucleus and the ICo. The asterisk in **B** indicates the small nucleus within MLd.O. Note that it is not as clearly visible as with the PV- and CR-like staining. **E–G:** high magnification views of areas boxed in **A**, **B** and **C**. **E:** Photomicrograph of MLd.I (inset **E** in panel **A**) showing the specific high density of labeled terminals in this region (some are indicated by arrow heads) and the absence of neuropil staining in intermediate sections. **F**Photomicrograph of MLd.I (inset **F** in panel **C**) showing the staining pattern in a more rostral section. Note the high density of labeled terminals and the difference in neuropil staining as well as the number of stained somata. **G:** Photomicrograph of ICo (inset **G** in panel **B**) showing the CB-LI staining of this region. **H:** Photomicrograph of PV-LI staining in ICo in an adjacent section (inset **H** in panel **B** – Figure 2) showing the absence of neuropil staining. Scale bar: A–D=100 µm; E–G=50 µm.

Summary of Staining Patterns

PV staining was commensurate with the whole of MLd, defined as that region of the torus receiving direct and indirect ascending auditory afferents [19], [20]. Within the PV-LI region, two regions based mainly on the apparent abundance of puncta could be differentiated. An inner region, which had less punctate staining, corresponded to a region that also exhibited a CR-LI-positive neuropil and matched the part of MLd where most of the terminal boutons showing CB-LI were concentrated. We have termed this the inner region MLd.I. An outer region of MLd (MLd.O), which surrounded the inner region, was characterized by PV-LI exhibiting a higher density of punctate staining than that of MLd.I. In contrast, MLd.O exhibited a CR-LI negative neuropil, but was rich in CR-positive fibers and also presented a few CB-LI-positive somata and a light CB-LI positive neuropil. Surrounding MLd is a CB-LI- and CR-LI- positive region (Figures 3 and 4) which is not stained with PV (Figure 4, H), does not receive ascending auditory projections and is, therefore, considered part of ICo. It is interesting that the set of CaBPs used in the current study clearly delineate two regions within MLd, as well as the ICo (Figure 5, E–H), whereas these boundaries do not always appear as easily identifiable in Nissl stained material (Figure 5, A–D) especially at the most caudal and rostral levels (Figure 5, A and D).

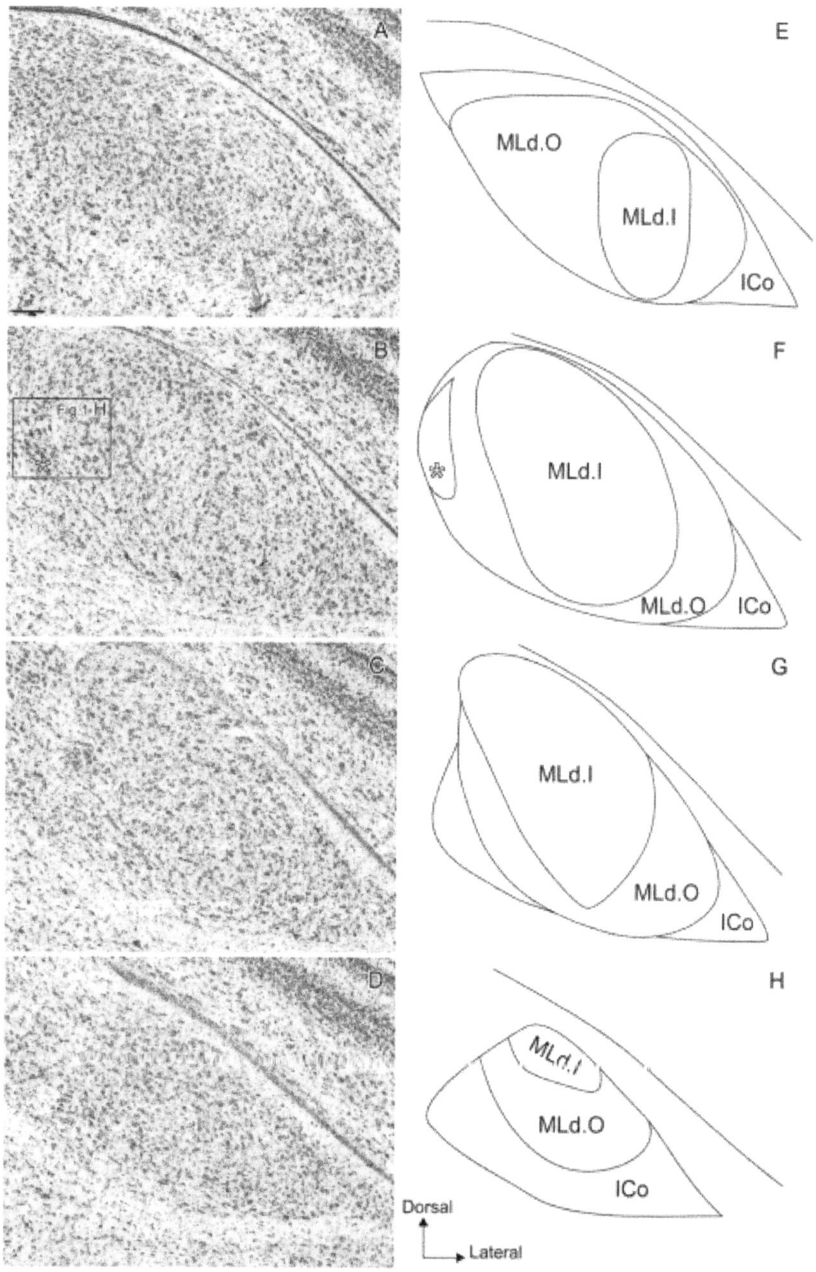

Figure 5: Subdivisions of MLd in Nissl stained material.

A–D: caudal (top) to rostral (bottom) coronal Nissl-stained sections through the right MLd. The asterisk in **B** indicates the small nucleus within MLd.O showing a different staining pattern in PV- and CR-LI adjacent sections. Note that it is clearly visible in Nissl-stained sections. **E–G:** Schematic drawings of the different regions based on PV-, CR- and CB-LI staining. The asterisk in **F** indicates the subnucleus delineated by the PV- and CR- LI staining and by Nissl staining. Note how the boundaries can be identified by naked eye for more intermediate sections (**F** and **G** and corresponding panels **B** and **C** respectively) while they are obscure in the more caudal and rostral ones (**E** and **H** and corresponding panels **A** and **D** respectively). Scale bar=100 μm.

CaBP staining patterns revealed no differences between males and females in the organization of the auditory midbrain, except for differences in PV staining patterns of DM (compare Figure 2 A–D with Figure 6). We did not quantify cell numbers in MLd in our various cases, but no striking differences were apparent either between males and females (see Figures 2A–D and 6) or between left and right MLds.

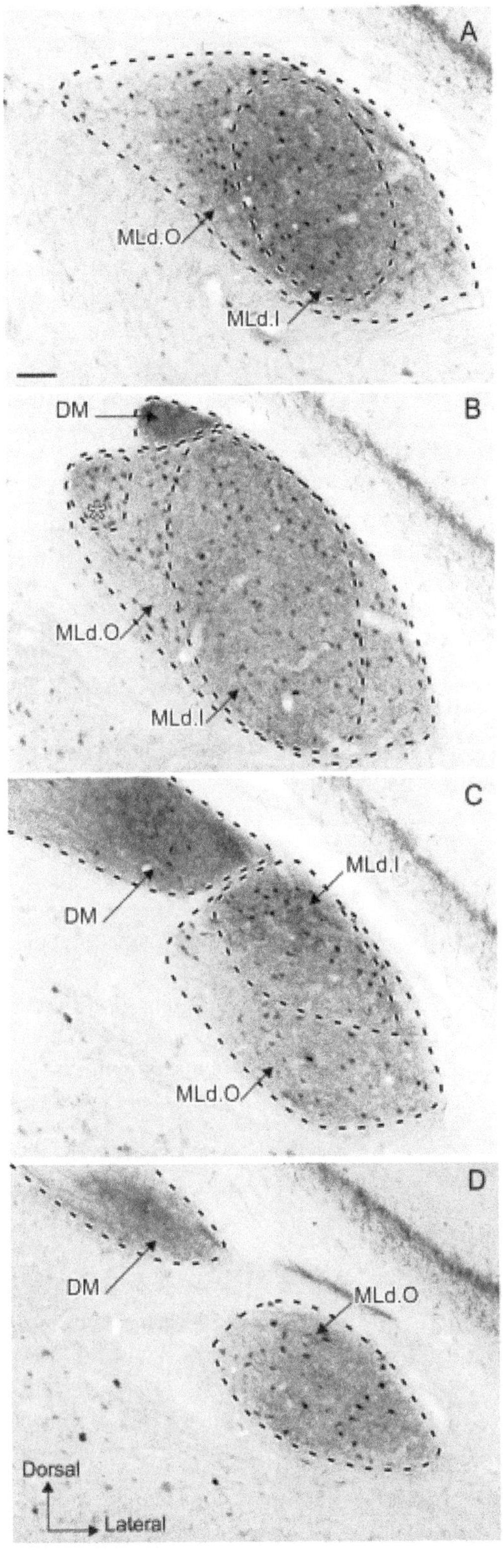

Figure 6: Parvalbumin-like immunoreactivity in males and females.

A–D: MLdCaudal (top) to rostral (bottom) coronal sections showing PV-LI through the right MLd delineating MLd.I and MLd.O within the nucleus in a male zebra finch. A comparison with Figure 2 A–D shows the absence of sexual dimorphism in the staining of nucleus MLd and the presence of sexual dimorphism in the staining of nucleus DM (see text). Scale bar=100 μm.

DISCUSSION

We have used CaBP immunostaining to identify the regional organization of MLd within the context of its ascending projections recently described [19], [20]. An inner and an outer region of MLd (MLd.I and MLd.O, respectively) can be distinguished based on the patterns of CaBP immunoreactivity, which also distinguish MLd proper from its surrounding ICo. The patterns of staining in the areas examined in the midbrain were similar in males and females, with the exception of DM. In females, only few DM somata were immunostained (Figure 2, B), while in males DM showed a strong PV-LI neuropil with few stained somata (Figure 6, A–D), as shown previously in the context of song system anatomy [65]. This is interesting because zebra finches – and songbirds in general – are known to present sexual dimorphism of certain brain areas. Adult females, for instance, do not possess a song system (interconnected nuclei, distinct from the auditory pathway, involved in both vocal learning and vocal motor output) as developed as that seen in males [66]. DM receives direct descending projections from the forebrain robust nucleus of the arcopallium [67]–[70] in both sexes, but only in males do projection neurons in RA and their terminal fields in DM stain with PV [65]. Sexual dimorphism has also been shown in the higher auditory center NCM, where Pinaud et al. [71], found that males had twice as many CB-LI positive cells as females.

Comparison with Other Avian Species

Most of what is known about anatomical subdivisions of the avian MLd, based on cytoarchitecture and/or neurochemistry, ascending projections from the brainstem or neurophysiological properties, applies to non-songbirds (chicken: [1]–[5]; guinea fowl: [6]; mallards: [7]; owl: [8]–[15]; pigeon: [16]–[18]). In comparison, data available for songbirds are fewer [19]–[24], [58]–[62], [72], [73]. Recent studies [19], [20] have shown that the projection patterns of the ascending inputs to the auditory torus in zebra finches differ from those described for non-songbirds, thereby challenging the validity of a general schema for MLd subdivisions [3], [13], [14], as well as the generally presumed subdivisions of MLd in songbirds [21], [22], [73]. While the terminal fields of NA and NL projections are segregated within MLd in chickens [2], [4], pigeons [17], [18] and barn owls [13], they extensively overlap in zebra finches. Thus, segregated terminal fields within MLd cannot be used in the zebra finch (and presumably not in the closely related Bengalese finch) to differentiate what in other species are called core and shell. Braun et al. [21], [22] and Zeng et al. [73] have attempted to identify the regional organization of MLd in zebra and Bengalese finches, respectively. Braun and her colleagues described the complementary staining patterns of PV and CB (and other markers) in the brain of young male zebra finches and implied that the PV positive staining was restricted to a core of MLd, while a shelf (or shell) or marginal zone of MLd was characterized by CB-positive immunoreactivity. This differentiation, which has also been referred to (and presumably accepted) by other authors, we contend blurs the real boundary of MLd. Specifically, we suggest that the CB positive region that they seem to consider part of their shell is actually part of ICo, since it corresponds to a similar CB-positive region defined in the present study, but one that is now known not to receive ascending auditory afferents and therefore not part of MLd. If this is correct, the 'core' defined by PV-positive staining in the studies of Braun et al. would comprise the entirety of MLd.

Zeng et al. [73], using antibodies to Met-enkephalin, substance P and serotonin, suggested that the MLd of Bengalese finches was equivalent to MLd of barn owls. Thus, an MLd core and shell in Bengalese finches was considered analogous to the core and both lateral and medial shells of the central nucleus of the inferior colliculus of barn owls [13]. Zeng et al. also considered that ICo was equivalent to the external nucleus of the inferior colliculus of mammals. In their study, the core of MLd can easily be identified by a lack of substance P, as was reported for pigeons [18], but the boundary between shell and ICo remained quite unclear (see Figure 8, p. 11 in Zeng et al. [73]). The results of Zeng et al., when compared to ours, suggest that their subdivisions are congruent with ours, but a re-examination of their neurochemical boundaries with regards to known projection patterns needs to be reassessed. The complementarity of the CB and PV staining patterns characteristic of ICo and MLd, respectively, is, however, strikingly clear in their study on the neurogenesis of core and shell areas in the chick brain [5]. Still, neither of their two studies included the use of an antibody against calretinin, which Puelles et al. [3] suggest is the appropriate marker for the core region of the central nucleus in chickens, in which a dark CR-positive plexus appears to match the projections of NL onto MLd in this species [2], [4], as it does in barn owls [11], [12], [14]. Since we have now traced the ascending projections to MLd and described their terminal fields within the nucleus in zebra finches [19], [20], we can try to correlate these results with the subdivisions observed using CaBPs in the present study. In doing so, it appears that the PV-positive staining demarcates the terminal fields of ascending projections of both NA and NL and the nuclei of the lateral lemniscus, and should therefore include all MLd subdivisions. Based on this hodological criterion, the CB-positive external zone should not be considered part of MLd, but rather of ICo, which is in agreement with the organization proposed by Zeng and his colleagues for Bengalese finches [73]. Moreover, within the PV-positive region in the present study of zebra finch MLd, two distinct regions could be delineated based on the density of puncta. Also, the central zone with less puncta anatomically matched the dark CR-positive central neuropil within MLd. The two MLd regions, inner and outer, may, or may not, represent two functionally different zones. For instance, in barn owls, core and shell regions are the recipients of NL and NA projections, respectively, and have specific neurophysiological properties that originate from separate time and intensity pathways (referred as ITD and ILD, respectively). These pathways eventually converge in the lateral shell, from where projections are sent to the external nucleus, ICX, where a map of auditory space emerges (for review, see [10]). As mentioned earlier, NA and NL terminal fields in zebra finch MLd are not strictly segregated, but rather overlap substantially. These inter-species differences may reflect different evolutionary demands on the auditory system in these two lineages. Barn owls, as nocturnal hunters, excel at sound localization [74], [75], while zebra finches, as songbirds, perform rather poorly in sound localizing tasks [76] (but see also [77]). This difference in itself could suggest that the functional organization of MLd in songbirds is different from that in barn owls. In any case, exhaustive neurophysiological studies in the zebra finch midbrain are required to establish proper functional subdivisions. The few studies that have investigated electrophysiological properties of neurons in the finch MLd have reported a dorsoventral tonotopic organization of the nucleus, with low frequencies being represented dorsally and high frequencies ventrally [59], as seen in other avian species and in the mammalian central nucleus of the inferior colliculus [78]. By comparing the recording loci of Woolley and Casseday (Figure 3, p. 139, [59]) with the staining patterns of the present study, it seems that these recording loci fall outside the external edges of both our inner CR-positive region and our PV-positive region with less puncta, suggesting that they were located in what we call the outer region of MLd. This conclusion must remain hypothetical without a double labeling of recording loci and CR-IR. Thus, whether MLd.I and MLd.O exhibit different physiological properties remains to be established. Unlike the case in barn owls, these regions in finches are probably unrelated to the encoding of ITDs and ILDs, but rather to the processing of biologically relevant vocalization signals, given the differences in the organization of ascending inputs [19], [20]. Woolley and Casseday [59], [60] and Logerot et al. [79], described neurons in zebra finch MLd with tuning properties indicative of the processing of complex acoustic signals, especially their temporal aspects. Woolley et al. [61] reported four functional groups in the midbrain of the zebra finch, each of them being involved in the extraction of different features of vocal sounds. They identified broadband neurons, narrow-band temporal neurons, wideband neurons and two-band excitatory based on the spectrotemporal receptive fields of these neurons. Thus, in songbirds, feature extraction from songs might actually be a more important function than sound localization, and could be necessary for accurate song recognition [77], although the likelihood of single units coding for songs seems remote. Rather, synchronized responses of populations of neurons are proposed to "create a neural representation of the temporal patterns of the song" ([62] p. 2510). Precise recording localizations of Woolley and Casseday [59], [60] and Logerot et al. [79] units in respect to the boundaries we have defined in the present study would be a valuable addition in understanding the role of MLd subdivisions in the finch. In terms of population encoding, Poirier et al. [72]investigated MLd's responses to the Bird's Own Song (BOS), conspecific (CON) and heterospecific vocalizations. They found lateralized processing to BOS and CON, with BOS selectivity in the right MLd and CON selectivity in the left MLd. No differences were found in the present study between the staining patterns of left and right MLd. Using IEG immunocytochemistry, Woolley and Doupe [80] found no differences in ZENK expression in response to familiar or unfamiliar songs in MLd. This further adds to the necessity of investigating neuronal properties in MLd within the context of the anatomical subdivisions and how these relate to ascending inputs.

Comparison with Other Tetrapods

In the present study we have deliberately eschewed a core and shell divisional schema for MLd of the zebra finch, because of potential interpretive problems associated with comparisons across species and authors: what is shell for some workers is core for others, and vice versa. Never the less, a core/shell (or belt) organization of the auditory midbrain is frequently assumed in the literature and is thought to be a conserved feature of tetrapods. The core is exclusively auditory by way of the topographic projections from lower brainstem auditory nuclei which result in a characteristic tonotopic organization of the nucleus. Moreover, the core conveys auditory information to the thalamus over lemniscal pathways. The belt is the site of ascending multimodal sensory information, including auditory, and receives descending projections from higher auditory centers.

In mammals, the core or central nucleus of the inferior colliculus (ICC) can be differentiated from the belt area (composed of dorsal (DC) and lateral (LC) cortices) on the basis of cytoarchitecture, auditory and somatosensory projections (for review see [81], [82]) or neurophysiological properties (for review see [83]). Numerous studies have shown the complementarity of parvalbumin and calbindin as well as calretinin staining, with PV-LI structures predominantly in the ICC and CR-LI and CB-LI structures predominant in the shell (bats: [54], [56]; chinchillas: [46]; gerbils: [51]; humans: [52], [53]; mice: [45], [55], [57]; rat: [41]–[43], [47]–[50]).

Similar observations have been reported in reptiles and amphibians, although the number of studies and species investigated are fewer. The torus semicircularis (auditory midbrain) of reptiles is composed of a central nucleus (Ce) –surrounded by laminar and superficial (L) nuclei. The cytoarchitecture, hodology and electrophysiological properties of these regions have been characterized [84]–[96]. The laminar nucleus has been proposed to correspond to part of the intercollicular nucleus of birds [97]. Belekhova et al., [37], [38] reported calcium-binding protein staining in the turtle midbrain. As is seen in mammals and birds, Ce was highly PV immunostained and CB-LI and CR-LI structures were mainly seen in the laminar nucleus. Interestingly, the staining patterns they observed in Ce were not homogeneous: the core region of the central nucleus (Cec) presented PV-LI staining while PV-, CB- and CR-LI structures were seen in the peripheral area of the central nucleus (Cep). Yan [39] and Yan et al. [40]investigated the pattern of staining in the midbrain torus of the gecko that revealed the presence of PV-, CB- and CR-LI structures in both the central and laminar nuclei. The staining patterns of these three CaBPs within the central nucleus showed distinct distributions, indicating subdivisions that could delineate some segregation of the ascending auditory projections. Whether a tonotopic organization of the gecko's torus exists is unknown, which makes it difficult to relate to the present findings in zebra finch. Clearly, detailed electrophysiological studies are needed before any clear conclusion can be drawn as to a similar organization of the reptilian torus and the mammalian and avian auditory midbrains.

In amphibians, three subdivisions of the torus semicircularis are recognized: principal nucleus (Tp), laminar nucleus (Tl) and magnocellular nucleus (Tmc). The morphology, ascending projection patterns and neurophysiological properties of these three areas are well documented [98]–[111]. As seen in sauropsids and mammals, there is an exclusively auditory area, Tp, and multisensory areas Tl and Tmc. Very few studies have reported patterns of calcium-binding protein immunoreactivity in the midbrain of amphibians and only the results for parvalbumin staining are available [35], [36]. In their study, Endepols et al. observed a clear cut boundary between Tp, which was strongly PV-positive and Tl, which was completely devoid of PV-LI. In Tmc, however, some PV-positive cell bodies were visible. Zeng et al. [36] reported that Tp neuropil showed a stronger parvalbumin staining than did Tl or Tmc.

These studies in various tetrapods show that the tonotopically organized, central nucleus is characteristically strongly immunostained and delineated with CaBPs. However, as we pointed out for birds, the existence of similar "anatomical" subdivisions cannot be taken to imply functional parallels between different species. First, as mentioned earlier, the pattern of auditory ascending projections in the zebra finch [19], [20] appears to be closer to that seen in mammals, in which there are topographically organized but overlapping terminal fields of brainstem projections (for review see [112]). But the regions defined by different CaBPs seen in the present study are somewhat closer to those described in the barn owl and chicken [3], [11], [12], [14], or in reptiles [37], where there are two distinct subdivisions within the central nucleus. These apparent mismatches between MLd subdivisions and the pattern of ascending auditory inputs raise the question of the functional significance of these differences in the zebra finch MLd. As stated above, NA and NL show overlapping terminal fields in both the inner and outer regions of MLd [19]. Contralateral and ipsilateral ascending projections of the LLV may, however, differentiate between these two regions (Figure S1). Ipsilaterally, LLV projections can be seen in both the inner and outer regions of MLd, while contralaterally, they appear to be restricted to the outer MLd (Materials and Methods S1; Figure S1). Biotinylated dextran amine injections into nucleus ovoidalis (Ov) also delineate both the inner and outer regions of MLd: retrogradely labeled somata are mainly present within MLd.I (Materials and Methods S1; Figure S2) but are also seen in MLd.O. Moreover, CB-LI and CR-LI structures defined a region just outside MLd that may correspond to the belt of other tetrapod ICs. However, our previous studies [19], [20] clearly showed that this region is not an apparent recipient of any ascending auditory brainstem projections and we therefore chose to classify this region as part of the ICo. Whether the outer region of MLd could be homologous to the belt region of other vertebrates cannot be ascertained because of the lack of studies focusing on somatosensory projections to the songbird auditory torus which could reveal an area in which multisensory inputs take place.

Supporting Information

Figure S1 A–D: caudal (top) to rostral (bottom) transverse sections showing projections to the contralateral MLd after BDA injection in right LLV. Note the presence of ascending auditory fibers and terminal fields mainly in the outer region of MLd. E–H: caudal (top) to rostral (bottom) transverse sections showing projections to the ipsilateral MLd after BDA injection in right LLV. Note that the ascending auditory fibers and terminal fields can be observed in both the inner and outer region of MLd. Scale bars = 100 mm.

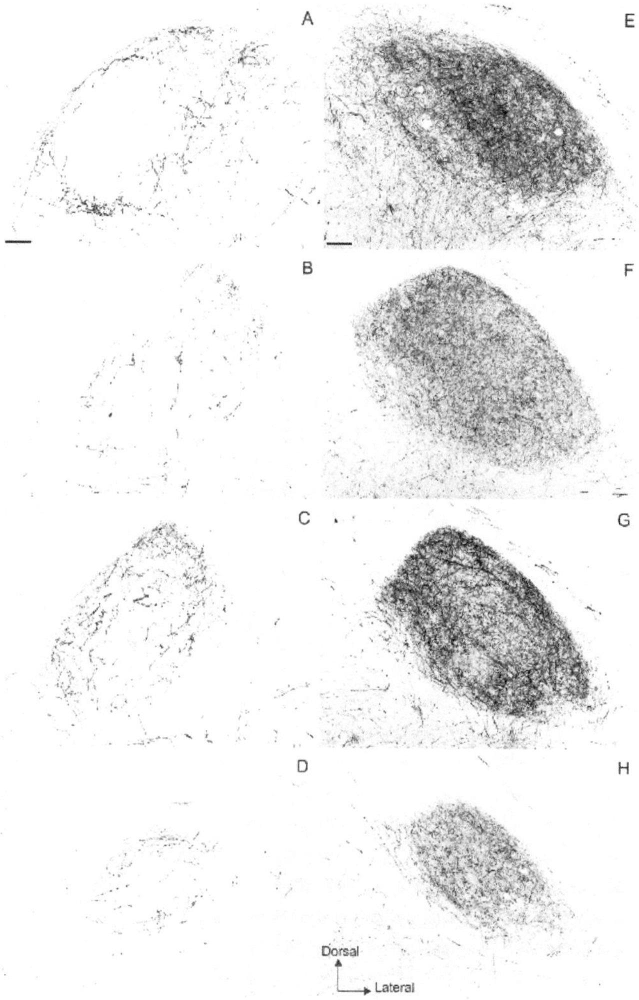

Figure S2 A–D: caudal (top) to rostral (bottom) transverse sections showing projections from the ipsilateral MLd after BDA injection in Ov. Note that retrogradely labeled somata are mainly visible and located within the inner MLd. Also note the absence of projections from the ICo. Scale bar = 100 mm. E–H: Schematic drawings of the different regions based on the PV-, CR- and CBLI stainings from the present study.

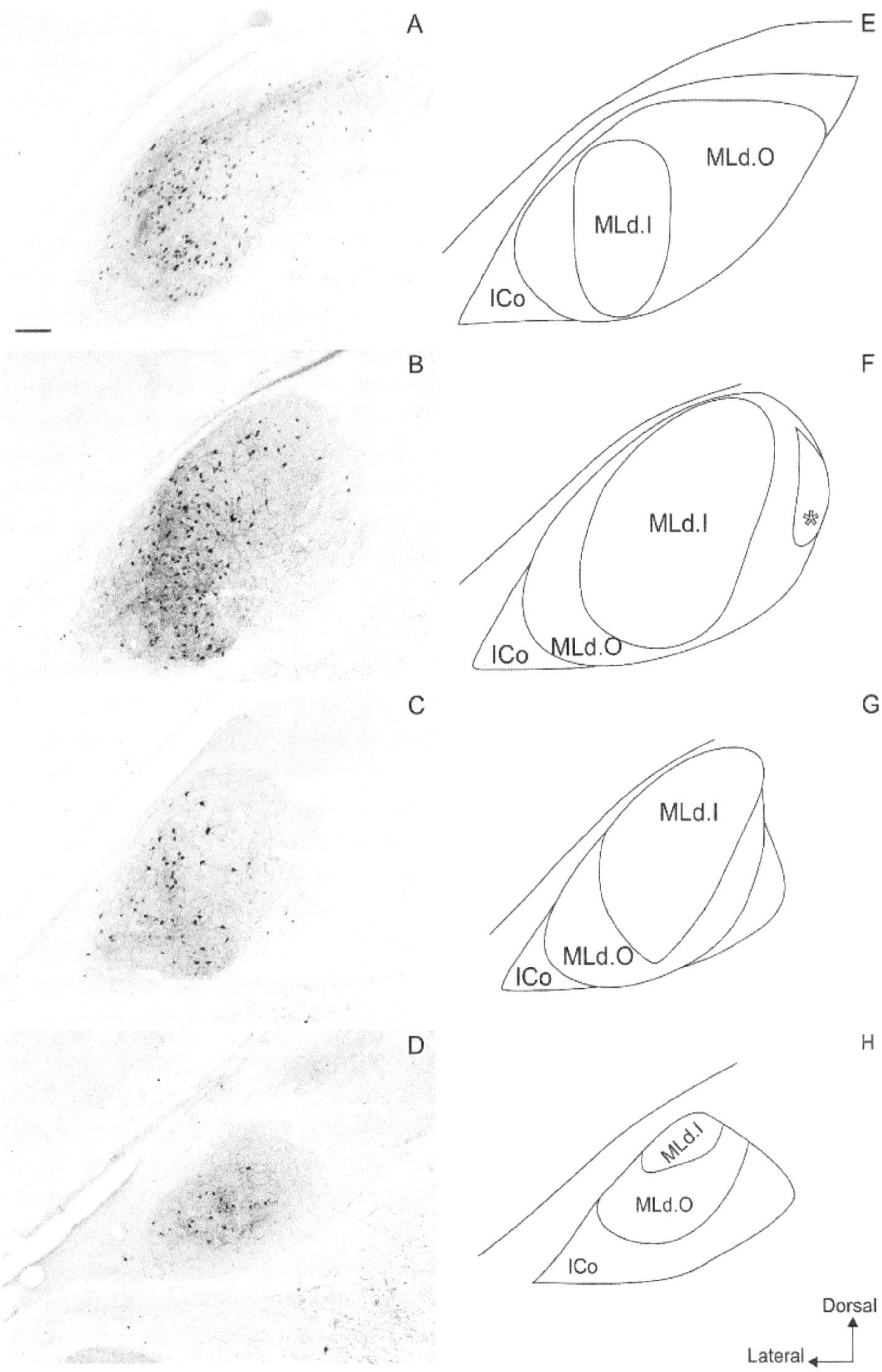

ACKNOWLEDGMENTS

We thank Silke Fuchs for technical assistance and producing the histological material used in this study.

REFERENCES

1. Coles RB, Aitkin LM (1979) The response properties of auditory neurones in the midbrain of the domestic fowl (Gallus gallus) to monaural and binaural stimuli. Journal of Comparative Physiology A 134: 241–251.
2. Conlee JW, Parks TN (1986) Origin of ascending auditory projections to the nucleus mesencephalicus lateralis pars dorsalis in the chicken. Brain Research 367: 96–113.
3. Puelles L, Robles C, Martínez-de-la-Torre M, Martínez S (1994) New subdivision schema for the avian torus semicircularis: neurochemical maps in the chick. The Journal of Comparative Neurology 340: 98–125.
4. Wang Y, Karten HJ (2010) Three subdivisions of the auditory midbrain in chicks (Gallus gallus) identified by their afferent and commissural projections. The Journal of Comparative Neurology 518: 1199–1219.
5. Zeng S, Lin Y, Yang L, Zhang X, Zuo M (2008) Comparative analysis of neurogenesis between the core and shell regions of auditory areas in the chick (Gallus gallus domesticus). Brain Research 1216: 24–37.
6. Scheich H, Langner G, Koch R (1977) Coding of narrow-band and wide-band vocalizations in the auditory midbrain nucleus (MLd) of the Guinea Fowl (Numida meleagris). Journal of Comparative Physiology A 117: 245–265.

7. Arends JJ (1981) Sensory and motor aspects of the trigeminal system in the mallards (Anas Platyrhynchos L.). PhD Thesis. Leiden, Netherlands: University of Leiden.

8. Knudsen EI (1983) Subdivisions of the inferior colliculus in the barn owl (Tyto alba). The Journal of Comparative Neurology 218: 174–186.

9. Knudsen EI, Konishi M (1978) Space and frequency are represented separately in auditory midbrain of the owl. Journal of Neurophysiology 41: 870–884.

10. Konishi M (2003) Coding of auditory space. Annual Review of Neuroscience 26: 31–55.

11. Kubke MF, Gauger B, Basu L, Wagner H, Carr CE (1999) Development of calretinin immunoreactivity in the brainstem auditory nuclei of the barn owl (Tyto alba). The Journal of Comparative Neurology 415: 189–203.

12. Takahashi TT, Carr CE, Brecha N, Konishi M (1987) Calcium binding protein-like immunoreactivity labels the terminal field of nucleus laminaris of the barn owl. The Journal of Neuroscience 7: 1843–1856.

13. Takahashi TT, Konishi M (1988) Projections of nucleus angularis and nucleus laminaris to the lateral lemniscal nuclear complex of the barn owl. The Journal of Comparative Neurology 274: 212–238.

14. Wagner H, Güntürkün O, Nieder Br (2003) Anatomical markers for the subdivisions of the barn owl's inferior-collicular complex and adjacent peri- and subventricular structures. The Journal of Comparative Neurology 465: 145–159.

15. Wagner H, Takahashi T, Konishi M (1987) Representation of interaural time difference in the central nucleus of the barn owl's inferior colliculus. The Journal of Neuroscience 7: 3105–3116.

16. Correia MJ, Eden AR, Westlund KN, Coulter JD (1982) Organization of ascending auditory pathways in the pigeon (Columbia livia) as determined by autoradiographic methods. Brain Research 234: 205–212.

17. Leibler LM (1975) Monaural and binaural pathways in the ascending auditory system of the pigeon. PhD Thesis. Cambridge, MA: Massachusetts Institute of Technology.

18. Wild JM (1995) Convergence of somatosensory and auditory projections in the avian torus semicircularis, including the central auditory nucleus. The Journal of Comparative Neurology 358: 465–486.

19. Krützfeldt NOE, Logerot P, Kubke MF, Wild JM (2010) Connections of the auditory brainstem in a songbird, Taeniopygia guttata. I. Projections of nucleus angularis and nucleus laminaris to the auditory torus. The Journal of Comparative Neurology 518: 2109–2134.

20. Wild JM, Krützfeldt NOE, Kubke MF (2010) Connections of the auditory brainstem in a songbird, Taeniopygia guttata. III. Projections of the superior olive and lateral lemniscal nuclei. The Journal of Comparative Neurology 518: 2149–2167.

21. Braun K, Scheich H, Heizmann CW, Hunziker W (1991) Parvalbumin and calbindin-D28K immunoreactivity as developmental markers of auditory and vocal motor nuclei of the zebra finch. Neuroscience 40: 853–869.

22. Braun K, Scheich H, Schachner M, Heizmann CW (1985) Distribution of parvalbumin, cytochrome oxidase activity and 14C-2-deoxyglucose uptake in the brain of the zebra finch. Cell and Tissue Research 240: 101–115.

23. Montagnese CM, Geneser FA, Krebs JR (1993) Histochemical distribution of zinc in the brain of the zebra finch (Taenopygia guttata). Anatomy and Embryology 188: 173–187.

24. Watson JT, Adkins-Regan E, Whiting P, Lindstrom JM, Podleski TR (1988) Autoradiographic localization of nicotinic acetylcholine receptors in the brain of the zebra finch (Poephila guttata). The Journal of Comparative Neurology 274: 255–264.

25. Wild JM (1997) The avian somatosensory system: The pathway from wing to Wulst in a passerine (Chloris chloris). Brain Research 759: 122–134.

26. Zeng S, Zhang X, Peng W, Zuo M (2004) Immunohistochemistry and neural connectivity of the Ov shell in the songbird and their evolutionary implications. The Journal of Comparative Neurology 470: 192–209.

27. Karten HJ (1967) The organization of the ascending auditory pathway in the pigeon (Columba livia) I. Diencephalic projections of the inferior colliculus (nucleus mesencephali lateralis, pars dorsalis). Brain Research 6: 409–427.

28. Wild JM (1987) Nuclei of the lateral lemniscus project directly to the thalamic auditory nuclei in the pigeon. Brain Research 408: 303–307.

29. Durand SE, Tepper JM, Cheng MF (1992) The shell region of the nucleus ovoidalis: a subdivision of the avian auditory thalamus. The Journal of Comparative Neurology 323: 495–518.

30. Proctor L, Konishi M (1997) Representation of sound localization cues in the auditory thalamus of the barn owl. Proceedings of the National Academy of Sciences of the United States of America 94: 10421–10425.

31. Andressen C, Blümcke I, Celio MR (1993) Calcium-binding proteins: selective markers of nerve cells. Cell and Tissue Research 271: 181–208.

32. Baimbridge KG, Celio MR, Rogers JH (1992) Calcium-binding proteins in the nervous system. Trends in Neurosciences 15: 303–308.

33. Persechini A, Moncrief ND, Kretsinger RH (1989) The EF-hand family of calcium-modulated proteins. Trends in Neurosciences 12: 462–467.

34. Grabarek Z (2006) Structural basis for diversity of the EF-hand calcium-binding proteins. Journal of Molecular Biology 359: 509–525.

35. Endepols H, Walkowiak W, Luksch H (2000) Chemoarchitecture of the anuran auditory midbrain. Brain Research Reviews 33: 179–198.

36. Zeng S, Tian C, Zhang X, Zuo M (2008) Neurogenic development of the auditory areas of the midbrain and diencephalon in the Xenopus laevis and evolutionary implications. Brain Research 1206: 44–60.

37. Belekhova MG, Chudinova TV, Repérant J, Ward R, Jay B, et al. (2010) Core-and-belt organisation of the

mesencephalic and forebrain auditory centres in turtles: expression of calcium-binding proteins and metabolic activity. Brain Research 1345: 84–102.

38. Belekhova MG, Kenigfest NB, Karamian OA, Vesselkin NP (2004) Distribution of calcium-binding proteins in the central and peripheral regions of the turtle mesencephalic center torus semicircularis. Doklady Biological Sciences 399: 451–454.

39. Yan K (2008) Calcium binding proteins and GAD immunoreactivity in the auditory system of Gekko gecko. MSc Thesis. College Park, MD: University of Maryland.

40. Yan K, Tang Y, Carr CE (2010) Calcium-binding protein immunoreactivity characterizes the auditory system of Gekko gecko. The Journal of Comparative Neurology 518: 3409–3426.

41. Celio MR (1990) Calbindin D-28k and parvalbumin in the rat nervous system. Neuroscience 35: 375–475.

42. Coleman JR, McDonald AJ, Pinek B, Zrull MC (1992) The inferior colliculus: Calbindin and parvalbumin immunoreactivity in neural grafts. Experimental Neurology 115: 142–145.

43. Friauf E (1994) Distribution of calcium-binding protein calbindin-D28k in the auditory system of adult and developing rats. The Journal of Comparative Neurology 349: 193–211.

44. Glezer II, Hof PR, Morgane PJ (1998) Comparative analysis of calcium-binding protein-immunoreactive neuronal populations in the auditory and visual systems of the bottlenose dolphin (Tursiops truncatus) and the macaque monkey (Macaca fascicularis). Journal of Chemical Neuroanatomy 15: 203–237.

45. Idrizbegovic E, Bogdanovic N, Canlon B (1999) Sound stimulation increases calcium-binding protein immunoreactivity in the inferior colliculus in mice. Neuroscience Letters 259: 49–52.

46. Kelley PE, Frisina RD, Zettel ML, Walton JP (1992) Differential calbindin-like immunoreactivity in the brain stem auditory system of the chinchilla. The Journal of Comparative Neurology 320: 196–212.

47. Lohmann C, Friauf E (1996) Distribution of the calcium-binding proteins parvalbumin and calretinin in the auditory brainstem of adult and developing rats. The Journal of Comparative Neurology 367: 90–109.

48. Paloff AM, Usunoff KG, Yotovski P, Hinova-Palova DV, Ovtscharoff WA (2004) Parvalbumin-like immunostaining in the cat inferior colliculus. Light and electron microscopic investigation. Acta Histochemica 106: 219–234.

49. Resibois A, Rogers JH (1992) Calretinin in rat brain: An immunohistochemical study. Neuroscience 46: 101–134.

50. Rogers JH, Resibois A (1992) Calretinin and calbindin-D28k in rat brain: Patterns of partial co-localization. Neuroscience 51: 843–865.

51. Seto-Ohshima A, Aoki E, Semba R, Emson PC, Heizmann CW (1990) Parvalbumin immunoreactivity in the central auditory system of the gerbil: A developmental study. Neuroscience Letters 119: 60–63.

52. Sharma V, Nag TC, Wadhwa S, Roy TS (2009) Stereological investigation and expression of calcium-binding proteins in developing human inferior colliculus. Journal of Chemical Neuroanatomy 37: 78–86.

53. Tardif E, Chiry O, Probst A, Magistretti PJ, Clarke S (2003) Patterns of calcium-binding proteins in human inferior colliculus: identification of subdivisions and evidence for putative parallel systems. Neuroscience 116: 1111–1121.

54. Vater M, Braun K (1994) Parvalbumin, calbindin D-28k, and calretinin immunoreactivity in the ascending auditory pathway of horseshoe bats. The Journal of Comparative Neurology 341: 534–558.

55. Zeng S, Lin Y, Tian C, Song K, Zhang X, et al. (2009) Evolutionary significance of delayed neurogenesis in the core versus shell auditory areas of Mus musculus. The Journal of Comparative Neurology 515: 600–613.

56. Zettel ML, Carr CE, O'Neill WE (1991) Calbindin-like immunoreactivity in the central auditory system of the mustached bat, Pteronotus parnelli. The Journal of Comparative Neurology 313: 1–16.

57. Zettel ML, Frisina RD, Haider S, O'Neill WE (1997) Age-related changes in calbindin D-28k and calretinin immunoreactivity in the inferior colliculus of CBA/CaJ and C57Bl/6 mice. The Journal of Comparative Neurology 386: 92–110.

58. Hsu A, Woolley SMN, Fremouw TE, Theunissen FE (2004) Modulation power and phase spectrum of natural sounds enhance neural encoding performed by single auditory neurons. The Journal of Neuroscience 24: 9201–9211.

59. Woolley SMN, Casseday JH (2004) Response properties of single neurons in the zebra finch auditory midbrain: response patterns, frequency coding, intensity coding, and spike latencies. Journal of Neurophysiology 91: 136–151.

60. Woolley SMN, Casseday JH (2005) Processing of modulated sounds in the zebra finch auditory midbrain: responses to noise, frequency sweeps, and sinusoidal amplitude modulations. Journal of Neurophysiology 94: 1143–1157.

61. Woolley SMN, Gill PR, Fremouw T, Theunissen FE (2009) Functional groups in the avian auditory system. The Journal of Neuroscience 29: 2780–2793.

62. Woolley SMN, Gill PR, Theunissen FE (2006) Stimulus-dependent auditory tuning results in synchronous population coding of vocalizations in the songbird midbrain. The Journal of Neuroscience 26: 2499–2512.

63. Karten HJ, Hodos W (1967) A stereotaxic atlas of the brain of the pigeon (Columba livia). Baltimore, MD: Johns Hopkins Press.

64. Puelles L, Martínez-de-la-Torre M, Paxinos G, Watson C, Martínez S (2007) The chick brain in stereotaxic coordinates. An atlas featuring neuromeric subdivisions and mammalian homologies. Amsterdam: Elsevier, Academic Press.

65. Wild JM, Williams MN, Suthers RA (2001) Parvalbumin-positive projection neurons characterise the vocal

premotor pathway in male, but not female, zebra finches. Brain Research 917: 235–252.

66. Nottebohm F, Arnold AP (1976) Sexual dimorphism in vocal control areas of the songbird brain. Science 194: 211–213.

67. Fukushima Y, Aoki K (2000) The role of the dorsomedial nucleus (DM) of intercollicular complex with regard to sexual difference of distance calls in Bengalese finches. Zoological Science 17: 1231–1238.

68. Nottebohm F, Kelley DB, Paton JA (1982) Connections of vocal control nuclei in the canary telencephalon. The Journal of Comparative Neurology 207: 344–357.

69. Vicario DS (1991) Organization of the zebra finch song control system: Functional organization of outputs from nucleusrobustus archistriatalis. The Journal of Comparative Neurology 309: 486–494.

70. Wild JM (1993) Descending projections of the songbird nucleus robustus archistriatalis. The Journal of Comparative Neurology 338: 225–241.

71. Pinaud R, Fortes AF, Lovell P, Mello CV (2006) Calbindin-positive neurons reveal a sexual dimorphism within the songbird analogue of the mammalian auditory cortex. Journal of Neurobiology 66: 182–195.

72. Poirier C, Boumans T, Verhoye M, Balthazart J, A (2009) Own-song recognition in the songbird auditory pathway: selectivity and lateralization. The Journal of Neuroscience 29: 2252–2258.

73. Zeng S, Li J, Zhang X, Zuo M (2007) Distinction of neurochemistry between the cores and their shells of auditory nuclei in tetrapod species. Brain, Behavior and Evolution 70: 1–20.

74. Knudsen EI, Blasdel GG, Konishi M (1979) Sound localization by the barn owl (Tyto alba) measured with the search coil technique. Journal of Comparative Physiology A 133: 1–11.

75. Payne RS (1971) Acoustic location of prey by barn owls (Tyto alba). The Journal of Experimental Biology 54: 535–573.

76. Park TJ, Dooling RJ (1991) Sound localization in small birds: absolute localization in azimuth. Journal of Comparative Psychology 105: 125–133.

77. Nelson BS, Suthers RA (2004) Sound localization in a small passerine bird: discrimination of azimuth as a function of head orientation and sound frequency. The Journal of Experimental Biology 207: 4121–4133.

78. Covey E, Carr CE (2005) The auditory midbrain in bats and birds. In: Winer JA, Schreiner CE, editors. The Inferior Colliculus. New York: Springer. pp. 493–536.

79. Logerot P, Wild JM, Kubke MF (2009) Auditory processing of conspecific vocalizations in the auditory midbrain of the zebra finch. Paper Presented At The Australasian Winter Conference On Brain Research, Queenstown, New Zealand, August 29–September 2.

80. Woolley SC, Doupe AJ (2008) Social context-induced song variation affects female behavior and gene expression. PLoS Biology 6: e62–e62.

81. Huffman RF, W. O (1990) The descending auditory pathway and acousticomotor systems: connections with the inferior colliculus. Brain Research Reviews 15: 295–323.

82. Oliver DL (2005) Neuronal organization in the Inferior Colliculus. In: Winer JA, Schreiner CE, editors. The Inferior Colliculus. New York: Springer. pp. 69–114.

83. Ehret G, Schreiner CE (2005) Spectral and Intensity Coding in the Auditory Midbrain. In: Winer JA, Schreiner CE, editors. The Inferior Colliculus. New York: Springer. pp. 312–345.

84. Browner RH (1983) The ascending connections of the torus semicircularis central nucleus in Chrysemys scripta elegans. Hearing Research 12: 139–143.

85. Browner RH, Kennedy MC, Facelle T (1981) The cytoarchitecture of the torus semicircularis in the red-eared turtle. Journal of Morphology 169: 207–223.

86. Browner RH, Rubinson K (1977) The cytoarchitecture of the torus semicircularis in the Tegu lizard, Tupinambis nigropunctatus. The Journal of Comparative Neurology 176: 539–557.

87. Butler AB, Bruce LL (1981) Nucleus laminaris of the torus semicircularis: Projection to spinal cord in reptiles. Neuroscience Letters 25: 221–225.

88. Drakontides AB, Browner RH (1986) Ultrastructural features of the ventromedial region of the laminar nucleus in the red-eared turtle (Chrysemys scripta elegans). The Journal of Comparative Neurology 248: 555–572.

89. Foster RE, Hall WC (1978) The organization of central auditory pathways in a reptile, Iguana iguana. The Journal of Comparative Neurology 178: 783–831.

90. Kennedy MC, Browner RH (1981) The torus semicircularis in a gekkonid lizard. Journal of Morphology 169: 259–274.

91. Khachunts AS (1983) Electrophysiological characteristics of representation of auditory and somatosensory systems in the turtle midbrain. Neurophysiology 14: 191–198.

92. Künzle H (1986) Projections from the cochlear nuclear complex to rhombencephalic auditory centers and torus semicircularis in the turtle. Brain research 379: 307–319.

93. Künzle H, Woodson W (1982) Mesodiencephalic and other target regions of ascending spinal projections in the turtle, Pseudemys scripta elegans. The Journal of Comparative Neurology 212: 349–364.

94. Manley JA (1971) Single unit studies in the midbrain auditory area of Caiman. Zeitschrift für Vergleichende Physiologie 71: 255–261.

95. Pritz MB (1974) Ascending connections of a midbrain auditory area in a crocodile, Caiman crocodilus. The Journal of Comparative Neurology 153: 179–197.

96. Vergne AL, Pritz MB, Mathevon N (2009) Acoustic communication in crocodilians: from behaviour to brain. Biological Reviews of the Cambridge Philosophical Society 84: 391–411.

97. Díaz C, Yanes C, Trujillo CM, Puelles L (2000) Cytoarchitectonic subdivisions in the subtectal midbrain of the lizard Gallotia galloti. Journal of Neurocytology 29: 569–593.

98. Bass AH, Rose GJ, Pritz MB (2005) Auditory midbrain of fish, amphibians, and reptiles: model systems for understanding auditory function. In: Winer JA, Schreiner CE, editors. The Inferior Colliculus. New York: Springer. pp. 459–492.
99. Edwards CJ, Kelley DB (2001) Auditory and lateral line inputs to the midbrain of an aquatic anuran: neuroanatomic studies in Xenopus laevis. The Journal of Comparative Neurology 438: 148–162.
100. Endepols H, Walkowiak W (2001) Integration of ascending and descending inputs in the auditory midbrain of anurans. Journal of Comparative Physiology A 186: 1119–1133.
101. Feng AS, Lin WY (1991) Differential innervation patterns of three divisions of frog auditory midbrain (torus semicircularis). The Journal of Comparative Neurology 306: 613–630.
102. Hermes DJ, Eggermont JJ, Aertsen AMHJ, Johannesma PIM (1981) Spectro-temporal characteristics of single units in the auditory midbrain of the lightly anaesthetised grass frog (Rana temporaria L.) Investigated with noise stimuli. Hearing Research 5: 147–178.
103. Lowe DA (1986) Organisation of lateral line and auditory areas in the midbrain of Xenopus laevis. The Journal of Comparative Neurology 245: 498–513.
104. Luksch H, Walkowiak W (1998) Morphology and axonal projection patterns of auditory neurons in the midbrain of the painted frog, Discoglossus pictus. Hearing Research 122: 1–17.
105. Mohneke R (1983) Tonotopic organisation of the auditory midbrain nuclei of the midwife toad (Alytes obstetricans). Hearing Research 9: 91–102.
106. Potter HD (1965) Mesencephalic auditory region of the bullfrog. Journal of Neurophysiology 28: 1132–1154.
107. Potter HD (1965) Patterns of acoustically evoked discharges of neurons in the mesencephalon of the bullfrog. Journal of Neurophysiology 28: 1155–1184.
108. Simmons AM, Sanderson MI, Garabedian CE (2000) Representation of Waveform Periodicity in the Auditory Midbrain of the Bullfrog, Rana catesbeiana. Journal of the Association for Research in Otolaryngology 1: 2–24.
109. Walkowiak W, Luksch H (1994) Sensory Motor Interfacing in Acoustic Behavior of Anurans. Integrative and Comparative Biology 34: 685–695.
110. Will U, Luhede G, Görner P (1985) The area octavo-lateralis in Xenopus laevis I. Cell and Tissue Research 239: 147–161.
111. Will U, Luhede G, Görner P (1985) The area octavo-lateralis in Xenopus laevis II. Cell and Tissue Research 239: 163–175.
112. Cant NB (2005) Projections from the cochlear nuclear complex to the inferior colliculus. In: Winer JA, Schreiner CE, editors. The Inferior Colliculus. New York: Springer. pp. 115–131.

CHAPTER 7

DECLINE IN ANTIGENICITY OF TUMOR MARKERS BY STORAGE TIME USING PATHOLOGY SECTIONS CUT FROM TISSUE MICROARRAYS

Alex D. Rygg, Adri C. T. van Duin, Brent A. Craven

INTRODUCTION

The partition coefficient is a physicochemical property that is important in a wide variety of applications. Physically, the partition coefficient represents the relative affinity of a chemical for two different solvents. Mathematically, it is defined as the concentration ratio of a chemical in two phases at equilibrium, as described by the Nernst distribution (or partition) law [1], [2]

$$\frac{[x]_A}{[x]_B} = constant = K_{x,A/B} \quad (1)$$

where $[x]$ is the concentration of a solute X in phase A or B, and $K_{x,A/B}$ is the A/B partition coefficient of X. While this parameter is important in a number of fields (e.g. environmental pollution [3], drug delivery [4], [5], and geochemistry [6]), we are interested in determining the partitioning behavior of feeding stimulants in the olfactory mucus of fish and the potential implications for underwater olfaction.

In mammalian olfaction, the air/mucus partition coefficient of odorants has been shown to dramatically influence odorant deposition patterns in the olfactory region of the nose, wherein highly-soluble odorants are deposited anteriorly in the sensory region and less-soluble odorants are deposited more uniformly [7]. Such odorant-dependent deposition patterns result in a "chromatographic" separation of odorants along the sensory epithelium [8]–[13], which has been shown to broadly correspond with the spatial organization of olfactory receptor neurons (ORNs) [14]–[17] in the sensory region of the nasal cavity [7], [18]. That is, as odorant-laden air flows through the olfactory region of the nose (e.g., see [19]), an odorant is deposited in a region containing ORNs that are sensitive to that specific class of odorant. Such "imposed" odorant deposition patterns are used by the "inherent" distribution of ORNs for improved olfactory discrimination [11], [13].

It is unknown whether a similar phenomenon occurs in fish as water-borne odors circulate through the olfactory chamber. Recent computational fluid dynamics (CFD) simulations of water flow in an anatomically-accurate reconstruction of the head and olfactory chamber of the hammerhead shark [20] were used to elucidate the external and internal hydrodynamics of olfaction during swimming. Simulations of odorant transport are planned, which require odorant partition coefficients. However, though values have been published for many different solvents (e.g., [4], [21]–[24]), water/mucus odorant partition coefficients do not exist.

The objective of this study is to use molecular dynamics simulation techniques [6], [25]–[28]to calculate the water/mucus partition coefficients for underwater odorants, namely chemicals known to elicit feeding behavior in fish (i.e., feeding stimulants). We begin by reviewing the morphology of the olfactory organ of a representative cartilaginous fish, the hammerhead shark, which contains numerous lamellae that are lined with sensory epithelium, covered by a thin, viscous mucus layer. A summary of the evidence for the existence of the olfactory mucus layer in fish is provided, followed by the formulation of a simplified model of olfactory mucus. This model is subsequently used in molecular dynamics simulations to calculate the water/mucus odorant partition coefficients in

Citation: Rygg AD, van Duin ACT, Craven BA (2013) Decline in Antigenicity of Tumor Markers by Storage Time Using Pathology Sections Cut From Tissue Microarrays PLoS ONE 8(9): e72271. doi:10.1371/journal.pone.0072271.

fresh and salt water. Finally, the implications of the results regarding fish olfaction are discussed.

METHODS

Physical Model

Ultrastructure of the Olfactory Epithelium.

The olfactory chamber of the hammerhead shark (Figure 1 A and B) contains two rows of olfactory lamellae that provide an increased surface area for chemical sensing [20], [29]. Functionally, as the shark swims, water flows through the olfactory chamber, as described by Rygg et al. [20], delivering odorant to the sensory epithelium that lines each lamella (Figure 1C). Previous studies [30]–[33] have characterized the sensory epithelium in elasmobranch fishes (sharks, rays, and skates). At the ultrastructural level, supporting cells separate the olfactory sensory neurons, which project a dendritic process to the epithelial surface that terminates in an expanded olfactory knob (Figure 1 C). Microvilli are present on both the supporting cells and the olfactory knobs of the sensory neurons. Non-sensory motile cilia originate from the supporting cells, and in elasmobranchs (unlike in teleosts) the olfactory sensory neurons are not ciliated [30]–[35].

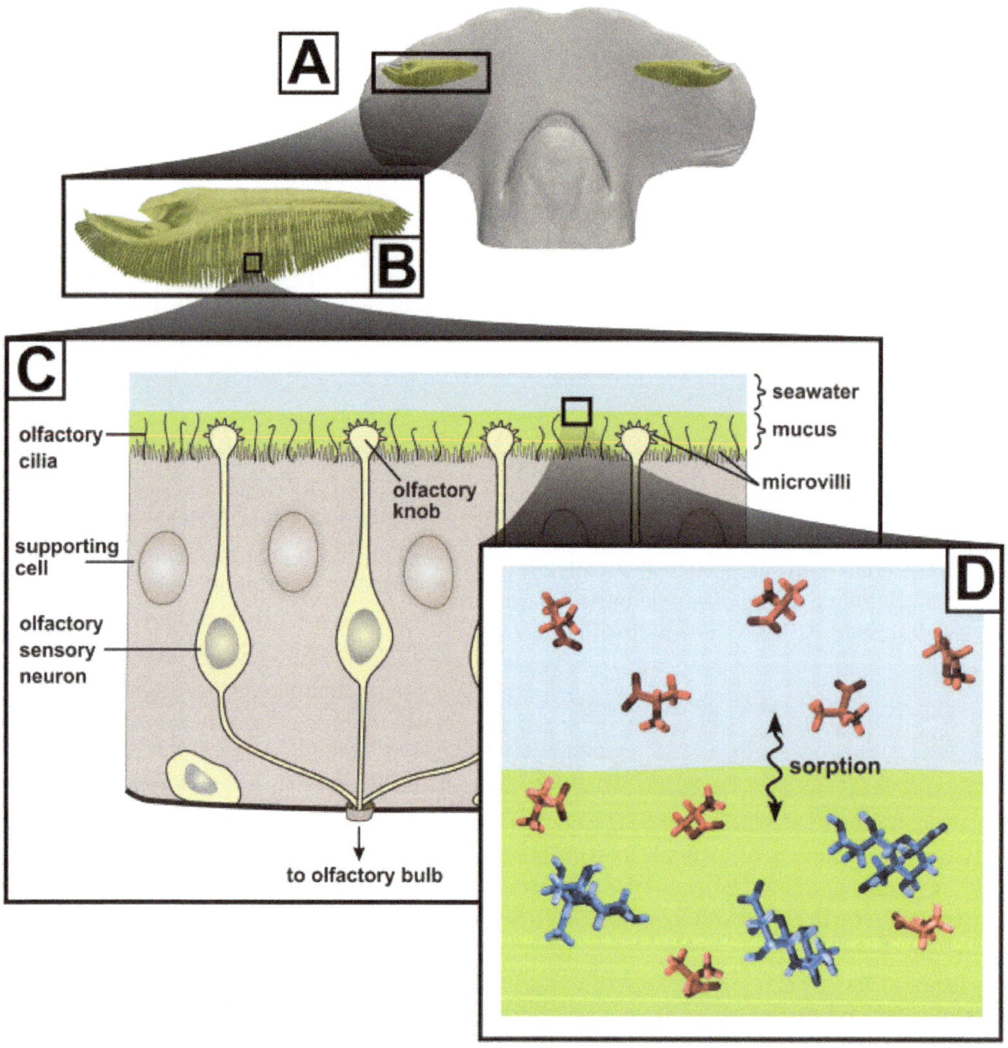

Figure 1: Multi-scale view of olfaction in the hammerhead shark.

The hammerhead shark (A) possesses two complex olfactory organs that contain numerous lamellae, as shown in B. The ultrastructure of the sensory epithelium that covers the lamellae is illustrated in C. At the nanoscale (D), sorption of odorant molecules (shaded in red) takes place at the seawater/ mucus interface. In the mucus phase, these odorant molecules likely interact with mucin sugar molecules (shaded in blue). Note: the panels are for illustrative purposes and are not drawn to scale.

Olfactory Mucus Layer

According to Getchell and Getchell [36], "the surface of the olfactory sensory epithelium of aquatic and terrestrial vertebrates is covered by a layer of mucus in which odorant molecules dissolve prior to reaching the site of olfactory stimulation, the cilia of the olfactory receptor neurons" (or the microvilli in elasmobranchs). Generally, the mucus layer serves a number of functions, including the protection of the olfactory epithelium from exposure to noxious chemicals, metabolism and removal of odorants, and to provide the biochemical microenvironment for olfactory transduction [37], [38]. In fish, olfactory mucus is produced by goblet cells [30], [31], [34], [36], [39], and an olfactory mucus layer has been observed on the olfactory lamellae of the sea trout [40], zebrafish [41], [42], freshwater minor carp [43], and the clearnose skate [34] (an elasmobranch).

In the respiratory system of terrestrial vertebrates, nasal mucus is comprised of a viscous superficial 'gel' layer and an underlying aqueous 'sol' (or periciliary) layer [44]–[46]. In contrast, the mucus that covers the olfactory epithelium in air-breathing animals consists of a thin, superficial watery layer and a thicker, underlying filamentous viscous layer [36]–[38], [47]–[49]. The superficial watery layer is thought to be produced by Bowman's glands [36], [37], [50]. However, Bowman's glands are not present in the olfactory mucosa of fish [30], [34], [36]. Further, water flowing through the nasal chamber would wash off such a superficial watery layer produced by other means. Therefore, at the macroscale, the olfactory mucus layer in fish may be well approximated by a filamentous viscous mucoid layer that is not washed off by low-speed water flowing through the olfactory chamber (e.g., see [20]).

Molecular Description of Olfactory Mucus

Olfactory mucus gets most of its properties from its high water content (~80–95% [45], [51]) and large macromolecules known as glycoproteins (or mucins), which give it the viscous consistency of a "gel" [52]. On a molecular level, mucins are typically 0.1 to 5 μm in length [51] and contain a polypeptide core that is largely glycosylated [45], [51]. Due to this heavy glycosylation, mucins are composed of approximately 75% carbohydrates and 25% amino acids [51]. Apomucin (i.e., the unglycosylated peptide core) is insoluble in water, and therefore it is the carbohydrate chains that confer hydrophilic properties to the protein and allow for hydration of the mucus [51], [53]. Common sugars found in the carbohydrate chains are fructose, galactose, N-acetylglucosamine, N-acetylgalactosamine, and N-acetylneuraminic acid (sialic acid) [45]. It is common for O-linked glycans (which are abundant in mucins) to be capped by sialic acid [54]. Sialic acid, being a negatively charged residue, may contribute to water uptake and retention. Although many of these properties have primarily been investigated in humans and other mammals, mucins from different organs and species have a similar general structure [51], and glycoproteins in fish mucus appear to be similar to those in mammals [52].

Molecular Models of Olfactory Mucus and Water

Given the foregoing molecular description, we developed a simplified molecular model of olfactory mucus for use in molecular dynamics simulations. Due to the complex composition of olfactory mucus, it is presently impractical to model all of the molecules that comprise the mucus phase. In addition, calculating solvation energies using molecular dynamics works best if the solvent is comprised of relatively small compounds [26]. Therefore, instead of trying to model the complete mucus phase, we aimed to model the most relevant interactions that occur between the mucus and odorant molecules.

To develop a realistic simplified molecular model of the mucus phase, we first assume that olfactory mucus in fish is similar in composition to the viscous mucus layer covering the mammalian olfactory epithelium (see Olfactory Mucus Layer). To further simplify the model, we approximate the mucus phase as being comprised of water and mucins, as water is the primary component of olfactory mucus and mucins are the most prominent macromolecule (see Molecular Description of Olfactory Mucus). Such a simplified water-mucin model retains the primary components of olfactory mucus that confer its physical properties, including a gel-like consistency necessary to prevent the mucus layer from washing off of the olfactory lamellae as water flows through the nasal chamber (e.g., see [20]).

Because the carbohydrate chains are responsible for water retention in mucus [45], [51], [53]and comprise ~75% of the mucins [51], odorant molecules have a high probability of interacting with the carbohydrates when they come into contact with the mucus phase. Specifically, N-acetylneuraminic acid (sialic acid) is a common terminal monosaccharide on the carbohydrate chains [54], and is therefore most likely to interact with odorant molecules, which are of the same order of size as N-acetylneuraminic acid molecules. Accordingly, based on the above approximations, the olfactory mucus phase was modeled as a solution of ~90% water and ~10% N-acetylneuraminic acid.

Finally, to compare differences between underwater environments, we constructed molecular models for both fresh water and salt water. The fresh water phase was straightforward, and consisted of a bath of ~ 450–550 water molecules. Modeling the salt water phase consisted of solvating each odorant in a bath of water molecules, then adding salt ions up to a salinity of 3.5%, a typical salinity for seawater [55]. Because the water and mucus phases have such similar compositions, we assumed an even distribution of salt between them. That is, in a salt water environment the olfactory mucus phase consisted of water, N-acetylneuraminic acid, and a salt concentration of 3.5%.

Odorant Chemicals

Unlike olfaction in air, where volatility strongly determines whether a chemical will be detected, underwater olfaction is facilitated by the presence of highly-soluble chemicals with low molecular weight. Amino acids, which are abundant in both tissue and blood [56], [57], have a low molecular weight, are highly water soluble, and are widely regarded as potent feeding stimulants for many different fish [57]–[64]. Thus, four amino acid odorants were selected for comparison in the present study, based on their reported prevalence as feeding stimulants.

According to Carr et al. [57], who analyzed the chemical composition of tissues in a diversity of marine organisms, alanine and glycine are major tissue components and the two most frequently reported feeding stimulants in a variety of fish. In addition, previous studies [65], [66] that utilized the electro-olfactogram (EOG) technique to determine olfactory sensitivity in elasmobranchs showed that hammerhead sharks (*Sphyrna tiburo* and *Sphyrna lewini*) are sensitive to a wide range of amino acids. While interspecific differences were evident, alanine was treated as the "standard" in both studies and was found to elicit a strong olfactory response with a low detection threshold, while glycine elicited a weak-to-moderate EOG response. In the present study, we aim to model amino acids that span a wide range of olfactory detection thresholds. Thus, in addition to alanine and glycine, based on the EOG results reported in [65], [66], cysteine and valine were chosen as amino acids that elicit a moderate-to-strong and weak olfactory response, respectively.

Molecular Dynamics

Mathematically, the water/mucus partition coefficient of a given molecule, $K_{water/mucus}$, is related to the difference between its solvation energies in each phase, as given by [25], [27]:

$$ln\left(K_{water/mucus}\right) = \frac{\Delta G_{mucus} - \Delta G_{water}}{RT} \quad (2)$$

where ΔG is the solvation energy of the odorant molecule in each phase, R is the ideal gas constant, and T is a reference temperature. Molecular dynamics simulations were used to calculate the solvation energies of each amino acid in the water and mucus phases. Figure 2shows a representative visualization of the computational box used in the molecular dynamics simulations, which contains an alanine molecule (the amino acid odorant) and N-acetylneuraminic acid surrounded by water (the simplified olfactory mucus phase). Similar molecular dynamics models were constructed for glycine, cysteine, and valine in both fresh water and salt water.

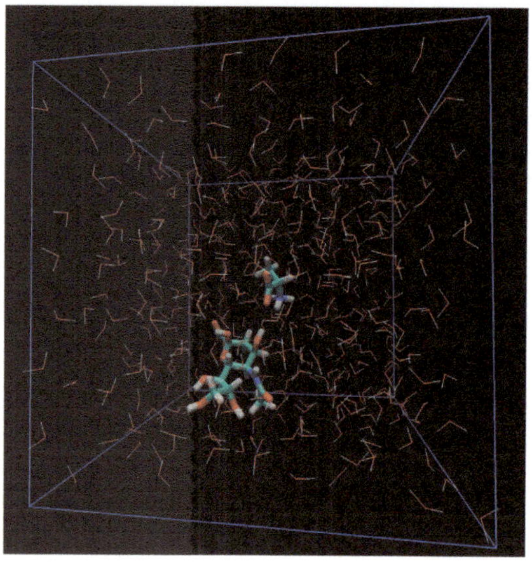

Figure 2: Molecular dynamics model of alanine in mucus.

The computational box contains an alanine molecule (the amino acid odorant) immersed in a simplified olfactory mucus phase, consisting of N-acetylneuraminic acid in a bath of water.

Simulations were performed using the open-source software package GROMACS, version 4.5.4 [67]. The Optimized Potentials for Liquid Simulations All-Atom (OPLS-AA) force field [68]–[71] was used for all molecules, along with the simple point charge water model with included self-energy correction (SPC/E) [72]. A cutoff radius of 1.0 nm was used for the short-range Coulomb interactions, while long-range electrostatics were calculated using the Particle-Mesh Ewald algorithm [73]. Periodic boundary conditions were applied to the computational box in all directions.

Solvation energy can be described as the change in Gibbs free energy when a molecule is transferred from a vacuum to a solvent. In general, the change in Gibbs free energy of a compound between two states, A and B, is given by the following equation [74]:

$$\Delta G_{BA} = G^B(p,T) - G^A(p,T) = \int_{\lambda_A}^{\lambda_B} \frac{\partial G(\lambda)}{\partial \lambda} d\lambda = \int_{\lambda_A}^{\lambda_B} \langle \frac{\partial \mathcal{H}}{\partial \lambda} \rangle_{NpT;\lambda} d\lambda \quad (3)$$

where G is the Gibbs free energy, $\mathcal{H}$ is the Hamiltonian, and λ is a coupling parameter that represents the state of the system. Here, $\lambda = 0$ corresponds to a system where the amino acid is completely decoupled from the solvent, while $\lambda = 1$ indicates that the amino acid is fully coupled to the rest of the system. Therefore, to calculate the solvation energy of a particular amino acid, Eq. (3) was integrated from $\lambda_A = 0$ to $\lambda_B = 1$. Thermodynamic integration was performed using the Bennett acceptance ratio (BAR) method [75].

Energy minimization of the system was performed using a steepest descent algorithm to a maximum force of 100 kJ mol^{-1} nm^{-1}. A second minimization using a low-memory Broyden-Fletcher-Goldfarb-Shanno (BFGS) approach [76] was then performed. The system subsequently underwent 1×10^{-10} s of constant volume/temperature (NVT) equilibration at a temperature of 300 K, followed by 1×10^{-10} s of constant pressure/temperature (NPT) equilibration at a pressure and temperature of 1 bar and 300 K, respectively. Production molecular dynamics simulations were then run at a constant pressure (1 bar) and temperature (300 K). A Parrinello-Rahman barostat [77], [78] was used, with a pressure coupling time constant of 5×10^{-13} s. A leap-frog stochastic dynamics integrator was utilized in the production molecular dynamics calculations, and temperature coupling was implicitly handled by the integrator. A time constant of 1×10^{-12} s was used for temperature coupling. Using a time step size of 2×10^{-15} s, simulations were run for 2.5×10^6 steps, or 5×10^{-9} s of simulated time.

Numerical Accuracy

The OPLS force field was chosen because it has been well validated for the types of molecules and phases that are being modeled in the present study. This force field has been validated with both experimental data and *ab initio* calculations [68]–[70]. Additionally, previous studies [25], [28], [79] have used OPLS to calculate solvation energies and phase behavior for systems involving water/chloroform and octanol/water. The solutes in these studies consisted of n-alkane, polar, nonpolar, alcohol, aromatic, and polychlorinated biphenyl molecules. Originally, OPLS was developed for the simulation of proteins in aqueous solutions [68], and has since been extended to include additional parameters for carbohydrates [70]. Consequently, the OPLS force field was selected in the present work for calculating the solvation energy of amino acids in aqueous solutions containing mucin sugars.

To verify the use of the OPLS-AA force field in our simulations, we calculated the Helmholtz solvation energy of alanine, glycine, cysteine, and valine in pure water using molecular dynamics and compared the values with those reported by Dixit et al. [80], who used the Finite Difference Poisson Boltzmann (FDPB) method (see Table 1). In general, the solvation energies were found to be comparable, with some discrepancy in the absolute values (~ 5–10%) that is attributable to the fact that the FDPB method is expected to be less accurate than the molecular dynamics method since the latter considers in more detail the packing of the molecules. Most importantly, however, similar trends in solvation energy were found among the chemicals with both methods (e.g., that cysteine and valine are more hydrophobic than alanine and glycine; see Table 1). Thus, in the absence of experimental data, such a strong comparison between two fundamentally different numerical methods verifies the use of the OPLS-AA force field in the present molecular dynamics simulations of amino acid solvation in aqueous solutions.

Table 1: OPLS-AA force field verification

	$\Delta A_{sol,OPLS}$	$\Delta A_{sol,FDPB}$ [80]	% Difference
Alanine	−295.44	−323.84	8.77%
Cysteine	−281.50	−311.37	9.59%
Glycine	−299.21	−347.06	13.79%
Valine	−288.63	−298.32	3.25%

Comparison of the Helmholtz solvation energies calculated using the OPLS-AA force field and the Finite Difference Poisson Boltzmann method ([80]).

In terms of accuracy with respect to the physical system, the present molecular dynamics results should not be considered exact due to the approximations made in developing a simplified molecular model of the olfactory mucus phase. Even so, because the simplified molecular model represents the most significant interactions occurring between the amino acid odorant molecules and the mucus phase, the results are expected to be representative of the physical system. Most important to the present study, we expect the relative differences between the calculated water/mucus odorant partition coefficients to be reliable.

RESULTS

Given the computed solvation energies from the molecular dynamics simulations, partition coefficients were calculated for the four amino acid odorants in both fresh water (Table 2) and salt water (Table 3). In each case, estimates of the numerical error were computed by splitting the simulation data into blocks and calculating the solvation energy for each block. Assuming the data blocks were independent, uncertainty estimates were calculated from the average variance over the blocks [81].

Table 2: Molecular dynamics results in fresh water

	Alanine	Cysteine	Glycine	Valine
$\Delta G_{freshwater}$, kJ/mol	-293.07 ± 0.21	-277.07 ± 0.17	-297.39 ± 0.13	-284.08 ± 0.22
ΔG_{mucus}, kJ/mol	-295.76 ± 0.29	-284.01 ± 0.19	-299.55 ± 0.24	-287.46 ± 0.23
$\Delta G_{mucus} - \Delta G_{freshwater}$, kJ/mol	-2.69 ± 0.50	-6.94 ± 0.36	-2.16 ± 0.37	-3.38 ± 0.45
$K_{freshwater/mucus}$	0.34 [0.28−0.42]	0.06 [0.05−0.07]	0.42 [0.36−0.49]	0.26 [0.22−0.31]

Solvation energies for each amino acid odorant in fresh water and mucus, which were used to calculate the water/mucus odorant partition coefficients.

Table 3: Molecular dynamics results in salt water

	Alanine	Cysteine	Glycine	Valine
$\Delta G_{saltwater}$, kJ/mol	-295.53 ± 0.22	-286.33 ± 0.29	-298.62 ± 0.23	-284.96 ± 0.21
ΔG_{mucus}, kJ/mol	-294.19 ± 0.24	-281.85 ± 0.28	-301.78 ± 0.30	-281.59 ± 0.22
$\Delta G_{mucus} - \Delta G_{saltwater}$, kJ/mol	1.34 ± 0.46	4.48 ± 0.57	-3.16 ± 0.53	3.37 ± 0.43
$K_{saltwater/mucus}$	1.71 [1.42−2.06]	6.03 [4.80−7.57]	0.28 [0.23−0.35]	3.86 [3.25−4.59]

Solvation energies for each amino acid odorant in salt water and mucus, which were used to calculate the salt water/mucus odorant partition coefficients.

The results indicate that the span of the calculated partition coefficients in each underwater environment is approximately one order of magnitude. In the fresh water case (Table 2), all of the partition coefficients are slightly less than one, meaning that all of the amino acids prefer the mucus phase. Moreover, we found that the values of the partition coefficients are correlated with the hydrophobicity of the amino acids. Glycine, which is the most hydrophilic odorant (i.e., it had the lowest value of $\Delta G_{freshwater}$), had the largest value of $K_{freshwater/mucus}$. Conversely, cysteine is the most hydrophobic of the four amino acids and also has the smallest partition coefficient. The same trend was similarly observed for alanine and valine. Thus, in fresh water, the more hydrophobic an amino acid, the more readily it is absorbed by the olfactory mucus phase.

In salt water (Table 3), we observed a reversal of the odorant partitioning behavior, where the most hydrophobic amino acids have the largest values of $K_{saltwater/mucus}$. Specifically, we found that the amino acids tend to prefer salt water to fresh water, as indicated by the lower values of $\Delta G_{saltwater}$ compared to $\Delta G_{freshwater}$. This may be explained by the fact that amino acids in their zwitterionic form likely interact with the salt ions in the water phase due to their internal charges. Additionally, the results indicate that adding salt to the mucus decreases the affinity of the amino acids for this phase – the exception is glycine, which is a very versatile molecule due to its short side chain.

To explain this decreased affinity for saline mucus, a radial distribution function (RDF) analysis was performed to determine the degree with which the salt ions interacts with the sugar molecule, N-acetylneuraminic acid. Figure 3 shows the RDF of the charged N-acetylneuraminic acid oxygen with the salt cations. The large peak at the small radial distance in this plot indicates that there is a high probability of finding the salt in the first coordination shell of the charged sugar site. The inset in Figure 3 also shows salt ions tending to cluster around the charged sugar site. Thus, it appears that the salt strongly favors and interacts with the sugar molecule. For comparison, a RDF of the charged N-acetylneuraminic acid oxygen with the water molecules was also computed (Figure 4), which shows characteristic coordination shells. However, the peak in the oxygen-water RDF is not nearly as large as that in the oxygen-salt RDF, indicating that the general sugar/water interactions are not nearly as strong as the sugar/salt interactions. Thus, it appears that the salt does indeed favor the sugar, and the addition of salt into the system has an appreciable effect on the chemical nature of the sugar molecule. In particular, it appears that the salt tends to increase the polarity and hydrophilic nature of the sugar. This essentially makes the saline mucus phase less preferable to the more hydrophobic amino acids, causing the reversal in odorant partitioning behavior observed in comparing Tables 2 and 3. Therefore, with the exception of glycine, the addition of salt into the system increases the affinity of the odorant molecules for the salt water phase, while also reducing their affinity for the saline mucus phase due to the interaction of the salt ions with N-acetylneuraminic acid. Compared with fresh water, this results in larger partition coefficients that tend to favor salt water over olfactory mucus.

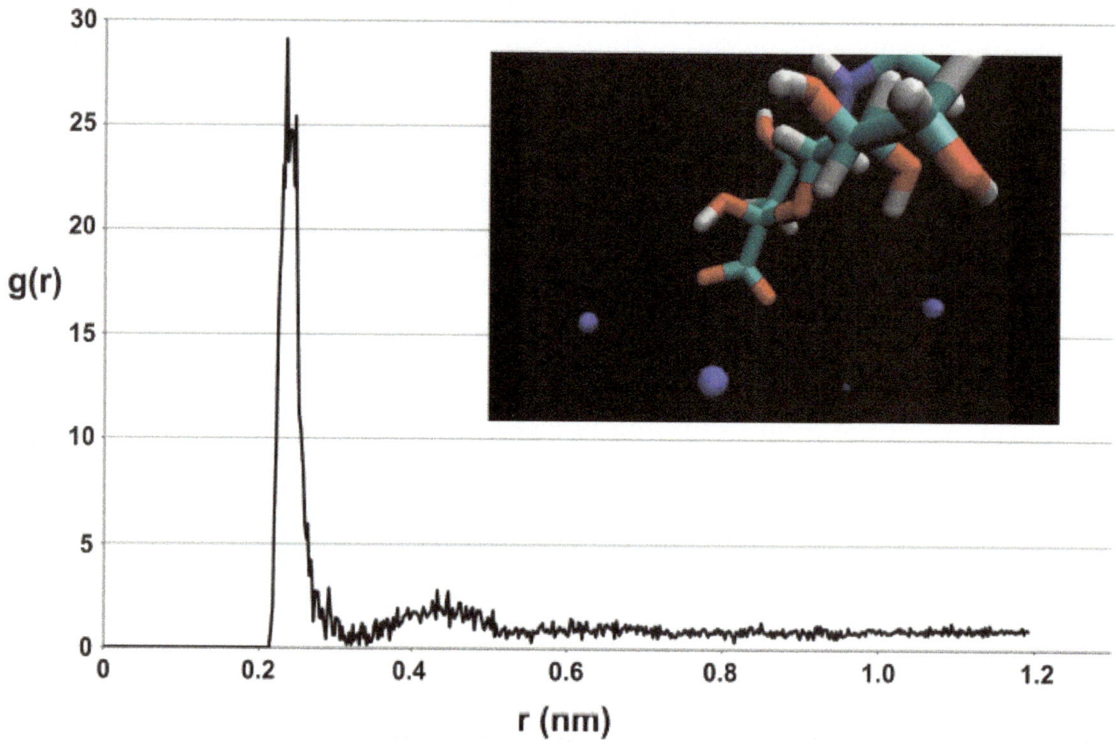

Figure 3: Oxygen-salt radial distribution function.

Radial distribution function of the charged N-acetylneuraminic acid oxygen with the salt cations. The inset shows the salt ions (blue spheres) tending to cluster around the charged sugar site.

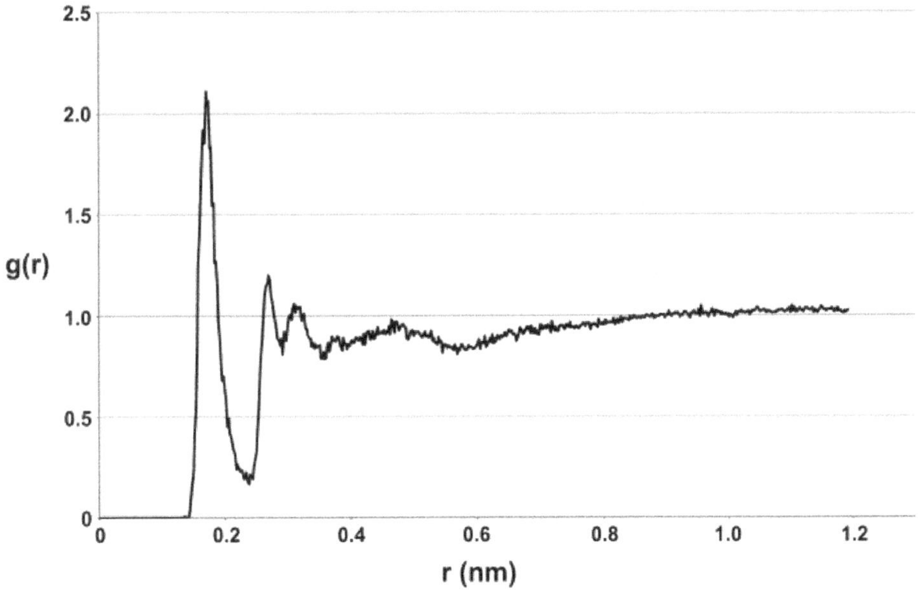

Figure 4: Oxygen-water radial distribution function.

Radial distribution function of the charged N-acetylneuraminic acid oxygen with the water molecules.

DISCUSSION

The present study quantified water/mucus partition coefficients for four ecologically-relevant feeding stimulants in fish that have been shown to span a wide range of olfactory detection thresholds. In fresh water, all of the amino acid odorants were shown to possess a partition coefficient slightly less than one, meaning that each of the odorants prefer the mucus phase to water. In contrast, we found a reversal in odorant partitioning behavior in salt water, where, with the exception of glycine, each of the feeding stimulants prefer the salt water phase to olfactory mucus (i.e., a partition coefficient greater than one). This was due to the interaction of the salt ions with the amino acid odorant molecules in the water phase and N-acetylneuraminic acid in the simplified olfactory mucus phase. Thus, because the water/mucus odorant partition coefficients were found to differ between fresh water and salt water, we anticipate slightly varied odorant deposition patterns in the fish olfactory organ depending on the salinity of the underwater environment.

However, in either case (fresh water and salt water), we found that the variation of the calculated partition coefficients was approximately one order of magnitude. This is in stark contrast to air/mucus odorant partition coefficients, which can span up to six orders of magnitude [7], [18], [21], [24]. As a result, odorant deposition patterns in the nose of air-breathing animals are strongly dependent on the relative magnitude of the air/mucus partition coefficient, leading to odorant-dependent "imposed" patterning (see Introduction). However, given the comparatively weak variation of the water/mucus partition coefficients calculated in the present study, we anticipate relatively similar deposition patterns for most amino acid odorants in the fish olfactory chamber.

Such a hypothesis is consistent with the fact that ORNs are randomly distributed throughout the olfactory epithelium of fish [82]–[87]. That is, in contrast to air-breathing mammals that possess an "inherent" spatial distribution of ORNs in the olfactory epithelium that is utilized in concert with "imposed" odorant-dependent deposition patterns for olfactory discrimination (see Introduction), there is no spatial organization of ORNs in the fish olfactory epithelium. Our results, which indicate that there is unlikely to be significant odorant-dependent deposition patterning in the fish olfactory chamber, may partially explain why "the fish peripheral olfactory organ is somewhat different from other animals" [87] in its lack of ORN spatial organization. In other words, living in an aquatic environment may preclude appreciable imposed patterning in the fish olfactory chamber due to a limited range of water/mucus odorant partition coefficients, thereby eliminating the utility of spatial ORN segregation in the olfactory epithelium for coding odorant identity. Future odorant transport simulations in the olfactory chamber of the hammerhead shark are planned to investigate this hypothesis.

REFERENCES

1. Nernst W (1891) The Distribution of a Substance Between Two Solvents and Between Solvent and Steam Room. Zeitschrift fur Physikalische Chemie 8: 110–139.
2. Negi A, Anand S (1985) A Textbook of Physical Chemistry. New Age International.
3. Gschwend P, Wu S (1985) On the Constancy of Sediment-Water Partition Coefficients of Hydrophobic Organic Pollutants. Environmental Science & Technology 19: 90–96. doi: 10.1021/es00131a011
4. Leo A, Hansch C, Elkins D (1971) Partition Coefficients and Their Uses. Chemical Reviews 71: 525–616. doi: 10.1021/cr60274a001
5. Khanvilkar K, Donovan M, Flanagan D (2001) Drug Transfer Through Mucus. Advanced Drug Delivery Reviews 48: 173–193. doi: 10.1016/s0169-409x(01)00115-6
6. van Duin A, Larter S (2001) Molecular Dynamics Investigation into the Adsorption of Organic Compounds

on Kaolinite Surfaces. Organic Geochemistry 32: 143–150. doi: 10.1016/s0146-6380(00)00143-1

7. Lawson M, Craven B, Paterson E, Settles G (2012) A Computational Study of Odorant Transport and Deposition in the Canine Nasal Cavity: Implications for Olfaction. Chemical Senses 37: 553–566. doi: 10.1093/chemse/bjs039

8. Mozell M (1964) Evidence for Sorption as a Mechanism of the Olfactory Analysis of Vapours. Nature 203: 1181–1182. doi: 10.1038/2031181a0

9. Mozell M (1966) The Spatiotemporal Analysis of Odorants at the Level of the Olfactory Receptor Sheet. The Journal of General Physiology 50: 25–41. doi: 10.1085/jgp.50.1.25

10. Mozell M (1970) Evidence for a Chromatographic Model of Olfaction. The Journal of General Physiology 56: 46–63. doi: 10.1085/jgp.56.1.46

11. Mozell M, Sheehe P, Hornung D, Kent P, Youngentob S, et al. (1987) "Imposed" and "Inherent" Mucosal Activity Patterns. Their Composite Representation of Olfactory Stimuli. The Journal of General Physiology 90: 625–650. doi: 10.1085/jgp.90.5.625

12. Mozell M, Kent P, Murphy S (1991) The Effect of Flow Rate Upon the Magnitude of the Olfactory Response Differs for Different Odorants. Chemical Senses 16: 631–649. doi: 10.1093/chemse/16.6.631

13. Kent P, Mozell M, Murphy S, Hornung D (1996) The Interaction of Imposed and Inherent Olfactory Mucosal Activity Patterns and their Composite Representation in a Mammalian Species Using Voltage-Sensitive Dyes. The Journal of Neuroscience 16: 345–353.

14. Vassar R, Ngai J, Axel R (1993) Spatial Segregation of Odorant Receptor Expression in the Mammalian Olfactory Epithelium. Cell 74: 309–318. doi: 10.1016/0092-8674(93)90422-m

15. Ressler KJ, Sullivan SL, Buck LB (1993) A Zonal Organization of Odorant Receptor Gene Expression in the Olfactory Epithelium. Cell 73: 597–609. doi: 10.1016/0092-8674(93)90145-g

16. Strotmann J, Wanner L, Helfrich T, Beck A, Breer H (1994) Rostro-Caudal Patterning of Receptor-Expressing Olfactory Neurones in the Rat Nasal Cavity. Cell and Tissue Research 278: 11–20. doi: 10.1007/s004410050189

17. Mombaerts P, Wang F, Dulac C, Chao S, Nemes A, et al. (1996) Visualizing an Olfactory Sensory Map. Cell 87: 675–686. doi: 10.1016/s0092-8674(00)81387-2

18. Yang G, Scherer P, Zhao K, Mozell M (2007) Numerical Modeling of Odorant Uptake in the Rat Nasal Cavity. Chemical Senses 32: 273–284. doi: 10.1093/chemse/bjl056

19. Craven B, Paterson E, Settles G (2010) The Fluid Dynamics of Canine Olfaction: Unique Nasal Airow Patterns as an Explanation of Macrosmia. Journal of The Royal Society Interface 7: 933–943. doi: 10.1098/rsif.2009.0490

20. Rygg A, Cox JPL, Abel R, Webb A, Smith N, et al. (2013) A Computational Study of the Hydrodynamics in the Nasal Region of a Hammerhead Shark (Sphyrna tudes): Implications for Olfaction. PLOS ONE 8: e59783. doi: 10.1371/journal.pone.0059783

21. Amoore J, Buttery R (1978) Partition Coefficient and Comparative Olfactometry. Chemical Senses 3: 57–71. doi: 10.1093/chemse/3.1.57

22. Sato A, Nakajima T (1979) Partition Coefficients of Some Aromatic Hydrocarbons and Ketones in Water, Blood and Oil. British Journal of Industrial Medicine 36: 231–234. doi: 10.1136/oem.36.3.231

23. Hornung D, Youngentob S, Mozell M (1987) Olfactory Mucosa/Air Partitioning of Odorants. Brain Research 413: 147–154. doi: 10.1016/0006-8993(87)90163-6

24. Kurtz D, Zhao K, Hornung D, Scherer P (2004) Experimental and Numerical Determination of Odorant Solubility in Nasal and Olfactory Mucosa. Chemical Senses 29: 763–773. doi: 10.1093/chemse/bjh079

25. Jorgensen W, Briggs J, Contreras M (1990) Relative Partition Coefficients for Organic Solutes from Fluid Simulations. Journal of Physical Chemistry 94: 1683–1686. doi: 10.1021/j100367a084

26. van Duin A, Larter S (1998) Application of Molecular Dynamics Calculations in the Prediction of Dynamical Molecular Properties. Organic Geochemistry 29: 1043–1050. doi: 10.1016/s0146-6380(98)00076-x

27. Lyubartsev A, Jacobsson S, Sundholm G, Laaksonen A (2001) Solubility of Organic Compounds in Water/Octanol Systems. A Expanded Ensemble Molecular Dynamics Simulation Study of log P Parameters. The Journal of Physical Chemistry B 105: 7775–7782. doi: 10.1021/jp0036902

28. Garrido N, Queimada A, Jorge M, Macedo E, Economou I (2009) 1-Octanol/Water Partition Coefficients of n-Alkanes from Molecular Simulations of Absolute Solvation Free Energies. Journal of Chemical Theory and Computation 5: 2436–2446. doi: 10.1021/ct900214y

29. Abel RL, Maclaine JS, Cotton R, Xuan VB, Nickels TB, et al. (2010) Functional Morphology of the Nasal Region of a Hammerhead Shark. Comparative Biochemistry and Physiology – Part A: Molecular & Integrative Physiology 155: 464–475. doi: 10.1016/j.cbpa.2009.10.029

30. Tucker D (1983) Fish Chemoreception: Peripheral Anatomy and Physiology. In: Northcutt R, Davis R, editors, Fish Neurobiology, The University of Michigan Press, volume 1: 311–350.

31. Theisen B, Zeiske E, Breucker H (1986) Functional Morphology of the Olfactory Organs in the Spiny Dogfish (Squalus acanthias L.) and the Small-spotted Catshark (Scyliorhinus canicula (L.)). Acta Zoologica 67: 73–86. doi: 10.1111/j.1463-6395.1986.tb00851.x

32. Zeiske E, Theisen B, Gruber S (1987) Functional Morphology of the Olfactory Organ of Two Carcharhinid Shark Species. Canadian Journal of Zoology 65: 2406–2412. doi: 10.1139/z87-362

33. Schluessel V, Bennett M, Bleckmann H, Blomberg S, Collin S (2008) Morphometric and Ultrastructural Comparison of the Olfactory System in Elasmobranchs: The Significance of Structure–Function Relationships

Based on Phylogeny and Ecology. Journal of Morphology 269: 1365–1386. doi: 10.1002/jmor.10661

34. Takami S, Luer C, Graziadei P (1994) Microscopic Structure of the Olfactory Organ of the Clearnose Skate, Raja eglanteria. Anatomy and Embryology 190: 211–230. doi: 10.1007/bf00234300
35. Meredith T, Caprio J, Kajiura S (2012) Sensitivity and Specificity of the Olfactory Epithelia of Two Elasmobranch Species to Bile Salts. The Journal of Experimental Biology 215: 2660–2667. doi: 10.1242/jeb.066241
36. Getchell M, Getchell T (1992) Fine Structural Aspects of Secretion and Extrinsic Innervation in the Olfactory Mucosa. Microscopy Research and Technique 23: 111–127. doi: 10.1002/jemt.1070230203
37. Getchell T, Margolis F, Getchell M (1984) Perireceptor and Receptor Events in Vertebrate Olfaction. Progress in Neurobiology 23: 317–345. doi: 10.1016/0301-0082(84)90008-x
38. Getchell M, Mellert T (1991) Olfactory Mucus Secretion. In: Getchell T, Doty R, Bartoshuk L, Snow J, editors, Smell and Taste in Health and Disease, Raven Press, New York. 83–95.
39. Cox JPL (2012) Ciliary Function in the Olfactory Organs of Sharks and Rays. Fish and Fisheries doi: –10.1111/j.1467–2979.2012.00476.x.
40. Bertmar G (1972) Scanning Electron Microscopy of Olfactory Rosette in Sea Trout. Cell and Tissue Research 128: 336–346. doi: 10.1007/bf00306974
41. Hansen A, Zeiske E (1993) Development of the Olfactory Organ in the Zebrafish, Brachydanio rerio. Journal of Comparative Neurology 333: 289–300. doi: 10.1002/cne.903330213
42. Hansen A, Zeiske E (1998) The Peripheral Olfactory Organ of the Zebrafish, Danio rerio: An Ultrastructural Study. Chemical Senses 23: 39–48. doi: 10.1093/chemse/23.1.39
43. Ghosh S, Chakrabarti P (2010) Histological and Scanning Electron Microscopic Organization and Functional Aspects of the Surface Olfactory Epithelium of the Freshwater Minor Carp, Puntius sophore (Hamilton). In: Proceedings of the Zoological Society. Springer, volume 63, 115–119.
44. Sleigh M (1989) Adaptations of Ciliary Systems for the Propulsion of Water and Mucus. Comparative Biochemistry and Physiology Part A: Physiology 94: 359–364. doi: 10.1016/0300-9629(89)90559-8
45. Quraishi M, Jones N, Mason J (1998) The Rheology of Nasal Mucus: A Review. Clinical Otolaryngology & Allied Sciences 23: 403–413. doi: 10.1046/j.1365-2273.1998.00172.x
46. Tomenzoli D (2005) Physiology of the Nose and Paranasal Sinuses. In: Imaging in Treatment Planning for Sinonasal Diseases, Springer. 29–34.
47. Menco B, Farbman A (1992) Ultrastructural Evidence for Multiple Mucous Domains in Frog Olfactory Epithelium. Cell and Tissue Research 270: 47–56. doi: 10.1007/bf00381878
48. Getchell T, Su Z, GetchellM(1993) Mucous Domains: Microchemical Heterogeneity in the Mucociliary Complex of the Olfactory Epithelium. In: Ciba Foundation Symposium 179 – The Molecular Basis of Smell and Taste Transduction. 27–50.
49. Reese T (1965) Olfactory Cilia in the Frog. The Journal of Cell Biology 25: 209–230. doi: 10.1083/jcb.25.2.209
50. Getchell M, Rafols J, Getchell T (1984) Histological and Histochemical Studies of the Secretory Components of the Salamander Olfactory Mucosa: Effects of Isoproterenol and Olfactory Nerve Section. The Anatomical Record 208: 553–565. doi: 10.1002/ar.1092080411
51. Bansil R, Stanley E, Lamont J (1995) Mucin Biophysics. Annual Review of Physiology 57: 635– 657.
52. Shephard K (1994) Functions for Fish Mucus. Reviews in Fish Biology and Fisheries 4: 401–429. doi: 10.1007/bf00042888
53. Sellers L, Allen A, Morris E, Ross-Murphy S (1988) Mucus Glycoprotein Gels. Role of Glycoprotein Polymeric Structure and Carbohydrate Side-Chains in Gel-Formation. Carbohydrate Research 178: 93–110. doi: 10.1016/0008-6215(88)80104-6
54. Varki A (1999) Essentials of Glycobiology. Cold Spring Harbor Laboratory Press.
55. Wiesenburg D, Little B (1987) A Synopsis of the Chemical/Physical Properties of Seawater. Ocean Physics and Engineering 12: 127–165.
56. Brigham M, Stein W, Moore S (1960) The Concentrations of Cysteine and Cystine in Human Blood Plasma. Journal of Clinical Investigation 39: 1633–1638. doi: 10.1172/jci104186
57. Carr W, Gleeson R, Derby C (1996) Stimulants of Feeding Behavior in Fish: Analyses of Tissues of Diverse Marine Organisms. The Biological Bulletin 190: 149–160. doi: 10.2307/1542535
58. Hara T (1975) Olfaction in Fish. Progress in Neurobiology 5: 271–335. doi: 10.1016/0301-0082(75)90014-3
59. Hara T (1982) Chemoreception in Fishes, volume 8. Elsevier Science Ltd.
60. Carr W, Derby C (1986) Chemically Stimulated Feeding Behavior in Marine Animals. Journal of Chemical Ecology 12: 989–1011. doi: 10.1007/bf01638992
61. Hara T (1992) Mechanisms of Olfaction. In: Hara T, editor, Fish Chemoreception, Chapman & Hall, volume 6: 150–170. doi: 10.1007/978-94-011-2332-7_8
62. Jones K (1992) Food Search Behaviour in Fish and the Use of Chemical Lures in Commercial and Sports Fishing. In: Hara T, editor, Fish Chemoreception, Chapman & Hall, volume 6: 288–320. doi: 10.1007/978-94-011-2332-7_14
63. Hara T (1994) Olfaction and Gustation in Fish: An Overview. Acta Physiologica Scandinavica 152: 207–217. doi: 10.1111/j.1748-1716.1994.tb09800.x
64. Hara T (1994) The Diversity of Chemical Stimulation in Fish Olfaction and Gustation. Reviews in Fish Biology and Fisheries 4: 1–35. doi: 10.1007/bf00043259
65. Tricas T, Kajiura S, Summers A (2009) Response of

the Hammerhead Shark Olfactory Epithelium to Amino Acid Stimuli. Journal of Comparative Physiology A: Neuroethology, Sensory, Neural, and Behavioral Physiology 195: 947–954. doi: 10.1007/s00359-009-0470-3

66. Meredith T, Kajiura S (2010) Olfactory Morphology and Physiology of Elasmobranchs. Journal of Experimental Biology 213: 3449–3456. doi: 10.1242/jeb.045849

67. Hess B, Kutzner C, van der Spoel D, Lindahl E (2008) GROMACS 4: Algorithms for Highly Efficient, Load-Balanced, and Scalable Molecular Simulation. Journal of Chemical Theory and Computation 4: 435–447. doi: 10.1021/ct700301q

68. Jorgensen W, Tirado-Rives J (1988) The OPLS [Optimized Potentials for Liquid Simulations] Potential Functions for Proteins, Energy Minimizations for Crystals of Cyclic Peptides and Crambin. Journal of the American Chemical Society 110: 1657–1666. doi: 10.1021/ja00214a001

69. Jorgensen W, Maxwell D, Tirado-Rives J (1996) Development and Testing of the OPLS All-Atom Force Field on Conformational Energetics and Properties of Organic Liquids. Journal of the American Chemical Society 118: 11225–11236. doi: 10.1021/ja9621760

70. Damm W, Frontera A, Tirado-Rives J, Jorgensen W (1998) OPLS All-Atom Force Field for Carbohydrates. Journal of Computational Chemistry 18: 1955–1970. doi: 10.1002/(sici)1096-987x(199712)18:16<1955::aid-jcc1>3.3.co;2-a

71. Kaminski G, Friesner R, Tirado-Rives J, Jorgensen W (2001) Evaluation and Reparametrization of the OPLS-AA Force Field for Proteins via Comparison with Accurate Quantum Chemical Calculations on Peptides. The Journal of Physical Chemistry B 105: 6474–6487. doi: 10.1021/jp003919d

72. Berendsen H, Grigera J, Straatsma T (1987) The Missing Term in Effective Pair Potentials. Journal of Physical Chemistry 91: 6269–6271. doi: 10.1021/j100308a038

73. Darden T, York D, Pedersen L (1993) Particle Mesh Ewald: An N log (N) Method for Ewald Sums in Large Systems. The Journal of Chemical Physics 98: 10089. doi: 10.1063/1.464397

74. Gomes M, Padua A (2007) Solubility and Molecular Modeling. In: Letcher T, editor, Developments and Applications in Solubility, Royal Society of Chemistry. 153–168.

75. Bennett C (1976) Efficient Estimation of Free Energy Differences from Monte Carlo Data. Journal of Computational Physics 22: 245–268. doi: 10.1016/0021-9991(76)90078-4

76. Nocedal J (1980) Updating Quasi-Newton Matrices with Limited Storage. Mathematics of Computation 35: 773–782. doi: 10.2307/2006193

77. Parrinello M, Rahman A (1981) Polymorphic Transitions in Single Crystals: A New Molecular Dynamics Method. Journal of Applied Physics 52: 7182–7190. doi: 10.1063/1.328693

78. Nosé S, Klein M (1983) Constant Pressure Molecular Dynamics for Molecular Systems. Molecular Physics 50: 1055–1076. doi: 10.1080/00268978300102851

79. Yang L, Ahmed A, SI S (2013) Comparison of Two Simulation Methods to Compute Solvation Free Energies and Partition Coefficients. Journal of Computational Chemistry 34: 284–293. doi: 10.1002/jcc.23127

80. Dixit S, Bhasin R, Rajasekaran E, Jayaram B (1997) Solvation Thermodynamics of Amino Acids: Assessment of the Electrostatic Contribution and Force-Field Dependence. Journal of the Chemical Society, Faraday Transactions 93: 1105–1113. doi: 10.1039/a603913h

81. GROMACS 4.6.1 Online Reference. Available: http://manual.gromacs.org/online.html. Accessed: 2013 Apr 22.

82. Riddle D, Oakley B (1991) Evaluation of Projection Patterns in the Primary Olfactory System of Rainbow Trout. The Journal of Neuroscience 11: 3752–3762.

83. Ngai J, Chess A, Dowling M, Necles N, Macagno E, et al. (1993) Coding of Olfactory Information: Topography of Odorant Receptor Expression in the Catfish Olfactory Epithelium. Cell 72: 667–680. doi: 10.1016/0092-8674(93)90396-8

84. Riddle D, Wong L, Oakley B (1993) Lectin Identification of Olfactory Receptor Neuron Subclasses with Segregated Central Projections. The Journal of Neuroscience 13: 3018–3033.

85. Chang Q, Caprio J (1996) Electrophysiological Evidence for the Broad Distribution of Specific Odorant Receptor Molecules across the Olfactory Organ of the Channel Catfish. Chemical Senses 21: 519–527. doi: 10.1093/chemse/21.5.519

86. Cao Y, Oh B, Stryer L (1998) Cloning and Localization of Two Multigene Receptor Families in Goldfish Olfactory Epithelium. Proceedings of the National Academy of Sciences 95: 11987–11992. doi: 10.1073/pnas.95.20.11987

87. Laberge F, Hara T (2001) Neurobiology of Fish Olfaction: A Review. Brain Research Reviews 36: 46–59. doi: 10.1016/s0165-0173(01)00064-9

CHAPTER 8

DETECTION AND CHARACTERIZATION OF AUTOANTIBODIES TO NEURONAL CELL-SURFACE ANTIGENS

Marleen H. van Coevorden-Hameete, Maarten J. Titulaer, Marco W. J. Schreurs, Esther de Graaff, Peter A. E. Sillevis Smitt and Casper C. Hoogenraad

Keywords: Autoantibodies, anti-neuronal antibodies, cell-surface antigens, diagnostic testing, autoimmune encephalitis

INTRODUCTION

Anti-neuronal autoimmune encephalitis (AIE) is a heterogeneous group of disorders characterized by autoantibodies that are directed at the extracellular domains of antigens in the synaptic or extra-synaptic plasma membrane. These antigens are often key players in synaptic transmission and neuronal excitability. Antibody binding to these antigens therefore directly leads to neuronal dysfunction. When the antibodies are removed, neuronal dysfunction is commonly reversed and patients often completely recover (van Coevorden-Hameete et al., 2014; Höftberger, 2015). This striking response to immunotherapy stresses the importance of early diagnosis and treatment of AIE. To achieve this, the availability of sensitive and specific tests to detect cell-surface autoantibodies is of key importance.

Whereas diagnostics in AIE is an emerging field, large experience exists with laboratory tests used for the detection of anti-neuronal antibodies in classical paraneoplastic neurological syndromes (PNS; Probst et al., 2014). Some, but not all, of the methods used in PNS diagnostics are also suitable to detect autoantibodies involved in AIE. The different requirements for diagnostic methods are mainly determined by two major differences between classical PNS antigens and AIE antigens. Classical PNS antigens are primarily located intracellular whereas AIE antigens are located in or on the plasma membrane. In addition, antibodies directed at classical PNS antigens are mostly recognizing linear epitopes, whereas surface antigens contain mostly conformational epitopes.

Core methods in PNS and AIE diagnostics are immunohistochemistry (IHC) on rat brain sections and indirect immunofluorescence (IIF) on primate cerebellum sections. In these assays all relevant antigens are present and accessible. For the detection of neuronal surface antigens also immunocytochemistry (ICC) of primary hippocampal neurons is used. Although these techniques are very useful as initial screening methods, they do not allow for the identification of the exact molecular target of the autoantibodies. In addition, these techniques require extensive experience and are labor-intensive. Therefore, for diagnostic purposes, highly specific confirmatory tests are needed. For PNS antigens immunoblotting with recombinant antigen is used most frequently as a confirmatory test (Willison et al., 2000). For surface antigens a radioimmunoassay (RIA) can be used to detect antibodies directed at a channel complex, such as voltage gated calcium channels (VGCC; Motomura et al., 1995). However, a RIA cannot discriminate between antibodies to different channel components that can be of clinical relevance, as is the case for antibodies directed to the voltage gated potassium channel (VGKC; Lai et al., 2010; Lancaster et al., 2011a; van Sonderen et al., 2016b). To test single neuronal surface antigens cell based assays (CBA) are the method of choice. In CBAs the natural environment and conformation of the antigen is mostly maintained (Willison et al., 2000).

Despite the fact that many of these techniques are currently used in AIE diagnostic and research laboratories, the methodology to detect cell-surface antibodies is not widely standardized. In this article we review the advantages and pitfalls of three different techniques for antibody detection: (1) IHC/IIF on adult rat/primate brain slices; (2) ICC on living cultured rat hippocampal neurons; and (3) CBAs for neuronal

Citation: van Coevorden-Hameete MH, Titulaer MJ, Schreurs MWJ, de Graaff E, Sillevis Smitt PAE and Hoogenraad CC (2016) Detection and Characterization of Autoantibodies to Neuronal Cell-Surface Antigens. Mol. Neurosci. 9:37. doi: 10.3389/fnmol.2016.00037.

membrane proteins (for an overview see Table 1). In addition we evaluate the use of immunoprecipitation and mass spectrometry analysis for the identification of novel cell-surface antigens.

Table 1: Laboratory techniques for the detection of neuronal cell-surface antibodies

	Number of patients reported	IHC	ICC of living neurons	CBA	Commercial CBA available	Sensitivity and specificity
NMDAR	>1000	Specific staining pattern hippocampus (AIE protocol) (Dalmau et al., 2007) and (Gresa-Arribas et al., 2014)	Surface labeling of excitatory synapses (Hughes et al., 2010)	Fixed (Dalmau et al., 2008) and (Gresa-Arribas et al., 2014)	Yes	*Sensitivity IHC:* CSF 100%, serum 92% (Gresa-Arribas et al., 2014) *Sensitivity fixed CBA:* CSF 100%, serum 86% (Gresa-Arribas et al., 2014) *Sensitivity IHC plus fixed CBA:* CSF 100%, serum 86% (Gresa-Arribas et al., 2014) *Specificity IHC plus fixed CBA:* CSF 100%, serum 100% (Gresa-Arribas et al., 2014)
LGI1	~250	Specific staining pattern of hippocampus (AIE protocol) (Lai et al., 2010)	Surface labeling of neurons, not further specified (Lai et al., 2010)	Fixed (with ADAM22/23 coexpression) (Lai et al., 2010) Fixed with added transmembrane part (van Sonderen et al., 2016c) Live (Irani et al., 2010a)	Yes	*Sensitivity IHC:* CSF 88%, serum 100% (van Sonderen et al., 2016c) *Sensitivity fixed CBA:* CSF 53%, serum 100% (van Sonderen et al., 2016c)
Caspr2	~100	Diffuse neuropil staining (AIE protocol) (Lancaster et al., 2011a)	Surface labeling of neurons, not further specified (Lancaster et al., 2011a)	Fixed (Lancaster et al., 2011a) Live (Irani et al., 2012)	Yes	*Sensitivity fixed CBA:* CSF 100%, serum 100% (van Sonderen et al., 2016a)
GlyR	~75	Neuropil of brainstem and spinal cord (PNS protocol) (Carvajal-González et al., 2014)	Not published	Live (Carvajal-González et al. 2014)	No	*Sensitivity live CBA:* CSF: PERM 100% (Carvajal-González et al., 2014), SPS-spectrum 0% (Martinez-Hernandez et al., 2016), serum: PERM 100% (Carvajal-González et al. 2014) *Sensitivity fixed CBA:* Serum 92–94% (disease controls) (Martinez-Hernandez et al., 2015) (Martinez-Hernandez et al. 2016)
$GABA_BR$	67	Diffuse neuropil staining (AIE protocol) (Lancaster et al., 2010) and (Höftberger et al., 2013)	Surface labeling of neurons, not further specified (Lancaster et al., 2010)	Fixed (Lancaster et al., 2010)	Yes	*Sensitivity fixed CBA:* CSF 100%, serum 67–93% (Lancaster et al., 2010); (Höftberger et al., 2013); and (Jeffery et al., 2013)
DNER	65	PC cytoplasm, punctate staining of molecular layer cerebellum (PNS protocol) (Graus et al., 1997) and (de Graaff et al., 2012)	Surface labeling of neurons overexpressing DNER (de Graaff et al., 2012)	Fixed (de Graaff et al., 2012) Live (Greene et al., 2014)	Yes	*Sensitivity fixed CBA:* Serum 100% (Probst et al., 2015) *Specificity fixed CBA:* Serum 100% (Probst et al., 2015)
AMPAR	64	Diffuse neuropil staining (AIE protocol) (Lai et al., 2009)	Surface labeling of excitatory synapses (Lai et al., 2009)	Fixed (Lai et al., 2009) and (Höftberger et al., 2015)	Yes	*Specificity fixed CBA:* CSF 100%, serum 70% (Höftberger et al., 2015)
DPPX	28	Diffuse neuropil staining (AIE protocol)	Surface labeling of both excitatory and inhibitory	Fixed (Boronat et al., 2013); (Balint et al., 2014),	Yes	Not available

		(Boronat et al., 2013); (Balint et al., 2014); and (Tobin et al., 2014)	synapses (Piepgras et al., 2015)	and (Tobin et al., 2014)		
DopamineR*	26	Staining of basal ganglia (Dale et al., 2012)	Surface labeling of neurons, not further specified (Dale et al., 2012)	Live (Dale et al., 2012)	No	Not available
mGluR1	16	PC cytoplasm, molecular layer cerebellum (PNS protocol) (Sillevis Smitt et al., 2000) and (Lopez-Chiriboga et al., 2016)	Not published	Fixed (Lopez-Chiriboga et al., 2016) and (Iorio et al., 2013)	Yes	Not available
IgLon5	10	Diffuse neuropil staining (AIE protocol) (Sabater et al., 2014)	Surface labeling of neurons, not further specified (Sabater et al., 2014)	Live (Sabater et al., 2014)	No	Not available
mGluR5	3	Diffuse neuropil staining (AIE protocol) (Lancaster et al., 2011b)	Surface labeling of neurons, not further specified (Lancaster et al., 2011b)	Fixed (Lancaster et al., 2011b)	Yes	Not available

*IHC, Immunohistochemistry; ICC, Immunocytochemistry; CBA, Cell Based Assay; PC, Purkinje cell; PERM, Progressive encephalomyelitis with rigidity and myoclonus; SPS, Stiff person syndrome; *Not confirmed by other laboratories.*

IMMUNOHISTOCHEMISTRY

The reactivity of antibodies present in patient serum or CSF against rat brain proteins can be tested with IHC. In this assay 5–9 μm thick complete rat brain slices are used. Therefore all possible antigens are available and accessible, and different brain regions can be assessed. This technique has been a core method for the detection of antibodies directed at intracellular antigens in PNS. For classical PNS antigens diagnostic laboratories mostly use IIF of primate cerebellum, for which a commercial kit is available.

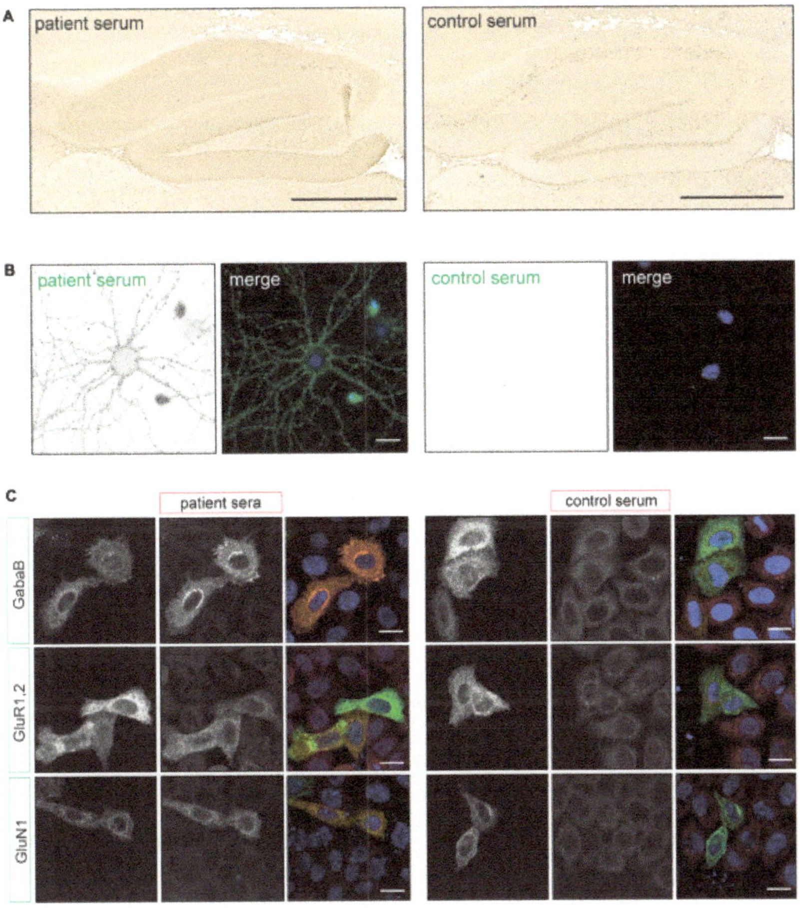

Figure 1: Examples of staining patterns. **(A)** Immunohistochemistry (IHC) of rat brain slices using the autoimmune encephalitis (AIE) protocol. The left picture shows neuropil staining of the hippocampus using anti-NMDA receptor (NMDAR) positive

patient serum. The right picture shows staining with a healthy control serum. Scale bars: 500 µm. (**B**) Live staining of cultured rat hippocampal neurons using anti-NMDAR positive patient or healthy control serum (green). The picture shows a punctate staining pattern along the dendrites. Scale bars: 20 µm. (**C**) Examples of staining patterns of fixed Cell Based Assays (CBA) for anti-GABA$_B$R, AMPAR and NMDAR antibodies. Transfected HeLa cells (green) show enhanced staining with patient serum (red) when compared to non-transfected cells and healthy control serum. Scale bars: 20 µm. Adapted from: De Bruijn and Titulaer (2016), Figure 12.1.

Although similar in many respects, the detection of synaptic surface antibodies requires a different pre-treatment of the rat brain tissue. For classical PNS antibodies brain tissue is snapfrozen, sliced with a cryostat and subsequently fixed with acetone or paraformaldehyde (PFA; Graus et al., 1997). For cell-surface antigens rat brains are fixed with PFA for 1 h at 4°C, cryoprotected in 40% sucrose for at least 24 h, snapfrozen in isopentane and subsequently sliced with a cryostat (Ances et al., 2005; Dalmau et al., 2007). By using this method of tissue preparation, antigens are well preserved and no antigen retrieval methods need to be used to obtain robust staining. The slices are incubated with serum or CSF and bound antibodies can be visualized with diaminobenzidine (DAB) peroxidase or fluorescently labeled secondary antibodies. For classical PNS antibodies, generally primate cerebellum is scored for specific staining patterns such as the distinct punctate anti-Tr/delta/notch-like epidermal growth factor-related receptor (DNER) pattern (Graus et al., 1997) or nuclear staining of anti-Hu antibodies (Sillevis Smitt et al., 2002). For cell-surface antigens, the hippocampus is scored for staining of the synapses containing gray matter, termed neuropil (Figure 1A). This neuropil staining is less robust when using the classical PNS pre-treatment of rat brain tissue. The different cell-surface antibodies can produce highly characteristic staining patterns on rat hippocampus (Dalmau et al., 2008; Montojo et al., 2015). With good quality IHC and experienced observers the recognition of these specific staining patterns may already lead to diagnosis.

Most synaptic proteins are highly homologous (for example rat-human homology on protein level for the NR1 subunit of the NMDA receptor (NMDAR) is 99.3% (source: NCBI). However, when screening for novel neuronal antigens it is important to keep in mind that due to interspecies differences some epitopes might be absent in rodents and are therefore missed on IHC.

IMMUNOCYTOCHEMISTRY ON LIVING PRIMARY HIPPOCAMPAL NEURONS

To assess antibody reactivity to extracellular epitopes live staining of cultured primary rat hippocampal neurons with patients' serum or CSF can be performed. In theory, this way only relevant extracellular epitopes will be detected, diminishing the background signal. Also, the effects of the protein crosslinking fixative PFA, on the antigenicity of the receptor will be circumvented (Peränen et al., 1993).

For this assay it is important to use neurons that are more than 14 days in culture and have developed axons and synapses. Serum or CSF is applied when the neurons are alive and are incubated for 30–45 min at 37°C. The secondary antibody can be applied on living neurons or after fixation under non-permeabilizing conditions (Hughes et al., 2010). In both cases only extracellular epitopes will be detected and result in a punctate staining pattern along the neurites (Figure 1B). In contrast with IHC, the staining patterns of antibodies directed at different surface antigens (e.g., NMDAR, GABA$_B$R) are indistinguishable (Dalmau et al., 2008; Lancaster et al., 2010). More information on the specific subcellular localization of the antigen could be determined by using co-staining with (excitatory or inhibitory) synaptic markers. However, it needs to be noted that binding of the patients antibodies to the antigen can alter the protein's localization. For the NMDA- and AMPAR it has been shown that receptors move out of the synaptic area and become internalized (Hughes et al., 2010; Mikasova et al., 2012; Moscato et al., 2014; Peng et al., 2015). Therefore after surface labeling such co-localization studies should be interpreted with caution.

CELL BASED ASSAYS

In a CBA a recombinant antigen is expressed by mammalian cells. The transfected cells are stained with patient serum or CSF using IIF. When the patient sample contains antibodies directed at this specific antigen, staining of the transfected cells is enhanced when compared to non-transfected cells (Figure 1C). In CBAs the antigen mostly maintains its tertiary structure and the appropriate post-translational modifications. This allows for the detection of antibodies directed at conformational epitopes.

Commercial CBAs, as well as most research laboratories, make use of human embryonic kidney (HEK) cells. HEK cells are a cell line suitable for membrane protein expression (Chaudhary et al., 2011). However, also HeLa or Chinese Hamster Ovary cells can be used as these cell lines attach more tightly to the culture plates than HEK cells and therefore wash off less easily during the staining procedure.

Controversy exists on the timing of fixation during the immunofluorescent staining procedure. With respect to the anti-NR1 CBA, some laboratories perform surface staining of live HEK cells with serum or CSF prior to fixation and permeabilization (Irani et al., 2010b; Ramberger et al., 2015), as in theory only relevant extracellular epitopes will be detected (as described in "Immunocytochemistry on Living Primary Hippocampal Neurons" Section). Other research groups fix and permeabilize the cells before immunostaining, as is also used in the commercial CBA. The only study to compare live vs. fixed CBA in an unselected way found a higher sensitivity of the fixed CBA (Gresa-Arribas et al., 2014), despite the theoretical expectations of the opposite. In addition, it needs to be noted that not all individual receptor subunits express equally well in cell lines. Some need co-expression of other subunits, auxiliary proteins or scaffolding molecules for proper receptor folding, assembly, ER export and surface expression (Leite et al., 2008; Irani et al., 2010b). This is especially important when performing live CBAs in which the receptors need to be located in the plasma membrane for antibodies to bind. It is therefore very well possible that the optimal choice between live vs. fixed CBA might be different for each receptor that is tested.

For both the fixed and live CBA one should also realize that the presence of a large number of ion channels in the plasma membrane for a longer period of time could lead to excitotoxicity and might require the addition of receptor blockers (e.g., ketamine for NMDAR) to the culture medium (Irani et al., 2010b; Ramberger et al., 2015)

Concerning the DNA constructs used for recombinant antigen expression in CBAs it is important to keep in mind that the addition of a molecular tag to a transmembrane protein for visualization purposes can affect protein trafficking and folding (Hughes et al., 2010). This could be overcome by using an untagged version in combination with cytoplasmic green fluorescent protein (GFP) to identify the transfected cells. However, in this case a commercial antibody to the antigen needs to be used to assess exact colocalization of antigen and patient antibody.

Mostly CBAs are scored with a subjective visual scoring system using epifluorescent microscopy. However, the staining intensity can vary considerably within one coverslip and accurate scoring depends heavily on the observers' experience. For this reason in most studies two independent blinded investigators perform the scoring. Some laboratories use a semi-quantitative scoring system ranging from 0 to 4 with an increasing strength of fluorescence intensity (Leite et al., 2008). However the value of this type of semi-quantitative scoring has never been validated. To get an idea of the antibody titres it is more reliable to perform serial dilutions on IHC (Gresa-Arribas et al., 2014).

Alternatively, the evaluation of CBAs using fluorescence-activated cell sorting (FACS) is less dependent on experience. In addition it could provide a quantitative method for determining antibody titres without the need of testing serial dilutions. CBA with FACS based scoring has been used for the detection of anti-aquaporin-4 antibodies in neuromyelitis optica (De Vidi et al., 2011) and anti-NMDAR (Amatoury et al., 2013). However, only one study compared visual scoring of CBA with FACS based analysis. This study showed lower sensitivity for anti-NMDAR antibodies when FACS was used instead of visual scoring (Ramberger et al., 2015).

Over the last years the sensitivity and specificity of CBAs using serum or CSF has become increasingly clear (see Table 1). Intrathecal antibody synthesis is high in anti-NMDA, -AMPA and $GABA_B$ receptor encephalitis (Lai et al., 2009; Lancaster et al., 2010; Dalmau et al., 2011), facilitating antibody detection in CSF. For anti-NMDAR antibodies, a permeabilized CBA has a sensitivity of 100% for CSF and 86% for serum (Gresa-Arribas et al., 2014). For anti-AMPAR antibodies this is 100% for CSF vs. 70% for serum (Höftberger et al., 2015), and for anti-$GABA_B$R 100% for CSF and 67–93% for serum (Lancaster et al., 2010; Höftberger et al., 2013; Jeffery et al., 2013). For anti-LGI1 antibodies sensitivity on IHC is 88% and 100% for CSF and serum respectively, whereas the commercial LGI1 CBA using CSF has only 53% sensitivity, probably reflecting lower intrathecal antibody synthesis (van Sonderen et al., 2016c). Special attention is required for patients undergoing plasma exchange at the moment of serum assessment, as antibodies may no longer be detectable in serum (Florance et al., 2009).

Over the last years high throughput screenings have been published, mainly in the field of psychiatry, in which the presence of anti-neuronal surface antibodies is tested using CBA with serum only. These studies have detected anti-NR1 antibodies in up to 10% of neuropsychiatric disorders, but also in healthy individuals (Zandi et al., 2011; Dahm et al., 2014; Hammer et al., 2014). However, these studies were confusing due to lumping of IgG with IgA/IgM antibody isotypes, incomplete testing or selection bias. Only IgG subclass antibodies directed at NR1 alone causes the disease described as anti-NMDAR encephalitis. The clinical relevance of IgM and IgA antibodies is so far unclear, as was also concluded from other articles studying psychiatric populations (Steiner et al., 2013). Anti-NMDAR encephalitis can present as an isolated first psychotic episode (Kayser et al., 2013), although the presence of anti-NMDAR encephalitis among first episode psychosis patients is likely to be (less than) 1%. This chance quickly increases if patients develop neurological symptoms or additional features such as fever or autonomic dysfunction. In studies testing for anti-NMDAR IgG in a purely psychiatric population using more than one method (CBA combined with IHC or ICC of living hippocampal neurons, or the combination of serum and CSF) no patients with only psychiatric features and anti-NMDAR encephalitis have been found (Masdeu et al., 2012; van Mierlo et al., 2015). The low *a priori* chance in patients with psychiatric disorders combined with a specificity of 97–99.4% for CBA of serum (Gresa-Arribas et al., 2014) results in a *post priori* chance of only 25–60% when testing serum only. These results indicate that high throughput screening studies in a population with low disease prevalence requires excellent specificity to be of value. Combining CBA with IHC or live neuron staining could for example increase the specificity (Gresa-Arribas et al., 2014).

IMMUNOPRECIPITATION AND MASS SPECTROMETRY ANALYSIS OF MEMBRANE ANTIGENS

Some patients have a clinical phenotype strongly suggesting an autoimmune etiology but test negative for all known surface antigens. If IHC and live ICC provide a strong indication for the presence of cell-surface antibodies one can try to identify the molecular target of the antibodies in order to develop a CBA. Classically, novel PNS antigens were identified using cDNA expression libraries by phage display (Hufton et al., 1999). Strikingly, only intracellular antigens with mostly linear epitopes have been identified using this technique, indicating that it is less suitable for conformational epitopes. Currently, most novel surface antigens are identified by performing immunoprecipitation with patient's serum or CSF followed by mass spectrometry analysis (IP-MS; Lai et al., 2009; Lancaster et al., 2010; de Graaff et al., 2012; Boronat et al., 2013; Petit-Pedrol et al., 2014; Sabater et al., 2014). Although in a seemingly straightforward procedure many factors are complicating the identification of a membrane antigen.

Firstly MS analysis is hampered by properties of the membrane proteins itself. They are expressed relatively low compared to cytosolic proteins. Due to their membrane spanning hydrophobic domains membrane proteins aggregate easily, leading to inefficient proteolytic cleavage. This leads to underrepresentation of membrane proteins in the sample (Helbig et al., 2010; Barrera and Robinson, 2011). Fractionation of membrane preparations, synaptosome isolation or surface biotinylation can be used to enrich (synaptic) membrane proteins in the input material. In order to reduce the detection of nonspecific cytosolic and nuclear proteins some labs perform surface labeling of primary hippocampal neurons and subsequently lyse the cells and precipitate IgG with the bound antigen (Boronat et al., 2013).

Secondly membrane proteins have the tendency to misfold when extracted by detergent. This leads to disruption of the conformational epitope and reduced antibody binding. Special attention is therefore required for the choice of detergent in order to optimize solubilization. Which detergent is suitable for membrane protein solubilization depends on the type of membrane protein that needs to be extracted (Privé, 2007). The fact that the membrane antigen is still unknown when performing IP-MS severely hampers the choice of detergent. A new amphipathic polymer that solubilizes membrane proteins in intact membrane patches might be a promising alternative (Dörr et al., 2016).

In general CSF contains less antibodies than serum, both in number and variety, and in case of intrathecal synthesis, the relative amount of specific antibodies is higher. Therefore the use of CSF in staining and immunoprecipitation is thought to provide cleaner results. However, CSF is usually less readily available than serum.

CONCLUSION AND RECOMMENDATIONS

The detection of synaptic cell-surface antibodies has significant consequences for the treatment and follow-up of AIE patients. It can confirm the autoimmune-mediated nature of the syndrome and can provide a clue for a possible underlying tumor. In order to successfully identify antibodies to surface antigens clinical assessment and patient selection by an experienced clinician is of key importance. For diagnostic purposes both serum and CSF should be tested by a combination of IHC and CBA to provide highest sensitivity and specificity. Live staining of cultured hippocampal neurons is labor intensive. The neurons used for diagnostic testing cannot be prepared beforehand and cannot be stored. However, live ICC of neurons can provide valuable additional information when the results from IHC and CBA are inconclusive.

Samples selected for IP-MS need to show robust results on both IHC and live ICC of hippocampal neurons. Preferentially patients with a similar staining pattern and clinical phenotype are grouped. If possible, two different serum samples from one patient can be used to perform IP-MS. Comparing two lists of one patient (or the lists of patients with a similar clinical phenotype and/or similar staining pattern on IHC) could facilitate the detection of novel antigens.

In the next years novel neuronal surface antigens will be identified, most likely by screening cohorts of patients with for example epilepsy or dementia. It is expected that these yet unknown patients will phenotypically show less encephalitis and more encephalopathy. As screening becomes more extensive, careful evaluation of specificity and pathogenicity of novel antibodies will be necessary. Given the low frequency of occurrence of most of these antibodies, meaningful clinical studies will require international collaboration.

FUNDING

This research was funded by NUTS-OHRA (1104-034), Hersenstichting (2012(1)-141).

CONFLICT OF INTEREST STATEMENT

MHvC-H has nothing to disclose. The work of MJT is supported by grants from the Netherlands Organisation for Scientific Research (NWO, Veni-incentive and Memorabel fellowship), the Dutch Epilepsy Foundations (NEF, project 14-19) and ErasmusMC fellowship. MJT received research funds for serving on a scientific advisory board of MedImmune LLC and a travel grant for lecturing in India from Sun Pharma, India. MWJS has received financial compensation for seminars and conference visits from Biognost, Inova and Thermo Scientific. EdG and PAESS received a research grant from Euroimmun for a patent for the use of DNER as an autoantibody test. CCH has nothing to disclose.

REFERENCES

1. Amatoury, M., Merheb, V., Langer, J., Wang, X. M., Dale, R. C., and Brilot, F. (2013). High-throughput flow cytometry cell-based assay to detect antibodies to N-methyl-D-aspartate receptor or dopamine-2 receptor in human serum. *J. Vis. Exp.* 81:e50935. doi: 10.3791/50935
2. Ances, B. M., Vitaliani, R., Taylor, R. A., Liebeskind, D. S., Voloschin, A., Houghton, D. J., et al. (2005). Treatment-responsive limbic encephalitis identified by neuropil antibodies: MRI and PET correlates. *Brain* 128, 1764–1777. doi: 10.1093/brain/awh526
3. Balint, B., Jarius, S., Nagel, S., Haberkorn, U., Probst, C., Blöcker, I. M., et al. (2014). Progressive encephalomyelitis with rigidity and myoclonus: a new variant with DPPX antibodies. *Neurology* 82, 1521–1528. doi: 10.1212/WNL.0000000000000372
4. Barrera, N. P., and Robinson, C. V. (2011). Advances in the mass spectrometry of membrane proteins: from individual proteins to intact complexes. *Annu. Rev. Biochem.* 80, 247–271. doi: 10.1146/annurev-biochem-062309-093307
5. Boronat, A., Gelfand, J. M., Gresa-Arribas, N., Jeong, H. Y., Walsh, M., Roberts, K., et al. (2013). Encephalitis and antibodies to dipeptidyl-peptidase-like protein-6, a subunit of Kv4.2 potassium channels. *Ann. Neurol.* 73, 120–128. doi: 10.1002/ana.23756
6. Carvajal-González, A., Leite, M. I., Waters, P., Woodhall, M., Coutinho, E., Balint, B., et al. (2014). Glycine receptor antibodies in PERM and related syndromes: characteristics, clinical features and outcomes. *Brain* 137, 2178–2192. doi: 10.1093/brain/awu142
7. Chaudhary, S., Pak, J. E., Pedersen, B. P., Bang, L. J., Zhang, L. B., Ngaw, S. M., et al. (2011). Efficient expression screening of human membrane proteins in transiently transfected Human Embryonic Kidney 293S cells. *Methods* 55, 273–280. doi: 10.1016/j.ymeth.2011.08.018
8. Dahm, L., Ott, C., Steiner, J., Stepniak, B., Teegen, B., Saschenbrecker, S., et al. (2014). Seroprevalence of autoantibodies against brain antigens in health and disease. *Ann. Neurol.* 76, 82–94. doi: 10.1002/ana.24189
9. Dale, R. C., Merheb, V., Pillai, S., Wang, D., Cantrill, L., Murphy, T. K., et al. (2012). Antibodies to surface

dopamine-2 receptor in autoimmune movement and psychiatric disorders. *Brain* 135, 3453–3468. doi: 10.1093/brain/aws256

10. Dalmau, J., Gleichman, A. J., Hughes, E. G., Rossi, J. E., Peng, X., Lai, M., et al. (2008). Anti-NMDA-receptor encephalitis: case series and analysis of the effects of antibodies. *Lancet Neurol.* 7, 1091–1098. doi: 10.1016/S1474-4422(08)70224-2
11. Dalmau, J., Lancaster, E., Martinez-Hernandez, E., Rosenfeld, M. R., and Balice-Gordon, R. (2011). Clinical experience and laboratory investigations in patients with anti-NMDAR encephalitis. *Lancet Neurol.* 10, 63–74. doi: 10.1016/S1474-4422(10)70253-2
12. Dalmau, J., Tüzün, E., Wu, H. Y., Masjuan, J., Rossi, J. E., Voloschin, A., et al. (2007). Paraneoplastic anti-N-methyl-D-aspartate receptor encephalitis associated with ovarian teratoma. *Ann. Neurol.* 61, 25–36. doi: 10.1002/ana.21050
13. De Bruijn, M. A. A. M., and Titulaer, M. J. (2016). Anti-NMDAR encephalitis and other glutamate and GABA receptor antibody encephalopathies. *Handb. Clin. Neurol.* 133, 199–217. doi: 10.1016/B978-0-444-63432-0.00012-8
14. CrossRef Full Text | Google Scholar
15. de Graaff, E., Maat, P., Hulsenboom, E., van den Berg, R., van den Bent, M., Demmers, J., et al. (2012). Identification of delta/notch-like epidermal growth factor-related receptor as the Tr antigen in paraneoplastic cerebellar degeneration. *Ann. Neurol.* 71, 815–824. doi: 10.1002/ana.23550
16. De Vidi, I., Boursier, G., Delouche, N., Portalès, P., Cadars, E., Bouthier, M., et al. (2011). Strategy for anti-aquaporin-4 auto-antibody identification and quantification using a new cell-based assay. *Clin. Immunol.* 138, 239–246. doi: 10.1016/j.clim.2010.11.012
17. Dörr, J. M., Scheidelaar, S., Koorengevel, M. C., Dominguez, J. J., Schäfer, M., van Walree, C. A., et al. (2016). The styrene-maleic acid copolymer: a versatile tool in membrane research. *Eur. Biophys. J.* 45, 3–21. doi: 10.1007/s00249-015-1093-y
18. Florance, N. R., Davis, R. L., Lam, C., Szperka, C., Zhou, L., Ahmad, S., et al. (2009). Anti-N-methyl-D-aspartate receptor (NMDAR) encephalitis in children and adolescents. *Ann. Neurol.* 66, 11–18. doi: 10.1002/ana.21756
19. Graus, F., Dalmau, J., Valldeoriola, F., Ferrer, I., Reñe, R., Marin, C., et al. (1997). Immunological characterization of a neuronal antibody (anti-Tr) associated with paraneoplastic cerebellar degeneration and Hodgkin's disease. *J. Neuroimmunol.* 74, 55–61. doi: 10.1016/s0165-5728(96)00205-6
20. Greene, M., Lai, Y., Baella, N., Dalmau, J., and Lancaster, E. (2014). Antibodies to Delta/notch-like epidermal growth factor-related receptor in patients with anti-Tr, paraneoplastic cerebellar degeneration and Hodgkin lymphoma. *JAMA Neurol.* 71, 1003–1008. doi: 10.1001/jamaneurol.2014.999
21. Gresa-Arribas, N., Titulaer, M. J., Torrents, A., Aguilar, E., McCracken, L., Leypoldt, F., et al. (2014). Antibody titres at diagnosis and during follow-up of anti-NMDA receptor encephalitis: a retrospective study. *Lancet Neurol.* 13, 167–177. doi: 10.1016/S1474-4422(13)70282-5
22. Hammer, C., Stepniak, B., Schneider, A., Papiol, S., Tantra, M., Begemann, M., et al. (2014). Neuropsychiatric disease relevance of circulating anti-NMDA receptor autoantibodies depends on blood-brain barrier integrity. *Mol. Psychiatry* 19, 1143–1149. doi: 10.1038/mp.2013.110
23. Helbig, A. O., Heck, A. J., and Slijper, M. (2010). Exploring the membrane proteome—challenges and analytical strategies. *J. Proteomics* 73, 868–878. doi: 10.1016/j.jprot.2010.01.005
24. Höftberger, R. (2015). Neuroimmunology: an expanding frontier in autoimmunity. *Front. Immunol.* 6:206. doi: 10.3389/fimmu.2015.00206
25. Höftberger, R., Titulaer, M. J., Sabater, L., Dome, B., Rózsás, A., Hegedus, B., et al. (2013). Encephalitis and GABAB receptor antibodies: novel findings in a new case series of 20 patients. *Neurology* 81, 1500–1506. doi: 10.1212/WNL.0b013e3182a9585f
26. Höftberger, R., van Sonderen, A., Leypoldt, F., Houghton, D., Geschwind, M., Gelfand, J., et al. (2015). Encephalitis and AMPA receptor antibodies: novel findings in a case series of 22 patients. *Neurology* 84, 2403–2412. doi: 10.1212/WNL.0000000000001682
27. Hufton, S. E., Moerkerk, P. T., Meulemans, E. V., de Bruïne, A., Arends, J. W., and Hoogenboom, H. R. (1999). Phage display of cDNA repertoires: the pVI display system and its applications for the selection of immunogenic ligands. *J. Immunol. Methods* 231, 39–51. doi: 10.1016/s0022-1759(99)00139-8
28. Hughes, E. G., Peng, X., Gleichman, A. J., Lai, M., Zhou, L., Tsou, R., et al. (2010). Cellular and synaptic mechanisms of anti-NMDA receptor encephalitis. *J. Neurosci.* 30, 5866–5875. doi: 10.1523/JNEUROSCI.0167-10.2010
29. Iorio, R., Damato, V., Mirabella, M., Vita, M. G., Hulsenboom, E., Plantone, D., et al. (2013). Cerebellar degeneration associated with mGluR1 autoantibodies as a paraneoplastic manifestation of prostate adenocarcinoma. *J. Neuroimmunol.* 263, 155–158. doi: 10.1016/j.jneuroim.2013.07.015
30. Irani, S. R., Alexander, S., Waters, P., Kleopa, K. A., Pettingill, P., Zuliani, L., et al. (2010a). Antibodies to Kv1 potassium channel-complex proteins leucine-rich, glioma inactivated 1 protein and contactin-associated protein-2 in limbic encephalitis, Morvan's syndrome and acquired neuromyotonia. *Brain* 133, 2734–2748. doi: 10.1093/brain/awq213
31. Irani, S. R., Bera, K., Waters, P., Zuliani, L., Maxwell, S., Zandi, M. S., et al. (2010b). N-methyl-D-aspartate antibody encephalitis: temporal progression of clinical and paraclinical observations in a predominantly non-paraneoplastic disorder of both sexes. *Brain* 133, 1655–1667. doi: 10.1093/brain/awq113
32. Irani, S. R., Pettingill, P., Kleopa, K. A., Schiza, N., Waters, P., Mazia, C., et al. (2012). Morvan syndrome:

clinical and serological observations in 29 cases. *Ann. Neurol.* 72, 241–255. doi: 10.1002/ana.23577

33. Jeffery, O. J., Lennon, V. A., Pittock, S. J., Gregory, J. K., Britton, J. W., and McKeon, A. (2013). GABAB receptor autoantibody frequency in service serologic evaluation. *Neurology* 81, 882–887. doi: 10.1212/WNL.0b013e3182a35271

34. Kayser, M. S., Titulaer, M. J., Gresa-Arribas, N., and Dalmau, J. (2013). Frequency and characteristics of isolated psychiatric episodes in anti-N-methyl-d-aspartate receptor encephalitis. *JAMA Neurol.* 70, 1133–1139. doi: 10.1001/jamaneurol.2013.3216

35. Lai, M., Hughes, E. G., Peng, X., Zhou, L., Gleichman, A. J., Shu, H., et al. (2009). AMPA receptor antibodies in limbic encephalitis alter synaptic receptor location. *Ann. Neurol.* 65, 424–434. doi: 10.1002/ana.21589

36. Lai, M., Huijbers, M. G., Lancaster, E., Graus, F., Bataller, L., Balice-Gordon, R., et al. (2010). Investigation of LGI1 as the antigen in limbic encephalitis previously attributed to potassium channels: a case series. *Lancet Neurol.* 9, 776–785. doi: 10.1016/S1474-4422(10)70137-X

37. Lancaster, E., Huijbers, M. G., Bar, V., Boronat, A., Wong, A., Martinez-Hernandez, E., et al. (2011a). Investigations of caspr2, an autoantigen of encephalitis and neuromyotonia. *Ann. Neurol.* 69, 303–311. doi: 10.1002/ana.22297

38. Lancaster, E., Martinez-Hernandez, E., Titulaer, M. J., Boulos, M., Weaver, S., Antoine, J. C., et al. (2011b). Antibodies to metabotropic glutamate receptor 5 in the Ophelia syndrome. *Neurology* 77, 1698–1701. doi: 10.1212/WNL.0b013e3182364a44

39. Lancaster, E., Lai, M., Peng, X., Hughes, E., Constantinescu, R., Raizer, J., et al. (2010). Antibodies to the $GABA_B$ receptor in limbic encephalitis with seizures: case series and characterisation of the antigen. *Lancet Neurol.* 9, 67–76. doi: 10.1016/S1474-4422(09)70324-2

40. Leite, M. I., Jacob, S., Viegas, S., Cossins, J., Clover, L., Morgan, B. P., et al. (2008). IgG1 antibodies to acetylcholine receptors in 'seronegative' myasthenia gravis. *Brain* 131, 1940–1952. doi: 10.1093/brain/awn092

41. Lopez-Chiriboga, A. S., Komorowski, L., Kümpfel, T., Probst, C., Hinson, S. R., Pittock, S. J., et al. (2016). Metabotropic glutamate receptor type 1 autoimmunity: clinical features and treatment outcomes. *Neurology* 86, 1009–1013. doi: 10.1212/WNL.0000000000002476

42. Martinez-Hernandez, E., Ariño, H., McKeon, A., Iizuka, T., Titulaer, M. J., Simabukuro, M. M., et al. (2016). Clinical and immunologic investigations in patients with stiff-person spectrum disorder. *JAMA Neurol.* doi: 10.1001/jamaneurol.2016.0133 [Epub ahead of print].

43. Martinez-Hernandez, E., Sepulveda, M., Rostásy, K., Höftberger, R., Graus, F., Harvey, R. J., et al. (2015). Antibodies to aquaporin 4, myelin-oligodendrocyte glycoprotein and the glycine receptor α1 subunit in patients with isolated optic neuritis. *JAMA Neurol.* 72, 187–193. doi: 10.1001/jamaneurol.2014.3602

44. Masdeu, J. C., González-Pinto, A., Matute, C., Ruiz De Azúa, S., Palomino, A., De Leon, J., et al. (2012). Serum IgG antibodies against the NR1 subunit of the NMDA receptor not detected in schizophrenia. *Am. J. Psychiatry* 169, 1120–1121. doi: 10.1176/appi.ajp.2012.12050646

45. Mikasova, L., De Rossi, P., Bouchet, D., Georges, F., Rogemond, V., Didelot, A., et al. (2012). Disrupted surface cross-talk between NMDA and Ephrin-B2 receptors in anti-NMDA encephalitis. *Brain* 135, 1606–1621. doi: 10.1093/brain/aws092

46. Montojo, M. T., Petit-Pedrol, M., Graus, F., and Dalmau, J. (2015). Clinical spectrum and diagnostic value of antibodies against the potassium channel related protein complex. *Neurologia* 30, 295–301. doi: 10.1016/j.nrl.2013.12.007

47. Moscato, E. H., Peng, X., Jain, A., Parsons, T. D., Dalmau, J., and Balice-Gordon, R. J. (2014). Acute mechanisms underlying antibody effects in anti-N-methyl-D-aspartate receptor encephalitis. *Ann. Neurol.* 76, 108–119. doi: 10.1002/ana.24195

48. Motomura, M., Johnston, I., Lang, B., Vincent, A., and Newsom-Davis, J. (1995). An improved diagnostic assay for Lambert-Eaton myasthenic syndrome. *J. Neurol. Neurosurg. Psychiatry* 58, 85–87. doi: 10.1136/jnnp.58.1.85

49. Peng, X., Hughes, E. G., Moscato, E. H., Parsons, T. D., Dalmau, J., and Balice-Gordon, R. J. (2015). Cellular plasticity induced by anti-α-amino-3-hydroxy-5-methyl-4-isoxazolepropionic acid (AMPA) receptor encephalitis antibodies. *Ann. Neurol.* 77, 381–398. doi: 10.1002/ana.24293

50. Peränen, J., Rikkonen, M., and Kääriäinen, L. (1993). A method for exposing hidden antigenic sites in paraformaldehyde-fixed cultured cells, applied to initially unreactive antibodies. *J. Histochem. Cytochem.* 41, 447–454. doi: 10.1177/41.3.8429208

51. Petit-Pedrol, M., Armangue, T., Peng, X., Bataller, L., Cellucci, T., Davis, R., et al. (2014). Encephalitis with refractory seizures, status epilepticus and antibodies to the GABAA receptor: a case series, characterisation of the antigen and analysis of the effects of antibodies. *Lancet Neurol.* 13, 276–286. doi: 10.1016/S1474-4422(13)70299-0

52. Piepgras, J., Höltje, M., Michel, K., Li, Q., Otto, C., Drenckhahn, C., et al. (2015). Anti-DPPX encephalitis: pathogenic effects of antibodies on gut and brain neurons. *Neurology* 85, 890–897. doi: 10.1212/WNL.0000000000001907

53. Privé, G. G. (2007). Detergents for the stabilization and crystallization of membrane proteins. *Methods* 41, 388–397. doi: 10.1016/j.ymeth.2007.01.007

54. Probst, C., Komorowski, L., de Graaff, E., van Coevorden-Hameete, M., Rogemond, V., Honnorat, J., et al. (2015). Standardized test for anti-Tr/DNER in patients with paraneoplastic cerebellar degeneration. *Neurol. Neuroimmunol. Neuroinflamm.* 2:e68. doi: 10.1212/NXI.0000000000000068

55. Probst, C., Saschenbrecker, S., Stoecker, W., and Komorowski, L. (2014). Anti-neuronal autoantibodies: current diagnostic challenges. *Mult. Scler. Relat.*

Disord. 3, 303–320. doi: 10.1016/j.msard.2013.12.001

56. Ramberger, M., Peschl, P., Schanda, K., Irschick, R., Hüftberger, R., Deisenhammer, F., et al. (2015). Comparison of diagnostic accuracy of microscopy and flow cytometry in evaluating N-methyl-D-aspartate receptor antibodies in serum using a live cell-based assay. *PLoS One*10:e0122037. doi: 10.1371/journal.pone.0122037
57. Sabater, L., Gaig, C., Gelpi, E., Bataller, L., Lewerenz, J., Torres-Vega, E., et al. (2014). A novel non-rapid-eye movement and rapid-eye-movement parasomnia with sleep breathing disorder associated with antibodies to IgLON5: a case series, characterisation of the antigen and post-mortem study. *Lancet Neurol.* 13, 575–586. doi: 10.1016/S1474-4422(14)70051-1
58. Sillevis Smitt, P., Grefkens, J., de Leeuw, B., van den Bent, M., van Putten, W., Hooijkaas, H., et al. (2002). Survival and outcome in 73 anti-Hu positive patients with paraneoplastic encephalomyelitis/sensory neuronopathy. *J. Neurol.* 249, 745–753. doi: 10.1007/s00415-002-0706-4
59. Sillevis Smitt, P., Kinoshita, A., De Leeuw, B., Moll, W., Coesmans, M., Jaarsma, D., et al. (2000). Paraneoplastic cerebellar ataxia due to autoantibodies against a glutamate receptor. *N. Engl. J. Med.* 342, 21–27. doi: 10.1056/nejm200001063420104
60. Steiner, J., Walter, M., Glanz, W., Sarnyai, Z., Bernstein, H. G., Vielhaber, S., et al. (2013). Increased prevalence of diverse N-methyl-D-aspartate glutamate receptor antibodies in patients with an initial diagnosis of schizophrenia: specific relevance of IgG NR1a antibodies for distinction from N-methyl-D-aspartate glutamate receptor encephalitis. *JAMA Psychiatry* 70, 271–278. doi: 10.1001/2013.jamapsychiatry.86
61. Tobin, W. O., Lennon, V. A., Komorowski, L., Probst, C., Clardy, S. L., Aksamit, A. J., et al. (2014). DPPX potassium channel antibody: frequency, clinical accompaniments and outcomes in 20 patients. *Neurology* 83, 1797–1803. doi: 10.1212/WNL.0000000000000991
62. van Coevorden-Hameete, M. H., de Graaff, E., Titulaer, M. J., Hoogenraad, C. C., and Sillevis Smitt, P. A. (2014). Molecular and cellular mechanisms underlying anti-neuronal antibody mediated disorders of the central nervous system. *Autoimmun. Rev.* 13, 299–312. doi: 10.1016/j.autrev.2013.10.016
63. van Mierlo, H. C., van Coevorden-Hameete, M. H., Munting, L. P., de Graaff, E., and de Witte, L. (2015). No evidence for the presence of neuronal surface autoantibodies in plasma of patients with schizophrenia. *Eur. Coll. Neuropsychopharmacol.* 25, 2326–2332. doi: 10.1016/j.euroneuro.2015.09.017
64. van Sonderen, A., Arino, H., Petit-Pedrol, M., Leypold, F. K., P Wandinger, K. P., Lancaster, E., et al. (2016a). The clinical spectrum of Caspr2-antibody associated disease. *Neurology* 86:S12.008.
65. van Sonderen, A., Schreurs, M. W., de Bruijn, M. A., Boukhrissi, S., Nagtzaam, M. M., Hulsenboom, E. S., et al. (2016b). The relevance of VGKC positivity in the absence of LGI1 and Caspr2 antibodies. *Neurology* 86, 1692–1699. doi: 10.1212/WNL.0000000000002637
66. van Sonderen, A., Thijs, R. D., Coenders, E. C., Jiskoot, L. C., Sanchez, E., de Bruijn, M. A. A. M., et al. (2016c). Anti-LGI1 encephalitis: clinical syndrome and long-term follow-up. *Neurology.*
67. Willison, H. J., Ang, W., Gilhus, N. E., Graus, F., Liblau, R., Vedeler, C., et al. (2000). EFNS task force report: a questionnaire-based survey on the service provision and quality assurance for determination of diagnostic autoantibody tests in European neuroimmunology centres. *Eur. J. Neurol.*7, 625–628. doi: 10.1046/j.1468-1331.2000.00158.x
68. Zandi, M. S., Irani, S. R., Lang, B., Waters, P., Jones, P. B., McKenna, P., et al. (2011). Disease-relevant autoantibodies in first episode schizophrenia. *J. Neurol.* 258, 686–688. doi: 10.1007/s00415-010-5788-9

CHAPTER 9

DIFFERENTIATION OF HUMAN PLURIPOTENT STEM CELLS INTO NEPHRON PROGENITOR CELLS IN A SERUM AND FEEDER FREE SYSTEM

Minyong Kang, Yong-Mahn Han

INTRODUCTION

The kidneys have crucial regulatory roles in the body, including control of fluid-electrolyte, acid-base and blood pressure, and the excretion of waste products. Kidneys rarely recover functions following irreversible damages [1], [2]. Like other common chronic diseases such as diabetes and hypertension that are associated with modern lifestyle, the prevalence of kidney disease is increasing worldwide [3]. Chronic kidney diseases that preserve the residual kidney function deteriorate into irreversible end-stage renal disease (ESRD) [4], [5]. Treatment options of ESRD are limited to dialysis or renal transplantation [6]. Because complications of long-term dialysis and shortage of donated organs are unsolved problems to the ESRD patients, chronic kidney disease is best treated properly before it progresses into ESRD [3]. Despite recent progress in renal medicine, recovery and de novo regeneration of kidneys are elusive [7]. Stem cell therapy is emerging as one of the new approaches for replenishing damaged renal tissues in the field of regenerative medicine [2], [8]–[11]. Based on the normal renal developmental steps, metanephros is the final step of nephrogenesis during gestation [12]–[14]. It consists of two structures derived from intermediate mesoderm, the ureteric bud (UB) and metanephric mesenchyme (MM) [14], [15]. While UB gives rise to non-nephron tissues such as collecting ducts and ureters, MM turns into all segments of nephrons and renal interstitium [13], [16]. Thus, MM cells are considered renal progenitor cells, cap mesenchymal cells (nephron progenitor) and metanephric stromal cells (stromal progenitor) [14]. To obtain nephron progenitor cells (NPCs) that are capable of regenerating nephron-consisting cells, two approaches have been tried. First, human renal progenitor (hRPCs) cells have been isolated from diverse regions of fetal and adult kidney [17]–[22]. hRPCs yielded significant therapeutic effects in mouse models of renal failure, including reduction of BUN/Creatinine levels and replacement of destroyed epithelial cells within nephrons [20], [22], [23]. Nonetheless, there are several limitations for clinical application of hRPCs, including ethical problems in the isolation of hRPCs from human donors, low isolation efficiency and incomplete culture system for expansion of hRPCs [24]. Second, as an alternative source of NPCs, human pluripotent stem cells (hPSCs) are highly attractive because they are able to differentiate into various specialized cell types. Unfortunately, differentiation of renal lineage cells have been performed primarily in mouse ESCs [25]–[29]. In the human systems, renal lineage cells expressing several developing kidney genes were differentiated after treatments with retinoic acid, activin A and BMP7 [30]. Poximal tubule-like cells were derived from hESCs in defined culture conditions with functional characterization [31]. In addition, a robust induction of intermediate mesoderm (IM) cells from hPSCs was accomplished with phenotypic characterization [32]. However, these cells were not kidney progenitor cells which have more therapeutic potential *in vivo* [21], [24]. Ureteric bud-committed kidney progenitor-like cells was recently derived from hPSCs *in vitro* and *in vivo* [33]. Nonetheless, differentiation of nephron-committed progenitor cells is needed for therapeutic usage aiming at damaged nephrons. In this study, we differentiated hPSCs into NPCs by step-wise approach in a serum- and feeder-free condition. These NPCs were able to turn into two cell types within nephrons, renal tubular epithelial-cells and glomerular podocytes *in vitro*.

Citation: Kang M, Han Y-M (2014) Differentiation of Human Pluripotent Stem Cells into Nephron Progenitor Cells in a Serum and Feeder Free System. PLoS ONE 9(4): e94888. doi:10.1371/journal.pone.0094888.

MATERIALS AND METHODS

Maintenance of Human Pluripotent Stem Cells

H9 human ES cell line (H9) and human induced pluripotent stem cell line derived from CRL-2097 fibroblasts (CRL-iPSCs) were cultured using techniques we developed in earlier research [34]. The ES medium consisted of DMEM/F12 mixed with 20% knockout serum replacement, 1% penicillin-streptomycin (PenStrep), 1% nonessential amino acids (NEAA), 2 mM L-glutamate, 0.1 mM β-mercaptoethanol and 10 ng/mL FGF2 (R&D Systems, Minneapolis, MN). All of these materials, except for the FGF2, were purchased from Invitrogen (Carlsbad, CA). Every five days, colonies of H9 and CRL-iPSCs were mechanically sliced into small pieces, detached from the culture dish after treatment with 10 mg/ml collagenase IV (Gibco, Carlsbad, CA), and then transferred on fresh MEF to maintain the pluripotency. For all experiments, hPSCs were used between passages 40 and 60 in this study.

Derivation of Nephron Progenitor Cells (NPCs) from hPSCs

We differentiated hPSCs into NPCs via a series of differentiations into stage-specific cell types of pluripotent, primitive streak (PS), intermediate mesoderm (IM) and NPCs. First, undifferentiated hESCs and hiPSCs were re-plated on Matrigel (1:40 dilution, BD Biosciences, Bedford, MA) coated 4-well culture dishes and cultured in mTeSR medium (Stemcell Technologies, Vancouver, BC, Canada) supplemented with 10 ng/ml FGF2 for four days under the feeder-free system. To induce PS cells derived from hPSCs, we modified the initial step of cardiomyocyte differentiation protocol previously described [35]. hPSCs were cultured in the basal differentiation serum-free media (RPMI-1640 medium containing 2% B27, 2 mM L-glutamine, 1% PenStrep) supplemented with both 100 ng/ml Activin A and 100 ng/ml Wnt3a (R&D Systems) for one day. For the next two days, hESCs were treated with 20 ng/ml BMP4 (Peprotech, Rocky Hill, NJ) and 10 ng/ml FGF2 while hiPSCs were treated with 20 ng/ml BMP4 and 10 ng/ml FGF2. For intermediate mesoderm induction from primitive streak, BMP4 was replaced with 50 ng/ml BMP7 (Peprotech) in the same basal medium supplemented with both 10 μM retinoic acid (RA; R&D Systems) and 10 ng/ml FGF2. In particular, hESCs were treated for six days while hiPSCs were treated for eight days with RA, BMP7 and FGF2 at this stage. In a final step for NPCs derivation, hPSC-derived IM cells were cultured in the medium supplemented with 150 ng/ml BMP7 and 50 ng/ml FGF2 without RA for 15 days. During differentiation into NPCs, basal culture medium was refreshed every two days.

Differentiation of NPCs into Renal Epithelial Cells Consisting of Nephrons

hPSC-derived NPCs were re-plated on fibronectin-coated dishes and stabilized in the same differentiation medium containing BMP7 (150 ng/ml) and FGF2 (50 ng/ml) for one day. They were incubated in renal epithelial cell growth medium (REGM™; Lonza, Allendale, NJ) supplemented with 50 ng/ml HGF (Peprotech) to develop into renal tubular epithelial cells (RTECs) for 21 days. For differentiation into glomerular podocytes, NPCs were cultured in VRAD medium, which consisted of DMEM/F12, 100 nM Vitamin D3 (Sigma-Aldrich, Saint Louis, Missouri), 100 μM RA and 10% FBS for seven days as previously described [19]. The medium was changed every two days during terminal differentiation.

In vitro Tubulogenic Assay

For *in vitro* tubulogenic assay, hPSCs-derived NPCs were detached from culture dishes after treatment with Acutase (Innovative Cell Technologies, San Diego, CA) for ten minutes. Cells were filtered with 40 μm-filter mesh and centrifuged at 300×g for three minutes. Cell pellets were suspended in the renal epithelial cell growth medium (REGM™) at a concentration of 2×10^5 cells/ml. The cell suspension was mixed with an equal volume of 200 μl collagen type I (BD biosciences) on ice for three-dimensional culture. After incubating collagen type I-cell mixtures on a 4-well dish at 37°C for 30 minutes for solidification of this mixture, 500 μl of REGM™ supplemented with 50 ng/ml HGF was gently added on the gels. Gels of collagen type I-cell mixtures were cultured in the REGM™ for 21 days. During cell culturing, the medium was changed every two days.

RNA Isolation and Real-time RT PCR

Total RNA was extracted from hESCs and their derivatives using TRIzol (Invitrogen), followed by treatment with DNase I (Invitrogen). Total RNA (1 μg) was used to synthesize cDNA using Moloney murine leukemia virus (M-MLV) reverse transcriptase (Enzynomics, Seoul, Korea) with oligonucleotides (oligo-dT). To analyze the transcriptional expression of stage-specific genes, quantitative real time RT-PCR (q-PCR) was conducted on Bio-Rad CFX manager (Bio-Rad Laboratories, Hercules, CA) with SyberGreen. The reaction used the following protocol: 95 °C for 10 minutes followed by 40 cycles of 95 °C for 15 seconds (denaturation), 60 °C for 15 seconds (annealing) and 72 °C for 30 seconds (synthesis). Primers of target genes were designed by primer design tools in PubMed (http://www.ncbi.nlm.nih.gov/tools/primer-blast) and were adjusted at a final concentration of 0.5 pmole. All reactions were duplicated to exclude technical errors. For relative quantification, the expression level of target genes was normalized to that of glyceraldehyde-3-phosphate dehydrogenase (GAPDH) gene. Differences between the samples and the control were analyzed using the formula $_{\Delta\Delta}$Ct. Relative expression of target genes was indicated as fold-changes compared with the control. All experiments for evaluating transcriptional expression by q-PCR were repeated three times for biological replication. Primers used in this study are summarized in Table S1.

Immunocytochemistry

Samples were washed with PBS and fixed with 4% formaldehyde (Sigma-Aldrich) for 20 minutes at room temperature (RT). After washing three times with PBS containing 0.1% Tween 20 (PBST), 0.3% Triton X-100 (Sigma-Aldrich) was used to permeabilize the cell membrane. After washing three times with PBST, samples were blocked with 5% donkey serum (Jackson ImmunoResearch Laboratories, West Grove, PA) for one hour at RT and then incubated with primary antibodies at 4 °C overnight. After rinsing three times with PBST, samples were incubated with secondary antibody (donkey anti-mouse IgG-, donkey anti-goat IgG-, and donkey anti-rabbit IgG-Alexa 488 or 594; Invitrogen) for one hour. After washing six times with PBST, samples were mounted in VECTASHIELD Mounting Medium containing DAPI for five minutes. Immunolocalized cells were observed on a fluorescence microscope or Zeiss LSM 510 confocal microscope. Notably, following a previous report's methods [33], quantification of the number of cells expressing the key markers of specific differentiation stage was performed by manual counting in three randomly chosen fields. Primary antibodies used in this study are described in Table S2.

RESULTS

To establish optimal conditions for differentiation into NPCs, hPSCs were differentiated into stage-specific cell types of pluripotent, primitive streak (PS), intermediate mesoderm (IM) and nephron progenitor cells (NPCs) by treating with different combinations of growth factors. A schematic diagram and stage-specific marker genes during the entire differentiation phases are in Figure 1A. Detailed procedures for differentiation of NPCs and its bidirectional derivatives are in Figure 1B.

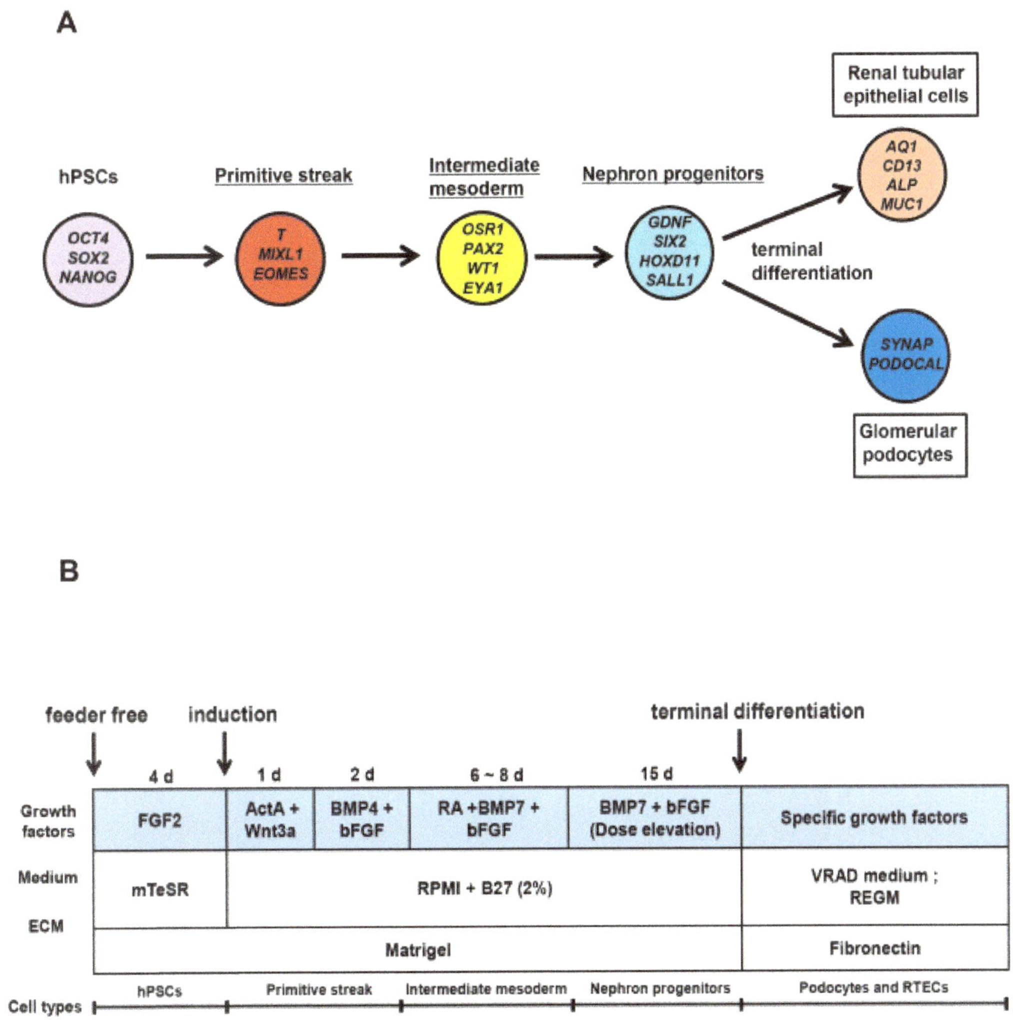

Figure 1: Overall protocol for differentiation of human pluripotent stem cells (hPSCs) into nephron progenitor cells (NPCs).

A. Illustration of developmental stage-specific marker genes during differentiation of NPCs and NPC-derived fully differentiated renal epithelial cells. B. Detailed procedures for hPSCs differentiation into NPCs and its derivatives.

Induction of hPSCs into Primitive Streak Cells

The initial stage of our protocol aimed at differentiating hPSCs toward PS population is based upon a reported method [35]. To determine optimal conditions for induction of hESCs to primitive streak cells, hESCs were incubated in medium supplemented with BMP4 and FGF2 (BF) for several days after treatments with Activin A and Wnt3a (AW) for one day. Transcriptional expression of *T* was enhanced at day 2 after addition of BMP4 and FGF2 (Figure 2A-a). Consecutive treatments with AW/BF showed higher transcription levels of PS genes such as *T*, *MIXL1*, and *EOMES* than treatments with two factors alone (AW or BF) (Figure 2A-b). However, AW/BF treatment did not up-regulate the transcription of other lineage marker genes such as *SOX17*, *FOXA2* (endoderm) and *PAX6*, *SOX1* (ectoderm) in hESCs-derivatives (Figure 2B-a, b). Immunostaining showed that consecutive treatments with AW/BF induced the expression of mesendodermal marker T and reduced the expression of pluripotent marker TRA1-81 and OCT4 in hESC-derived PS cells compared to undifferentiated hESCs (Figure 2C).

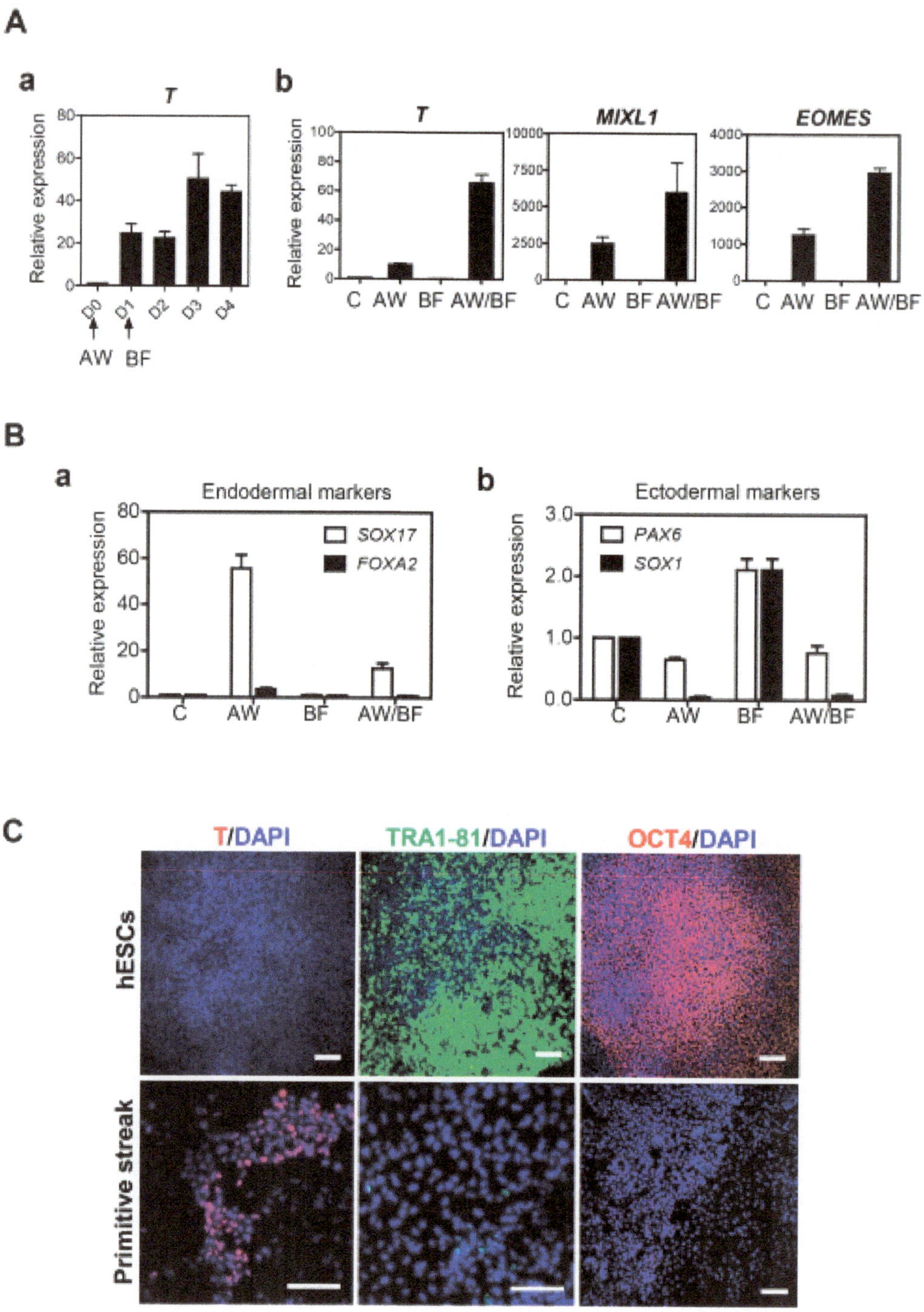

Figure 2: Induction of hESCs into primitive streak (PS) cells.

A. (a) Optimal duration for PS induction was determined by transcription level of *T* compared with undifferentiated hESCs before treatments. Relative gene expression was normalized to GAPDH, and the values of fold-changes are represented by mean ± S.E.M (n=3). (b) Comparison of expression levels of PS specific genes by combinatorial treatments with exogenous factors of Activin A, Wnt3a (AW) and BMP4, FGF2 (BF), in hESC-derived PS cells. Untreated samples were designated as (C). Relative transcriptional levels were normalized to GAPDH, and the bars show mean ± S.E.M (n=3). B. (a) Determination of heterogeneity with other germ layers such as definitive endoderm (DE) and ectoderm by evaluating transcriptional expression of (a) DE and (b) ectoderm marker genes in hESC-derived PS cells. C. Immunofluorescence of T (red), TRA1-81 (green), and OCT4 (red) expression in the cells of induction day 0 (undifferentiated hESCs) and day 3 (primitive streak). Scale bars=200 μm.

In hiPSCs, transcriptional expression of T was activated at day 3 after treatments with AW/BF (Figure S1A-a). In the same culture condition, the expression of T was enhanced while the expression of TRA1-81 was remarkably reduced in immunocytochemistry (Figure S1A-b). Higher concentration of BMP4 (50 ng/ml) was required to activate transcription of PS marker genes, but did not induce the transcriptional expression of endoderm and ectodermal genes (Figure S1A-c, d).

Specification of Intermediate Mesoderm from PS Cells

Intermediate mesoderm (IM) specified from PS stage is the most important step toward renal lineage differentiation [14]. Initially, the expression level of *OSR1*, a key upstream molecule in the renal development [15], was analyzed during IM cells differentiation. When hESC-derived PS cells were cultured in the basal medium supplemented with retinoic acid (RA), BMP7 (B7) and FGF2 (F2) for several days, the transcriptional level of *OSR1* was enhanced at day 6 after the treatment (Figure 3A-a). Combined treatment with RAB7F2 was more effective on transcriptional activation of *OSR1* than other treatment groups (Figure 3A-b). Of note, RA treatment resulted in the transcriptional activation of *OSR1* gene in a dose-dependent manner when comparing three different concentrations of RA, 0.1, 1, and 10 μM (Figure 3A-c). While hESC-derived PS cells did not express OSR1 (Figure 3B-a), the proportion of OSR1-positive cells was approximately 35% in hESC-derived IM cells in immunocytochemistry (Figure 3B-b). Other IM marker genes such as *PAX2*, *SALL1* and *EYA1* were detected at the transcription levels (Figure 3C). Interestingly, hESC-derived IM cells did not express *WT1* when compared to human fetal kidney (HFK) (Figure 3C-b). Expression of PAX2 and SALL1 were also detected in hESC-derived IM cells in immunocytochemistry (Figure 3D-a, b).

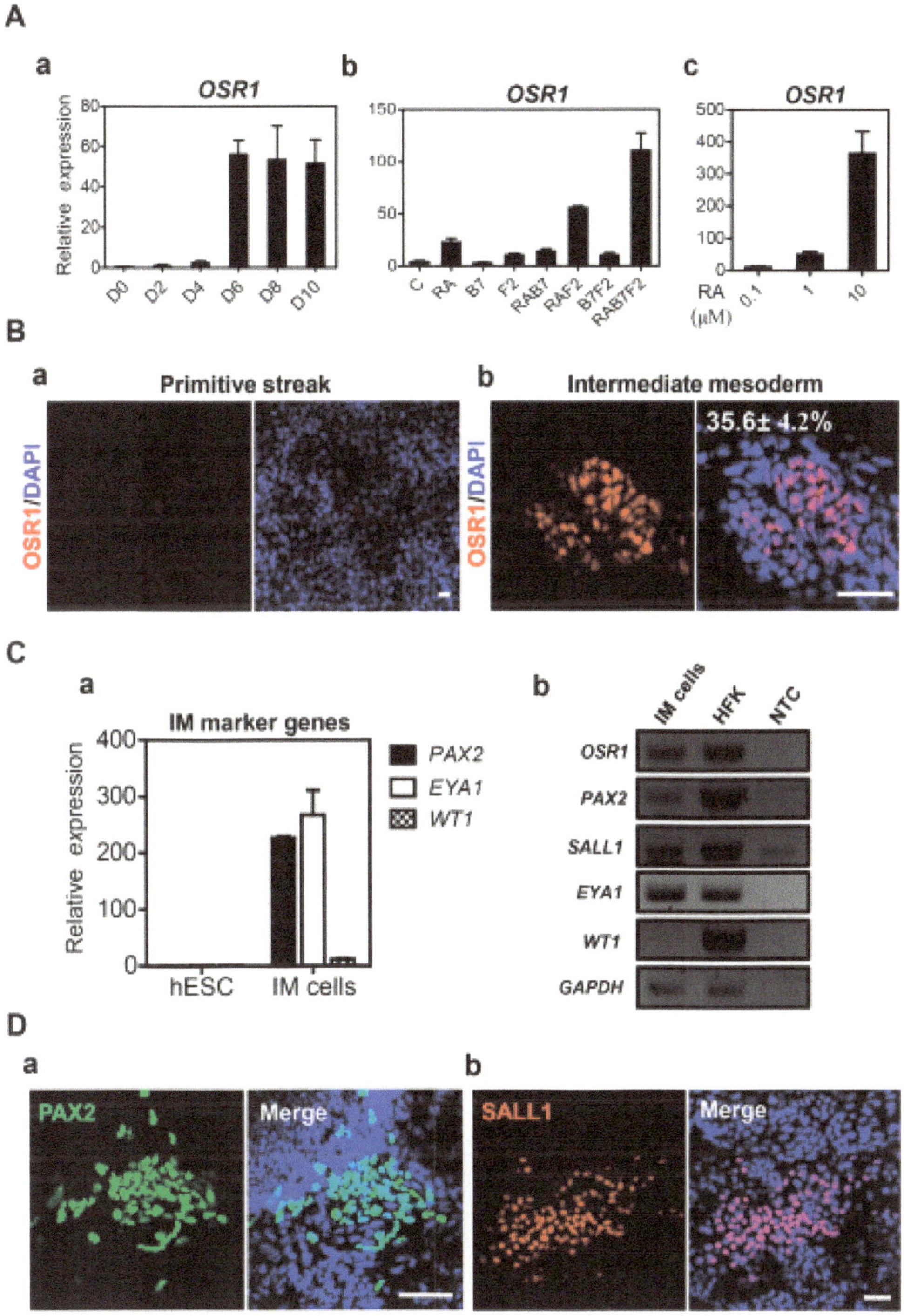

Figure 3: Specification of intermediate mesoderm (IM) from the hESC-derived PS cells.

A. (a) Optimal timing for IM induction was determined by transcriptional expression level of *OSR1*, comparing with expression values of undifferentiated hESCs, in hESC-derived cells. Relative gene expression was normalized to GAPDH, and the values of fold-changes are represented by mean ± S.E.M (n=3). (b) Comparison of *OSR1* transcripts by combinatorial treatments with exogenous growth factors of retinoic acid (RA), BMP7 (B7) and FGF2 (F2). Untreated samples were designated as (C). Transcriptional expression levels were normalized to GAPDH, and results of fold-change are indicated as mean ± S.E.M (n=3). (c) Comparison of *OSR1* transcription levels by the concentration of RA treatment, including 0.1, 1 and 10 μM. Relative gene expression was normalized to GAPDH. The values of fold-changes are represented by mean ± S.E.M (n=3). B. Immunocytochemistry for representative expression of OSR1 (red) in (a) hESC-derived PS and (b) IM cells. Quantification of the number of cells expressing the key markers of specific differentiation stage was performed by manual counting in three randomly chosen fields. Scale bars=50 μm. C. Transcriptional expression of various IM marker genes were evaluated by (a) real time RT-PCR and (b) RT-PCR in hESC-derived IM cells. Human fetal kidney (HFK) cDNA was used as positive control. Relative transcriptional levels were normalized to GAPDH, and the bars show mean ± S.E.M (n=3). D. Immunostaining of PAX2 (green) and SALL1 (red) at the end of IM induction in hESC-derivatives. Scale bars=100 μm.

In hiPSCs, transcriptional expression of *OSR1* was enhanced at day 8 after treatments with RAB7F2 (Figure S1B-a). Similar to hESCs, RA treatment effectively activated *OSR1* gene expression in a dose dependent manner (Figure S1B-b). Other IM marker gene *PAX2* was also transcriptionally activated in hiPSC-derived IM cells (Figure S1B-c). Immunocytochemistry showed remarkable expressions of IM markers, including OSR1, PAX2, and SALL1 in hiPSC-derived IM cells (Figure S1B-d). Of note, approximately 25% of cells were positive for OSR1 after IM induction (Figure S1B-d).

Differentiation of IM cells into NPCs and its Characterization

For derivation of NPCs, IM cells were cultured in the basal medium containing high doses of BMP7 (150 ng/ml) and FGF2 (50 ng/ml) without RA. Transcripts of a key NPC marker gene *SIX2* was gradually up-regulated after day 3 of high doses BMP7/F2 treatments in hESC-derivatives (Figure 4A-a). Transcriptional expressions of other marker genes such as *GDNF*, *HOXD11* and *WT1* in addition to *CITED1*, *OSR1*, *PAX2*, *SALL1* and *EYA1* were enhanced in hESC-derived NPCs (Figure 4A-b, c). Immunocytochemistry showed that approximately 38% of SIX2-positive cells were obtained in hESC-derivatives after NPCs induction (Figure 4B). Other NPCs markers PAX2, SALL1 and WT1 were also markedly detected in hESC-derived NPCs (Figure 4C). PAX2 and SALL1 were co-expressed with SIX2 in hESC-derived NPCs (Figure 4D-a, b). Notably, WT1-expressing cells were appeared at day 6 of NPCs induction and the proportion of these cells increased in a time-dependent manner (Figure 4E).

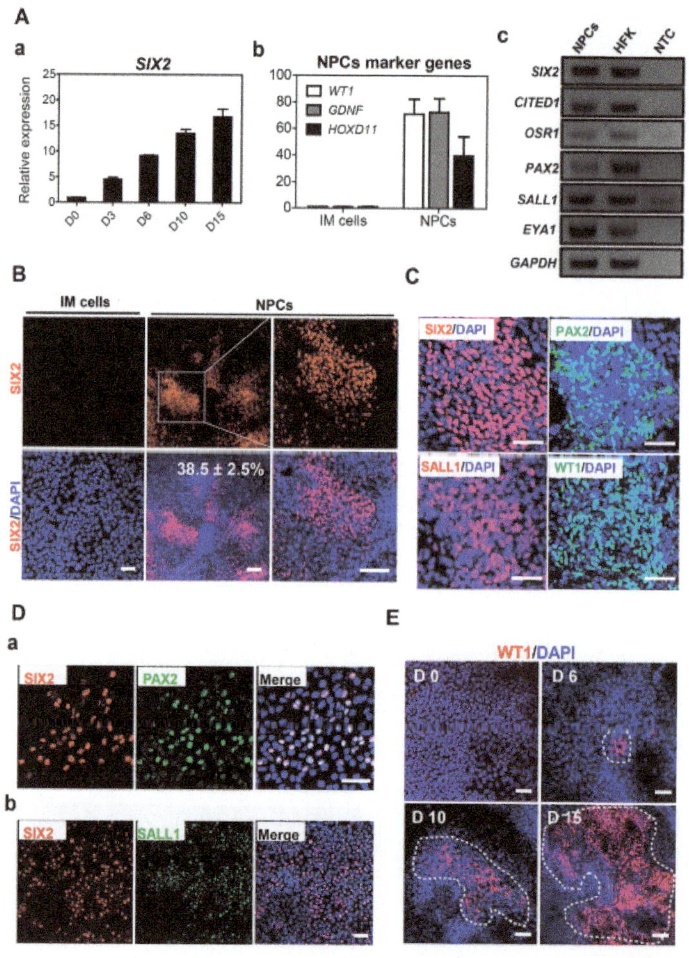

Figure 4: Differentiation of hESC-derived IM cells into NPCs.

A. (a) Time course of the transcriptional expression of key NPCs marker *SIX2* in hESC-derived NPCs. Appropriate duration of NPCs induction was determined by relatively higher transcriptional expression of *SIX2* than other days. Transcription of other NPCs marker genes were examined by (b) real time RT-PCR and (c) RT-PCR in hESC-derived NPCs. Human fetal kidney (HFK) cDNA was used as positive control. Relative transcriptional levels were normalized to GAPDH, and the bars show mean ± S.E.M (n=3). B. SIX2 expression rate was compared between hESC-derived IM cells and NPCs. Quantification of the number of cells expressing the key markers of specific differentiation stage was performed by manual counting in three randomly chosen fields. Scale bars=200 μm. C. Several NPCs markers, including SIX2 (red), PAX2 (green), SALL1 (red) and WT1 (green) were notably detected in hESC-derived NPCs. Scale bars=100 μm. D. Co-expression of other NPCs markers such as PAX2 (green) and SALL1 (green) with SIX2 (red) in hESC-derived NPCs in immunofluorescence. Scale bars=100 μm. E. Immunocytochemistry for WT1 expression during NPCs induction in hESC-derivatives. WT1 expression (red) was evaluated at four different time points of NPCs induction (D0, D6, D10 and D15 of NPCs induction after IM stage). WT1-positive regions are designated by white lines. Scale bars=100 μm.

To determine whether hESC-derived NPCs primed into other lineages cells, we evaluated marker genes expression of common derivatives from three lineages in transcription levels. Transcripts of several marker genes of other lineages, including metanephric stroma/ureteric bud (*FOXD1* and *HOXB7*), bone (*RUNX2* and *COL1A1*), vascular endothelium (*PECAM1* and *TIE2*), smooth muscle (*MYH11* and *CALPONIN*), liver (*ALB* and *AAT*), and neuron (*TUJ1* and *MAP2*) were not detectable in hESC-derived NPCs (Figure 5). These results indicate that our differentiation protocol is suitable to induce NPCs without contamination with other lineages cells derived from definitive endoderm, mesoderm and ectoderm.

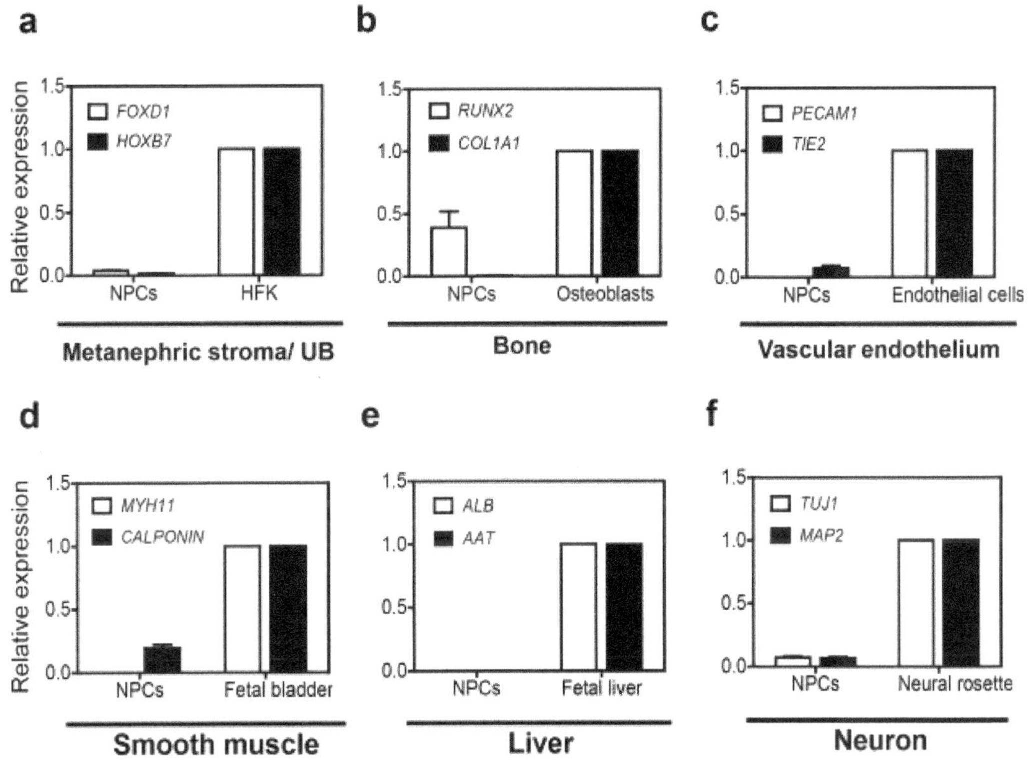

Figure 5: Evaluation of transcriptional activation of other inducible lineages markers in hESC-derived NPCs.

Transcriptional expression of (a) *FOXD1* and *HOXB11* (metanephric stroma/ureteric bud), (b) bone (*RUNX2* and *COL1A1*), (c) vascular endothelium (*PECAM1* and *TIE2*), (d) smooth muscle (*MYOSIN11* and *CALPONIN*), (e) liver (*ALB* and *AAT*), and (f) neuron (*TUJ1* and *MAP2*) were analyzed by q-PCR in hESC-derived NPCs. Relative expression values were normalized to GAPDH, and fold-changes are shown by mean ± S.E.M (n=3).

Similar to hESCs, several NPC-markers such as SIX2, PAX2, SALL1 and WT1 were notably expressed in hiPSC-derivatives (Figure S1C). The proportion of SIX2-positive cells was approximately 30% in hiPSC-derivatives (Figure S1C-b). Co-expression of PAX2 and SIX2 were also observed in these NPCs (Figure S1C-c).

Differentiation Potential of hPSC-derived NPCs toward Renal Tubular Cells and Glomerular Podocytes

In defined culture condition following previously reported protocols [19], hPSC-derived NPCs were able to differentiate into renal tubular epithelial cell (RTECs) and glomerular podocytes. After RTEC induction for 21 days, hESC-derivatives expressed E-CADHERIN, ZO1 and KRT18 (Figure 6A), representing mesenchymal-epithelial transition (MET). NPCs also formed tube-like structures in three dimensional culture condition (Figure 6B). Tube-like structures were stained with an epithelium-specific maker KRT18 as well as F-actin representing apicobasal polarization of RTECs within tubular structures (Figure 6B). These RTECs showed transcriptional activation of RTEC marker genes, *SLC12A3*, *CD13* and *AQP1*, whereas un-induced NPCs did not express these genes (Figure 6C). Additionally, RTECs expressed makers of proximal (ALP, AQP1 and CD13) and distal tubular cells (MUC1), while un-induced NPCs did not express RTEC markers in immunocytochemistry (Figure 6D). After podocytes induction, hESC-derivatives expressed podocyte-specific genes *SYN* and *NEPHRIN* in transcription levels (Figure 6E) as well as SYN and PDXL in protein levels, compared to un-induced NPCs (Figure 6F). Of note, these cells showed aborized morphology on high magnification view (Figure 6F). In addition, approximately 70% of SYN-expressing cells were obtained in hESC-derivatives after podocytes induction.

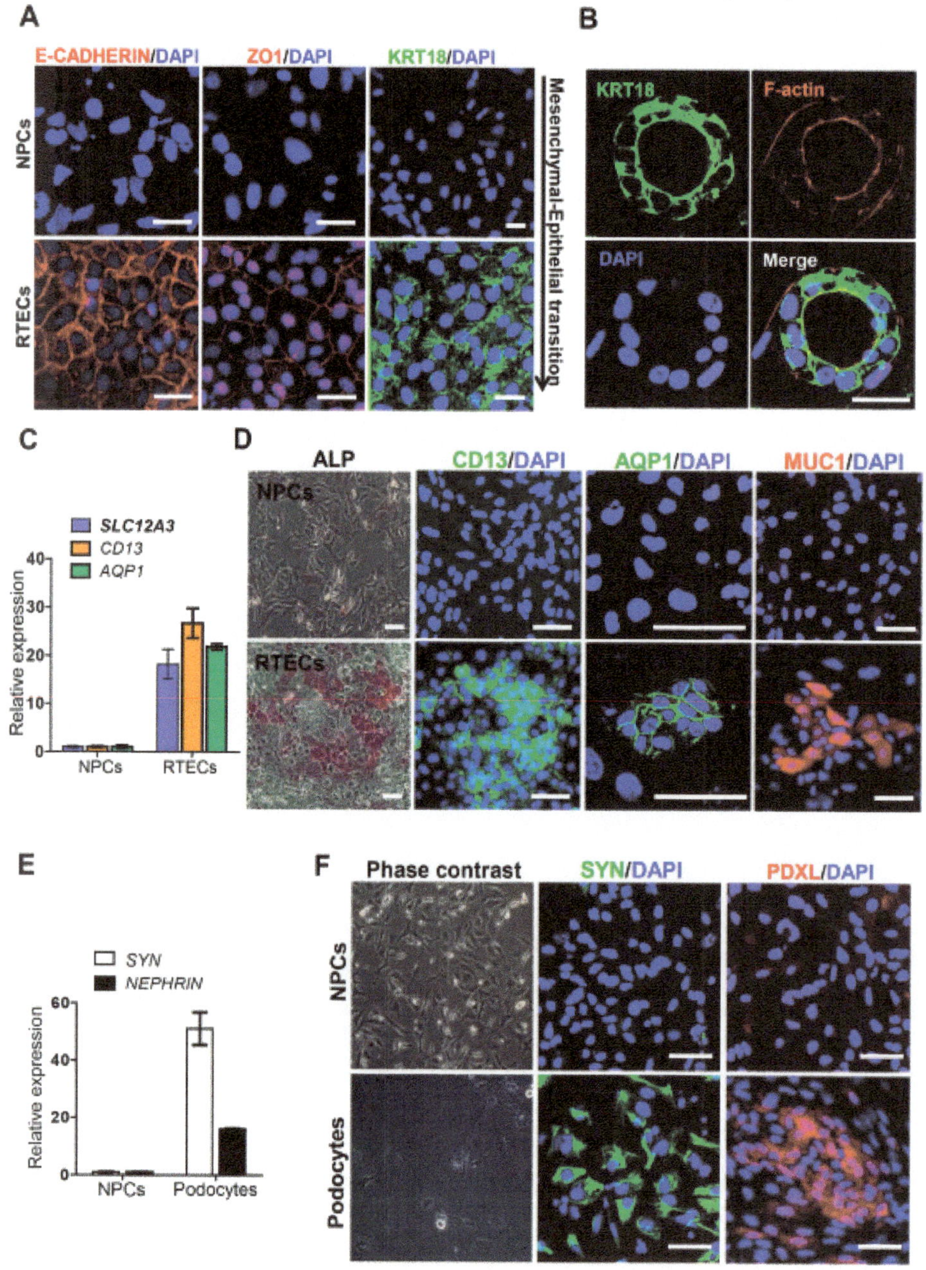

Figure 6: Differentiation potential of hESC-derived NPCs into fully differentiated cells within nephrons.

A. Expression of epithelial markers such as E-CADHERIN, ZO1 and KRT18 in hESC-derived renal tubular epithelial cells (RTECs) compared with un-induced NPCs in immunocytochemistry, representing mesenchymal-epithelial transition. Scale bars=50 μm. B. *In vitro* tubulogenesis of hESC-derived NPCs, cultured as three dimensional system mixed with collagen type I in renal epithelial cells growth medium (REGM™) for 21 days, which were analyzed by immunofluorescence with an epithelial marker KRT18 (green) and F-actin (red) for showing apicobasal polarization of RTECs in tubular structures. Scale bars=50 μm. C. Transcriptional expression of RTEC-specific genes (*SLC12A3*, *CD13* and *AQP1*) was examined by real time RT-PCR. Relative expression levels were normalized to GAPDH, and the bars show mean ± S.E.M (n=3). D. Expression of proximal renal tubular markers (ALP, alkaline phosphatase; AQP1, aquaporin1; CD13) and distal renal tubular marker MUC1 in hESC-derived RTECs compared with un-induced NPCs in immunocytochemistry. Scale bars=100 μm. E. Transcriptional expression of podocyte-specific genes (*SYN* and *NEPHRIN*) was evaluated by real time RT-PCR. Relative expression levels were normalized to GAPDH, and the bars show mean ± S.E.M (n=3). F. Phase contrast image and immunocytochemistry of podocyte-specific markers such as SYN (green) and PDXL (red) in hESC-derived glomerular podocytes compared with un-induced NPCs. Scale bars=100 μm.

In hiPSCs, markers of MET (E-CADHERIN, ZO1 and KRT18) and RTECs (ALP, CD13 and AQP1) were observed after 21 days of RTEC induction in immunocytochemistry (Figure S2A and S2B). These NPCs formed KRT18-positive tubule-like structures with apicobasal polarization in three dimensional cultures (Figure S2C). In addition, hiPSC-derivatives expressed podocyte-specific markers SYN and PDXL after podocytes induction (Figure S2D). Similar to hESCs, the proportion of SYN-positive cells was about at 70% in hiPSC-derivatives.

DISCUSSION

In contrast to other solid organs, kidneys consist of more than 10 specialized cell types in complex organization as functional units [11]. Thus, establishment of multipotent nephron progenitor cells (NPCs) is the most appropriate strategy to regenerate damaged renal cells within nephrons because progenitor cells can give rise to any cell types after administration into damaged tissues [9], [10], [21], [36]. Unfortunately, differentiation protocols of hPSCs into renal lineage-progenitor cells remain undefined. To our knowledge, this is the first report describing *in vitro* differentiation of hPSCs into NPCs in a chemically defined serum- and feeder-free system via developmental stage-dependent manner.

In normal kidney developmental processes, metanephric mesenchyme (MM) contain a population of renal progenitor cells expressing specific transcription factors, including *SIX2*, *SALL1*, *CITED1*, *GDNF* and *HOXD11* analogues in addition to *OSR1*, *PAX2*, *EYA1*, *WT1* that continuously appear following the IM stage [12], [16], [24], [37]. Because mutations of these genes resulted in failure of proper nephrogenesis [38]–[42], the expression of these transcription factors is critical for efficient induction of NPCs from hPSCs in our protocol. Interestingly, although WT1 is initially expressed in IM stage and persistently expressed during MM induction as a key transcription factor for *in vivo* nephrogenesis [43], [44], WT1 did not appear at the end of IM induction in this study. Instead, transcriptional activation of *WT1* and the proportion of WT1-positive cells in immunocytochemistry were increased after NPCs induction. These results indicate that there are temporal differences in the expression pattern of WT1 during renal lineage differentiation between *in vitro* and *in vivo*.

To differentiate hPSCs into NPCs through the consecutive developmental stages of PS and IM, different combinations of growth factors were optimized in this study. BMP7 is a transcription factor for IM and metanephric mesenchymal (MM) specification from the early stage of mesoderm [37]. Thus, BMP7 was used as a key exogenous factor during induction of IM cells from PS. We believe that RA is also needed for IM differentiation because it is secreted from the paraxial mesoderm and acts as an important signaling factor for specification of primitive streak into IM [25], [27], [30], [45], [46]. In contrast to the recent study suggesting that retinoic acid (RA) is not needed to induce OSR1-expressing IM cells [32], RA addition was highly effective in inducing IM in a dose dependent manner in this study. There are several factors that may lead to these different outcomes. First, Mae *et al.* used a low concentration of RA (0.1 μM), whereas we used a higher concentration of RA (10 μM) that was more effective on IM induction compared to 0.1 and 1 μM RA. Second, they used a different growth factors combination (100 ng/ml BMP7+3 μM CHIR99021+0.1 μM RA) from that which we used (150 ng/ml BMP7+10 ng/ml FGF2+10 μM RA) during IM induction. Finally, they used cell lines (a hiPSC line, 253G1; a hESC line, khES3) different from that which we used (a hiPSC line, CRL-2097; a hESC line, H9). We presume that these differences contribute to the differing the effect of RA on IM induction from hPSCs.

For NPCs induction, high doses of BMP7 (150 ng/ml) and FGF2 (50 ng/ml) were added for the specification of NPCs from IM cells because ureteric bud-secreting factors BMP7 and FGF2 have been known as the most important signaling factors to proliferate and sustain self-renewal potential of renal progenitor cells in MM [12], [16]. Notably, hiPSCs showed relatively lower efficiency of IM and NPCs differentiation compared to hESCs. These discrepancy may be attributed to epigenetic memory and alteration of iPSCs, making some iPSCs more resistant to exogenous signaling cues for differentiation into specific lineages [47].

There are several limitations in this study. First, our results showed only about 35% induction efficiency for SIX2-positive NPCs. However, a specific isolation of NPCs population with higher efficiency will be needed when considering clinical applications. To achieve this, we can examine the effects of many other growth factors on hPSC differentiation into NPCs by using high-throughput screening system and finding optimal combinations of NPC-inducing factors. Alternatively, we can identify the ideal markers to recover hPSC-derived NPCs to improve their purity. Second, we conducted only *in vitro* experiments that do not fully recapitulate *in vivo*conditions. To reduce the unknown hazards from implanted cells, *ex vivo* and *in vivo*experiments are needed to confirm that hPSC-derived NPCs can integrate into kidney structures without serious problems such as teratoma formation. In addition, evaluating the clinical efficacy of hPSC-derived NPCs will require *in vivo* renal failure models. Such additional experiments offer the potential of expanding knowledge in the field of regenerative medicine.

CONCLUSIONS

In summary, we differentiated hPSCs into NPCs that were further specified into RTECs and podocytes in a serum- and feeder-free system. This protocol can be useful for generating alternative sources of cell therapy as well as *in vitro* platform for the investigation of human kidney diseases at the molecular and cellular levels.

Supporting Information

Figure S1 Induction of hiPSCs into NPCs. A. Induction of PS cells. (a) Optimal timing of transcriptional expression of *T* during PS cells induction from hiPSCs by AW/BF serial treatments. Undifferentiated hiPSCs were used as control. Relative gene expression was normalized to GAPDH and fold-change values are represented by mean ± S.E.M (n=3). (b) Immunostaining of T (red) and TRA1-81 (green) expression in hiPSC-derived PS cells. Scale bars=200 μm. Comparison of transcriptional activation of (c) PS marker genes and (d) other lineage markers, including *SOX17* (definitive endoderm) and *PAX6* (ectoderm), between different concentrations of BMP4 (0, 20 and 50 ng/ml). B. Specification of IM cells. (a) Appropriate time point of IM-induction was determined by transcriptional activation levels of *OSR1* in hiPSC-derivatives. Relative gene expression was normalized to GAPDH, and fold-changes are represented by mean ± S.E.M (n=3), compared with expression values of undifferentiated hiPSCs. (b) Comparison of *OSR1* expression levels by concentration of retinoic acid (RA) treatment, including 0.1, 1 and 10 μM in hiPSC-derived cells. Untreated samples were used as control. Relative gene expression was normalized to GAPDH. The values of fold-changes are shown by mean ± S.E.M (n=3). (c) Transcriptional expression of several IM marker genes such as *OSR1* and *PAX2* were evaluated by real time RT-PCR in hiPSCs-derived IM cells. No factors indicate un-treated control. Relative gene expression was normalized to GAPDH, and fold-changes are represented by represented by mean ± S.E.M (n=3). (d) Immunocytochemistry for the expression of key IM markers, including OSR1 (red), PAX2 (green) and SALL1 (red) in hiPSC-derived IM cells. Scale bars=100 μm. C. Immunocytochemistry analysis for SIX2 expression in (a) hiPSC-derived IM cells and (b) NPCs. Quantification of the number of cells expressing the key markers of specific differentiation stage was performed by manual counting in three randomly chosen fields. Scale bars=100 μm. (c) Immunocytochemistry of other NPCs markers such as PAX2 (green), SALL1 (red) and WT1 (green). Scale bars=100 μm.

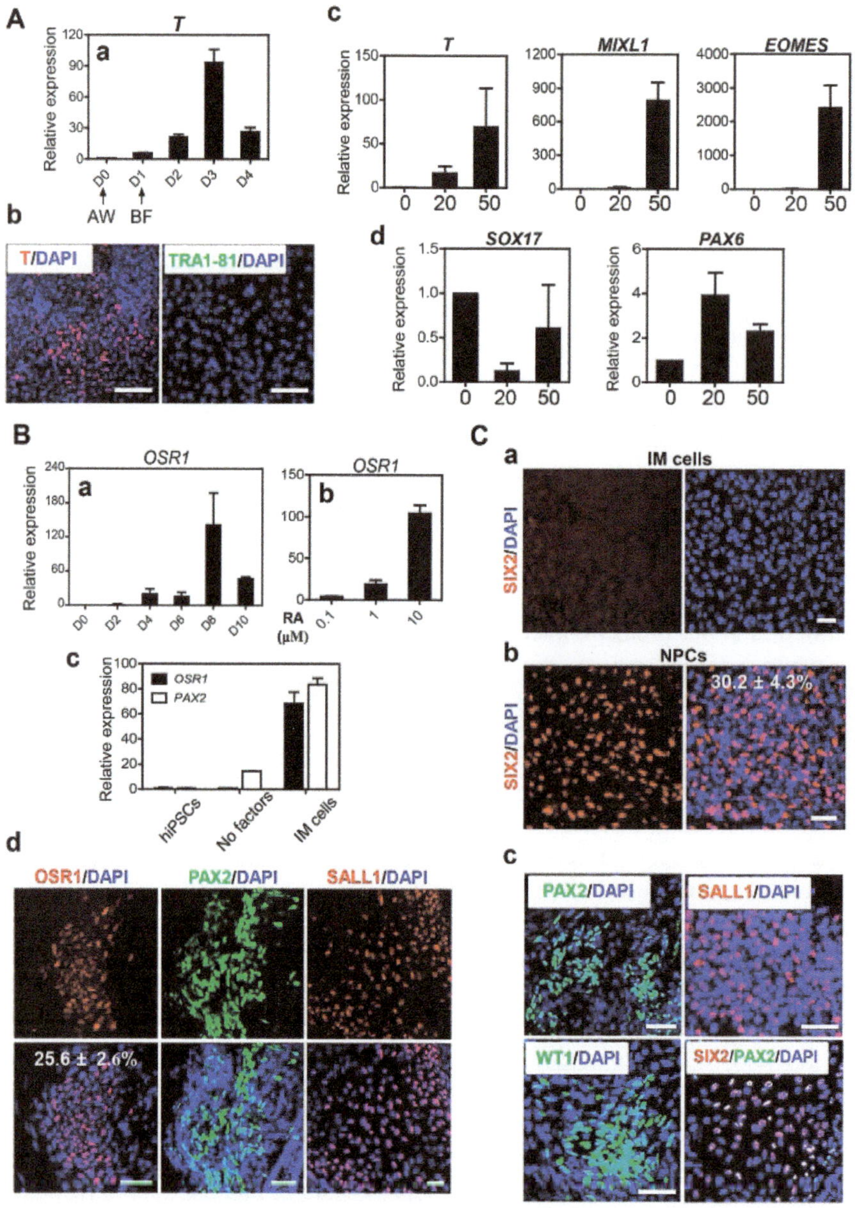

Figure S2. Differentiation of hiPSC-derived NPCs into fully differentiated nephron-consisting cells. A. Evaluation of epithelial markers expression, including E-CADHERIN, ZO1 and KRT18 in hiPSC-derived RTECs by immunocytochemistry, indicating mesenchymal-epithelial transition. Scale bars=50 μm. B. Expression of proximal renal tubular markers (ALP, AQP1 and CD13) and distal renal tubular marker MUC1 in hiPSC-derived RTECs in immunocytochemistry. Scale bars=100 μm. C. Immunocytochemistry for KRT18 (green) and F-actin (red) of 3D tubule-like structures formed by culturing hiPSC-derived NPCs with collagen type I-cells mixtures in REGM™ for 21 days. Scale bars=50 μm. D. Expression of glomerular podocyte-specific markers such as SYN (green) and PDXL (red) in hiPSC-derived glomerular podocytes in immunofluorescence. Scale bars=100 μm.

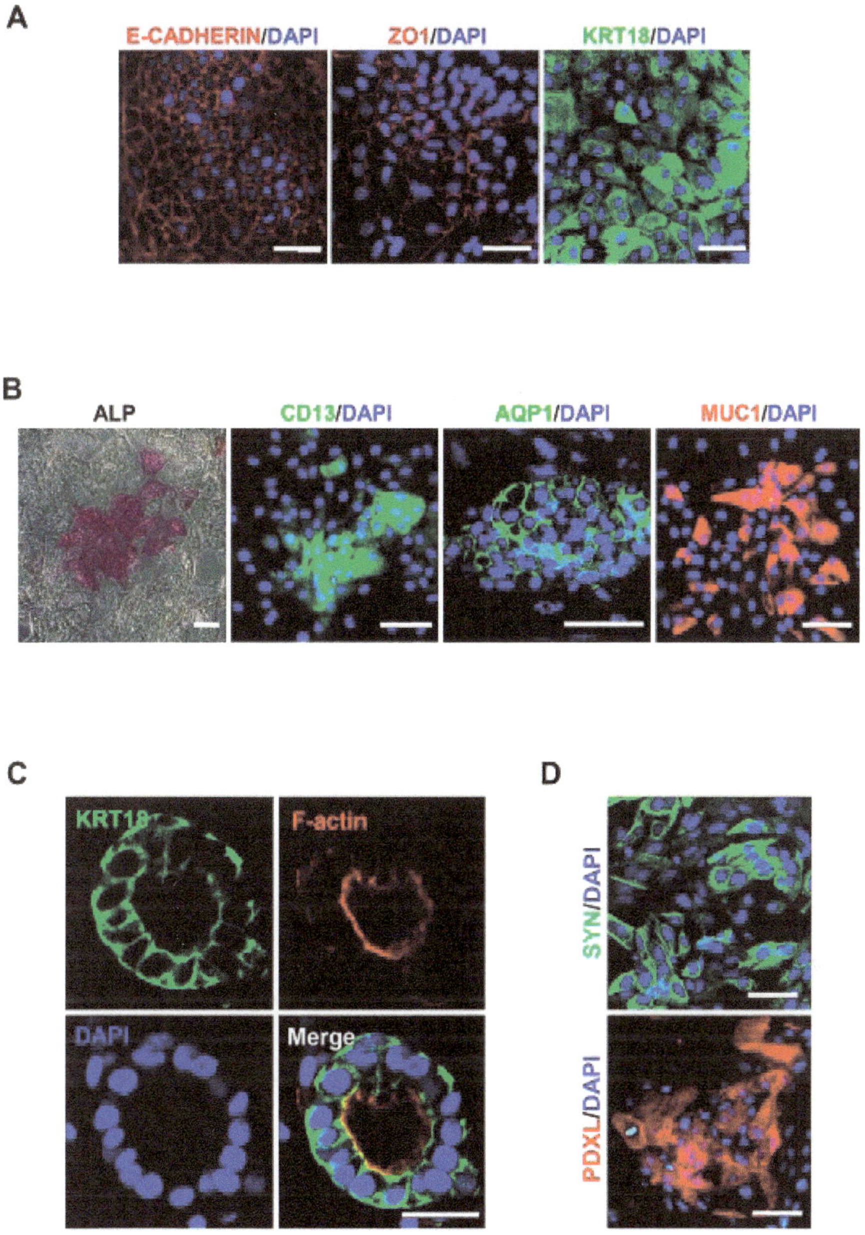

Table S1 The information of real time and RT-PCR primers.

Gene	Accession number	Forward sequence	Reverse sequence	Product size (bp)
GAPDH	NM_001256799.1	ctt cgc tct ctg ctc ctc ct	gtt aaa agc agc cct ggt ga	152
T	NM_031944	cag tgg cag tct cag gtt aag aag ga	cgc tac tgc agg tgt gag caa	122
MIXL1	NM_003181	tcc agg atc cag gta tgg tt	cgt ttc agt tcc agg agc ac	123
EOMES	NM_005442	atg ctg aag agt ata gta aag aca	aac acc acc aag tcc atc	128
SOX17	NM_031439	aaa gac cca ggg tac cta aa	agg aag aca aat tct cac agc ag	255
FOXA2	NM_021784	ctg agc gag atc tac cag tgg a	agt cgt tga agg aga gcg agt	103
PAX6	NM_000280.3	agc cca gta taa gcg gga gt	cta gcc agg ttg cga aga ac	135
SOX1	NM_005986.2	cac aac tcg gag atc agc aa	ggt act tgt aat ccg ggt gc	133
OSR1	NM_145260	cgg aga gtg agt gga gag	tga agc aga tac agg gat tac a	122
PAX2	NM_003987	acg ccc att aaa gca cag	tta cag aga aag agc caa caa a	149
SALL1	NM_002968	agc gaa gcc tca aca ttt cca atc c	aat tca aag aac tcg gca cag cac c	147
EYA1	NM_000503	gat gtc aag tgt cag taa gga t	aag tga ggt ggt agg aga g	133
WT1	NM_000378	tgt gtg ttg tgt tgt gtt t	tgt caa aga gca aat cat tat ca	105
SIX2	NM_016932	ctt gcc acc gtt cat tct	gga cca gga cac aga gta	103
GDNF	NM_000514	caa gaa gca gca gtt acc a	gag cag aaa gga cag aga ag	89
HOXD11	NM_021192.2	tgg aac gcg agt ttt tct tt	ctg cag acg gtc tct gtt ca	149
CITED1	NM_001144886	gct gct aat gcc aag tgt	gcc cgt ctc ttt gta agt aac	90
FOXD1	NM_004472.2	tgc ggg tcc ctc tat tta tg	taa cgc ctg gac ctg aga at	190
HOXB7	NM_004502.3	gtg gac tgt ggg tct gga ct	gaa cac gcg agt ggt agg tt	114
SCL12A3	NM_000339.2	gga ctt tgt ggg cac ctt	ggc atc ctc tgc ttg tgg	84
CD13	NM_001150.2	atc tct tac gca cat cag g	tcc agt tct ctt cgt cgt a	90
AQP1	NM_198098.2	cct cct ggc tat tga cta ca	ggt tgc tga agt tgt gtg t	86
SYN	NM_007286.5	agc cca agg tga ccc cga at	ccc tgt cac gag gtg ctg gc	162
NEPHRIN	NM_004646.3	tgg tct aca gcc ttc tac a	ctt tgt cag cca gtc cac	80
RUNX2	NM_001024630.3	gac agc ccc aac ttc ctg t	ccg gag ctc agc aga ata at	159
COL1A1	XM_005257059.1	act tgc ttg aag acc cat gc	ggt gtt tga gca ttg cct tt	196
PECAM1	NM_000517	tgc gaa tcg atc agt gga	acc ggg gct atc acc ttc	209
TIE2	XM_005251563.1	cct tag tga cat tct tcc	gca aaa atg tcc acc tgg	243
MYH11	NM_002474.2	cag ttc gaa agg gat ctc ca	gta gct gct tga tgg ctt cc	220
CALPONIN	NM_001299	agg ctc cgt gaa gaa gat ca	cca cgt tca cct tgt ttc ct	215
ALBUMIN	NM_000477	tgc aca gaa tcc ttg gtg aa	ttc acg agc tca aca agt gc	173
AAT	NM_000295	gaa gtc aag gac acc gag ga	gct ggc aga cct tct gtc tt	261
TUJ1	NM_006086.3	ggg cct ttg gac atc tct tc	cct ccg tgt agt gac cct tg	90
MAP2	XM_005246567.1	gtg gcg gac gtg tga aaa ttg ag	ctg gat ctg cct ggg gac tgt g	205

Table S2 The information of primary antibodies used for immunostaining.

Antibody	Host	Dilution factor	Industry
T	Goat	1:200	R&D Systems
TRA1-81	Mouse	1:100	Millipore
OSR1	Rabbit	1:40	Sigma-Aldrich
PAX2	Rabbit	1:200	Abcam
SALL1	Rabbit	1:400	Abcam
WT1	Rabbit	1:200	Abcam
SIX2	Mouse	1:200	Abnova
E-CADHERIN	Mouse	1:50	BD Pharmingen
ZO1	Rabbit	1:400	Millipore
KRT18	Mouse	1:200	Abcam
CD13	Rabbit	1:200	Abcam
AQP1	Rabbit	1:300	Abcam
MUC1	Mouse	1:200	Abcam
SYNAPTOPODIN	Mouse	1:200	PROGEN Biotechnik
PODOCALYXIN (TRA1-60)	Mouse	1:100	Millipore

Table S3 Abbreviations used in this study.

Abbreviation	Description
hPSCs	Human pluripotent stem cells
hESCs	Human embryonic stem cells
hiPSCs	Human induced pluripotent stem cells
PS	Primitive streak
DE	Definitive endoderm
IM	Intermediate mesoderm
NPCs	Nephron progenitor cells
MM	Metanephric mesenchyme
RTECs	Renal tubular epithelial cells
SYNAPTOPODIN	SYN
PODOCALYXIN	PDXL
AW	Activin and Wnt3a
BF	BMP4 and FGF2
RA	Retinoic acid
B7	BMP7
F2	FGF2
REGM™	Renal epithelial cells growth medium

ACKNOWLEDGMENTS

We appreciate Ms. Sora Oh and Ms. Younghee Ju for maintenance of human pluripotent stem cells, Mr. Dongkyu Kim for generation of human induced pluripotent stem cells derived from CRL-2097 fibroblasts.

REFERENCES

1. Hopkins C, Li J, Rae F, Little MH (2009) Stem cell options for kidney disease. J Pathol 217: 265–281. doi: 10.1002/path.2477
2. Brodie JC, Humes HD (2005) Stem cell approaches for the treatment of renal failure. Pharmacol Rev 57: 299–313. doi: 10.1124/pr.57.3.3
3. Stenvinkel P (2010) Chronic kidney disease: a public health priority and harbinger of premature cardiovascular disease. J Intern Med 268: 456–467. doi: 10.1111/j.1365-2796.2010.02269.x
4. Coresh J, Selvin E, Stevens LA, Manzi J, Kusek JW, et al. (2007) Prevalence of chronic kidney disease in the United States. JAMA 298: 2038–2047. doi: 10.1001/jama.298.17.2038
5. Keith DS, Nichols GA, Gullion CM, Brown JB, Smith DH (2004) Longitudinal follow-up and outcomes among a population with chronic kidney disease in a large managed care organization. Arch Intern Med 164: 659–663. doi: 10.1001/archinte.164.6.659
6. Grassmann A, Gioberge S, Moeller S, Brown G (2005) ESRD patients in 2004: global overview of patient numbers, treatment modalities and associated trends. Nephrol Dial Transplant 20: 2587–2593. doi: 10.1093/ndt/gfi159
7. Benigni A, Morigi M, Remuzzi G (2010) Kidney regeneration. Lancet 375: 1310–1317. doi: 10.1016/s0140-6736(10)60237-1
8. Yokoo T, Kawamura T, Kobayashi E (2008) Kidney organogenesis and regeneration: a new era in the treatment of chronic renal failure? Clin Exp Nephrol 12: 326–331. doi: 10.1007/s10157-008-0062-5
9. Yokoo T, Fukui A, Matsumoto K, Okabe M (2008) Stem cells and kidney organogenesis. Front Biosci 13: 2814–2832. doi: 10.2741/2888
10. Harari-Steinberg O, Pleniceanu O, Dekel B (2011) Selecting the optimal cell for kidney regeneration: fetal, adult or reprogrammed stem cells. Organogenesis 7: 123–134. doi: 10.4161/org.7.2.15783
11. Yokote S, Yokoo T (2013) Organogenesis for kidney regeneration. Curr Opin Organ Transplant 18: 186–190. doi: 10.1097/mot.0b013e32835f070d
12. Davies JA (2002) Morphogenesis of the metanephric kidney. ScientificWorldJournal 2: 1937–1950. doi: 10.1100/tsw.2002.854
13. Faa G, Gerosa C, Fanni D, Monga G, Zaffanello M, et al. (2012) Morphogenesis and molecular mechanisms involved in human kidney development. Journal of Cellular Physiology 227: 1257–1268. doi: 10.1002/jcp.22985
14. Little MH, McMahon AP (2012) Mammalian kidney development: principles, progress, and projections. Cold Spring Harb Perspect Biol 4..
15. Dressler GR (2006) The cellular basis of kidney development. Annu Rev Cell Dev Biol 22: 509–529. doi: 10.1146/annurev.cellbio.22.010305.104340
16. Michos O (2009) Kidney development: from ureteric bud formation to branching morphogenesis. Curr Opin Genet Dev 19: 484–490. doi: 10.1016/j.gde.2009.09.003
17. Bussolati B, Bruno S, Grange C, Buttiglieri S, Deregibus MC, et al. (2005) Isolation of renal progenitor cells from adult human kidney. Am J Pathol 166: 545–555. doi: 10.1016/s0002-9440(10)62276-6
18. Sagrinati C, Netti GS, Mazzinghi B, Lazzeri E, Liotta F, et al. (2006) Isolation and characterization of multipotent progenitor cells from the Bowman's capsule of adult human kidneys. J Am Soc Nephrol 17: 2443–2456. doi: 10.1681/asn.2006010089
19. Ronconi E, Sagrinati C, Angelotti ML, Lazzeri E, Mazzinghi B, et al. (2009) Regeneration of glomerular podocytes by human renal progenitors. J Am Soc Nephrol 20: 322–332. doi: 10.1681/asn.2008070709
20. Lindgren D, Bostrom AK, Nilsson K, Hansson J, Sjolund J, et al. (2011) Isolation and characterization of progenitor-like cells from human renal proximal tubules. Am J Pathol 178: 828–837. doi: 10.1016/j.ajpath.2010.10.026
21. Romagnani P, Lasagni L, Remuzzi G (2013) Renal progenitors: an evolutionary conserved strategy for kidney regeneration. Nat Rev Nephrol 9: 137–146. doi: 10.1038/nrneph.2012.290
22. Harari-Steinberg O, Metsuyanim S, Omer D, Gnatek Y, Gershon R, et al. (2013) Identification of human nephron progenitors capable of generation of kidney structures and functional repair of chronic renal disease. EMBO Mol Med 5: 1556–1568. doi: 10.1002/emmm.201201584
23. Lazzeri E, Crescioli C, Ronconi E, Mazzinghi B, Sagrinati C, et al. (2007) Regenerative potential of embryonic renal multipotent progenitors in acute renal failure. J Am Soc Nephrol 18: 3128–3138. doi: 10.1681/asn.2007020210
24. Pleniceanu O, Harari-Steinberg O, Dekel B (2010) Concise review: Kidney stem/progenitor cells: differentiate, sort out, or reprogram? Stem Cells 28: 1649–1660. doi: 10.1002/stem.486
25. Kim D, Dressler GR (2005) Nephrogenic factors promote differentiation of mouse embryonic stem cells into renal epithelia. J Am Soc Nephrol 16: 3527–3534. doi: 10.1681/asn.2005050544
26. Morizane R, Monkawa T, Itoh H (2009) Differentiation of murine embryonic stem and induced pluripotent stem cells to renal lineage in vitro. Biochem Biophys Res Commun 390: 1334–1339. doi: 10.1016/j.bbrc.2009.10.148
27. Bruce SJ, Rea RW, Steptoe AL, Busslinger M, Bertram JF, et al. (2007) In vitro differentiation of murine embryonic stem cells toward a renal lineage. Differentiation 75: 337–349. doi: 10.1111/j.1432-0436.2006.00149.x
28. Ren X, Zhang J, Gong X, Niu X, Zhang X, et al. (2010)

Differentiation of murine embryonic stem cells toward renal lineages by conditioned medium from ureteric bud cells in vitro. Acta Biochim Biophys Sin (Shanghai) 42: 464–471.

29. Nishikawa M, Yanagawa N, Kojima N, Yuri S, Hauser PV, et al. (2012) Stepwise renal lineage differentiation of mouse embryonic stem cells tracing in vivo development. Biochem Biophys Res Commun 417: 897–902. doi: 10.1016/j.bbrc.2011.12.071

30. Batchelder CA, Lee CC, Matsell DG, Yoder MC, Tarantal AF (2009) Renal ontogeny in the rhesus monkey (Macaca mulatta) and directed differentiation of human embryonic stem cells towards kidney precursors. Differentiation 78: 45–56. doi: 10.1016/j.diff.2009.05.001

31. Narayanan K, Schumacher KM, Tasnim F, Kandasamy K, Schumacher A, et al. (2013) Human embryonic stem cells differentiate into functional renal proximal tubular-like cells. Kidney Int 83: 593–603. doi: 10.1038/ki.2012.442

32. Mae S, Shono A, Shiota F, Yasuno T, Kajiwara M, et al. (2013) Monitoring and robust induction of nephrogenic intermediate mesoderm from human pluripotent stem cells. Nat Commun 4: 1367. doi: 10.1038/ncomms2378

33. Xia Y, Nivet E, Sancho-Martinez I, Gallegos T, Suzuki K, et al. (2013) Directed differentiation of human pluripotent cells to ureteric bud kidney progenitor-like cells. Nat Cell Biol 15: 1507–1515. doi: 10.1038/ncb2872

34. Park SW, Jun Koh Y, Jeon J, Cho YH, Jang MJ, et al. (2010) Efficient differentiation of human pluripotent stem cells into functional CD34+ progenitor cells by combined modulation of the MEK/ERK and BMP4 signaling pathways. Blood 116: 5762–5772. doi: 10.1182/blood-2010-04-280719

35. Paige SL, Osugi T, Afanasiev OK, Pabon L, Reinecke H, et al. (2010) Endogenous Wnt/beta-catenin signaling is required for cardiac differentiation in human embryonic stem cells. PLoS One 5: e11134. doi: 10.1371/journal.pone.0011134

36. Yokote S, Yamanaka S, Yokoo T (2012) De novo kidney regeneration with stem cells. J Biomed Biotechnol 2012: 453519. doi: 10.1155/2012/453519

37. Reidy KJ, Rosenblum ND (2009) Cell and molecular biology of kidney development. Semin Nephrol 29: 321–337. doi: 10.1016/j.semnephrol.2009.03.009

38. Dressler GR (1995) Transcription factors in renal development: the WT1 and Pax-2 story. Semin Nephrol 15: 263–271.

39. Sanyanusin P, Schimmenti LA, McNoe LA, Ward TA, Pierpont ME, et al. (1995) Mutation of the PAX2 gene in a family with optic nerve colobomas, renal anomalies and vesicoureteral reflux. Nat Genet 9: 358–364. doi: 10.1038/ng0495-358

40. Sanchez MP, Silos-Santiago I, Frisen J, He B, Lira SA, et al. (1996) Renal agenesis and the absence of enteric neurons in mice lacking GDNF. Nature 382: 70–73. doi: 10.1038/382070a0

41. Xu PX, Adams J, Peters H, Brown MC, Heaney S, et al. (1999) Eya1-deficient mice lack ears and kidneys and show abnormal apoptosis of organ primordia. Nat Genet 23: 113–117.

42. Susa K, Kita S, Iwamoto T, Yang SS, Lin SH, et al. (2012) Effect of heterozygous deletion of WNK1 on the WNK-OSR1/SPAK-NCC/NKCC1/NKCC2 signal cascade in the kidney and blood vessels. Clin Exp Nephrol 16: 530–538. doi: 10.1007/s10157-012-0590-x

43. Hsu HJ, Lin G, Chung BC (2004) Parallel early development of zebrafish interrenal glands and pronephros: differential control by wt1 and ff1b. Endocr Res 30: 803. doi: 10.1081/erc-200044044

44. Kreidberg JA (2010) WT1 and kidney progenitor cells. Organogenesis 6: 61–70. doi: 10.4161/org.6.2.11928

45. Dressler G (2002) Tubulogenesis in the developing mammalian kidney. Trends Cell Biol 12: 390–395. doi: 10.1016/s0962-8924(02)02334-6

46. Bollig F, Perner B, Besenbeck B, Kothe S, Ebert C, et al. (2009) A highly conserved retinoic acid responsive element controls wt1a expression in the zebrafish pronephros. Development 136: 2883–2892. doi: 10.1242/dev.031773

47. Bilic J, Izpisua Belmonte JC (2012) Concise review: Induced pluripotent stem cells versus embryonic stem cells: close enough or yet too far apart? Stem Cells 30: 33–41. doi: 10.1002/stem.700

CHAPTER 10

MASS SPECTROMETRY COMBINED WITH HIGH PERFORMANCE IMMUNOCHEMISTRY

Katrin Bomans, Antje Lang, Veronika Roedl, Lisa Adolf, Kyrillos Kyriosoglou, Katharina Diepold, Gabriele Eberl, Michael Mølhøj, Ulrike Strauss, Christian Schmalz, Rudolf Vogel, Dietmar Reusch, Harald Wegele, Michael Wiedmann, Patrick Bulau

INTRODUCTION

Host cell proteins (HCPs) carry potential clinical safety risks for patients treated with biologics. On the one hand, HCP might cause an immune response (due to their "non-self" nature), adjuvant activity, and theoretically also function in the human body [1–3]. Furthermore, HCPs with protease activity have the potential to impact product stability [4]. Consequently, regulatory guidelines mandate the setting of HCP specifications [5].

Thus, one key aspect of any biologics manufacturing is to reduce HCP to levels considered acceptable in the final drug [6]. The HCP composition is impacted by the proteome complexity of the utilized host expression system [7–9], the manner in which the therapeutic protein is expressed [10–13], and the purification process itself [10,12]. Moreover, all methods for analytical HCP characterization face challenges due to the dynamic range of HCP abundance at proteome and final drug level.

Several analytical techniques have been used for the detection, identification, and quantification of HCPs [1,3,14,15]. To perform bio-process and release analytics, immunoassays like protein gel blots and multicomponent generic or process-specific enzyme-linked immunosorbent assays (ELISA) are most commonly used to detect and monitor HCPs [16–18]. The ELISA technique is typically applied for HCP analysis, mostly due to the good precision of the method and also that it provides quantitative results for setting control limits and specifications. However, generic ELISAs do not offer complete coverage for all process-specific HCPs and process-specific ELISAs might be not qualified to evaluate the HCP content after process changes [3,16–18]. Two-dimensional gel electrophoresis combined with fluorescent staining is also applied for the detection and quantification of HCPs [19,20]. The technique is semi-quantitative, has a limited dynamic range, and needs mass spectrometry for HCP identification.

Approaches involving liquid chromatography coupled to mass spectrometry (LC-MS) provide alternative solutions for product characterization within the biopharmaceutical industry [21–25].. Advances in two dimensional LC-MS (2D–LC-MS) have enabled the analysis of low-abundance analytes in complex protein mixtures [26–28]. Recently, the identification and quantification of HCPs in biotherapeutics by 2D–LC-MS was demonstrated [29,30].

In the present study, an approach employing affinity chromatography to capture HCPs, highly sensitive LC-MSMS, and high throughput immunoassay testing for the enrichment, identification and quantification of HCPs in biotherapeutics was developed. This test system allowed us to identify and monitor Bacterial Alkaline Phosphatase in a biopharmaceutical purification process.

RESULTS

Increased levels of HCPs were detected in the manufacturing process for a recombinant protein derived from *E. coli* by ELISA and RP-HPLC analysis. At final drug substance level, several batches with HCP levels minimal greater than the release specification of 30 ppm were observed by a process-specific ELISA system. RP-HPLC analysis with UV detection is routinely applied to monitor product variants at the final drug substance level and at various purifications steps (Figure 1).

Citation: Bomans K, Lang A, Roedl V, Adolf L, Kyriosoglou K, Diepold K, et al. (2013) Mass Spectrometry Combined with High Performance Immunochemistry. PLoS ONE 8(11): e81639. doi:10.1371/journal.pone.0081639.

At the final drug substance level no significant differences in product purity where observed for batches with elevated HCP levels (Figure 2A). The first chromatographic purification step of the recombinant protein is accomplished by metal chelate chromatography (purification step 1). At this stage several product variants (marked by asterisks) can be observed in the obtained elution pool (Figure 2B).

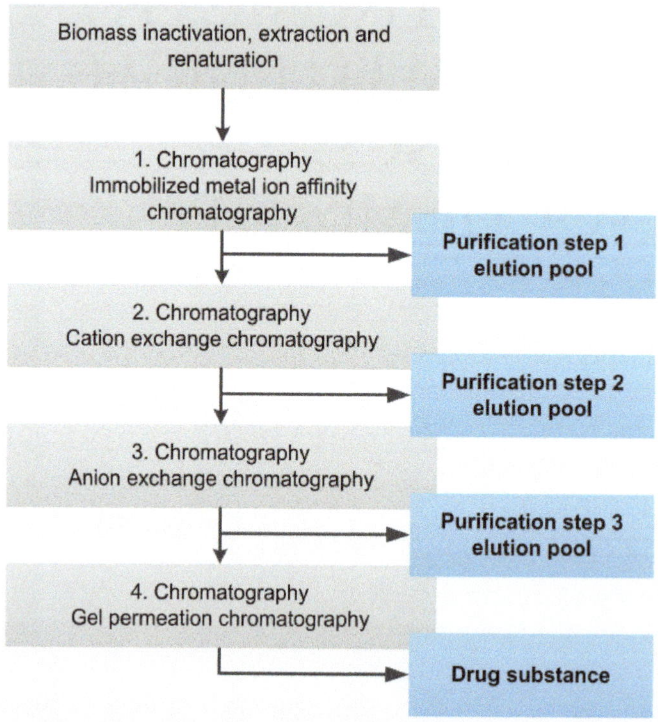

Figure 1: Scheme of the investigated protein purification processes.

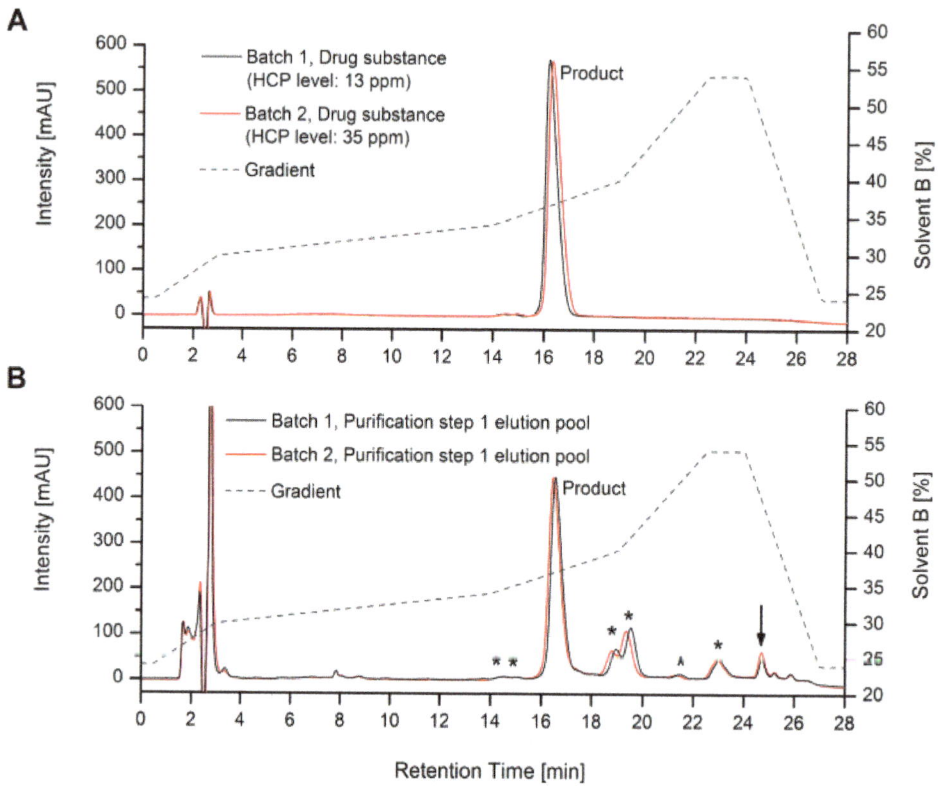

Figure 2: Monitoring of product variants (*) by RP-HPLC.

Batches with different HCP content at drug substance level (A) and the product elution pool after metal affinity purification step 1 (B). Batch differences are marked by an arrow.

In general, no significant differences in product variants where observed for batches with elevated HCP levels at purification step 1 level. However, a slight but distinct increase in peak intensity of the product variant with a retention time of 25 min could be observed for batches with elevated HCP levels (Figure 2B; marked by an arrow). The existence of elevated product variants or HCP levels was further suggested by SDS-PAGE analysis of the respective HPLC fractions (retention time window: 24-26 min), in which an increased content of a protein species with a molecular weight of around 23 kDa was observed for batches with elevated HCP levels (Figure 3). The unknown protein was identified as *E. coli* Alkyl hydroperoxide reductase subunit C (see Table 1) by nano-ESI-MS peptide mapping after in tryptic-gel digestion combined with database searching (mass spectrometric data not shown). Additionally, various potential host cell proteins, not detected by RP-HPLC analysis, were visualized by SDS-PAGE analysis of total purification step 1 elution pool (Figure 4). The dominant HCP with a molecular weight of around 50 kDa was identified as Bacterial Alkaline Phosphatase (BAP; see Table 1) by the procedure as described above (data not shown) and located in the injection peak of the RP-HPLC chromatogram by HPLC fractionation (retention time window: 2-4 min, Figure 2B). The SDS-PAGE analysis of purification step 1-3 elution pools suggest a complete HCP removal by the applied purification process (Figure 4). Nevertheless, tryptic peptide mapping combined with comprehensive online liquid chromatography mass spectrometry (LC-MS/MS) was utilized to identify low abundant HCPs of the different elution pools. Protein identification by database searching was successful to identify various bacterial proteins present in the elution pools of the purifications steps 1 and 2. The identified HCPs are summarized in Table 1. Although the analysis was performed with a highly sensitive LTQ Orbitrap Velos electrospray mass spectrometer, only one bacterial protein (BAP) was verified in the elution pool of purification step 3 and no HCPs were detected at the final drug substance level (Table 1). Since the deployed process-specific ELISA system does demonstrate low abundant HCP levels at final bulk stage (Figure 2), we introduced HCP enrichment by affinity chromatography using the ELISAs polyclonal antibodies in our sample preparation protocol to detect bacterial proteins of low abundance (see details in materials and methods). In order to judge if the HCP enrichment step does significantly enrich or deplete individual HCPs, purification step 1 elution pool was again analyzed with and without applying the affinity enrichment procedure. The identified proteins (identification score ≥ 20; peptides with an FDR <1%) are listed in Table 2(Repeatability results are summarized in Table S1). All abundant bacterial proteins of the purification step 1 elution pool were also detected after applying the HCP enrichment step. Although the identification scores of some bacterial proteins do suggest alterations of the relative protein abundances only minor effects on protein sequence coverage were observed. In addition, an increasing number of identified HCPs was demonstrated as a consequence of the affinity enrichment procedure. Thus, from a qualitative point of view, the results achieved do not suggest significant alterations of the HCP profile related to the affinity enrichment step.

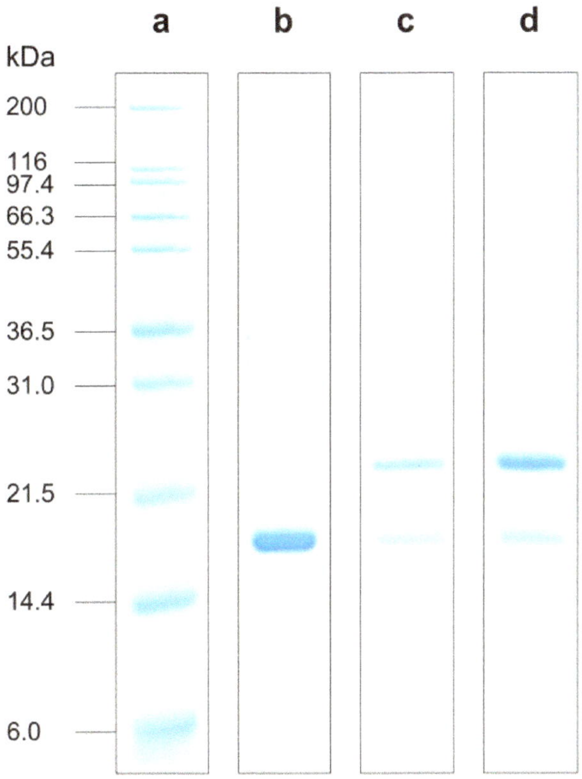

Figure 3: SDS-PAGE analysis of RP-HPLC fractions.

(a) Mark12™ Standard; (b) Reference material, drug substance level; (c) RP-HPLC fraction (24-26 min, Figure 2B) of purification step 1 elution pool, HCP content at drug substance level: 13 ppm; (d) RPHPLC fraction (24-26 min, Figure 2B) of purification step 1 elution pool, HCP content at drug substance level: 35 ppm.

Table 1: Overview of identified HCPs at different purification (P.) steps

			P. step 1		**P. step 2**		**P. step 3**		**Drug substance**	
ACC	**Identified *E. coli*protein**	**MW [kDa]**	**SC**	**COV [%]**	**SC**	**COV [%]**	**SC**	**COV [%]**	**SC**	**COV [%]**
P00634	Alkaline phosphatase	49.4	**458**	92	**210**	88	**36**	27	*n.d.*	*n.d.*
P0A6Y8	Chaperone protein dnaK	69.1	**250**	80	**151**	61	*n.d.*	*n.d.*	*n.d.*	*n.d.*
P23843	Periplasmic oligopeptide-binding protein	60.9	**214**	78	**107**	68	*n.d.*	*n.d.*	*n.d.*	*n.d.*
P0A6P1	Elongation factor Ts	30.4	**163**	76	**87**	60	*n.d.*	*n.d.*	*n.d.*	*n.d.*
P0A6P9	Enolase	45.6	**116**	69	**70**	50	*n.d.*	*n.d.*	*n.d.*	*n.d.*
P0A877	Tryptophan synthase alpha chain	28.7	**103**	87	**42**	51	*n.d.*	*n.d.*	*n.d.*	*n.d.*

P0AE08	Alkyl hydroperoxide reductase subunit C	20.8	**97**	84	**74**	84	*n.d.*	*n.d.*	*n.d.*	*n.d.*
P0AFM2	Glycine betaine-binding periplasmic protein	36.0	**92**	79	**<20**	20	*n.d.*	*n.d.*	*n.d.*	*n.d.*
P0ABK5	Cysteine synthase A	34.5	**84**	76	**22**	29	*n.d.*	*n.d.*	*n.d.*	*n.d.*
P77395	Uncharacterized protein ybbN	31.8	**68**	58	**52**	62	*n.d.*	*n.d.*	*n.d.*	*n.d.*
	Total number of identified HCPs (score >20)		**76**		**16**		**1**		**0**	

Database query was conducted by analyzing LC-MS/MS CID spectra using Proteome Discoverer V1.3 and a false discovery rate FDR < 1%. The Top 10 HCPs were sorted according to the score value at purification step 1 level. ACC, accession number (http://www.uniprot.org/); SC, score; MW, theoretical molecular weight; COV, Sequence coverage; n.d., not detected.

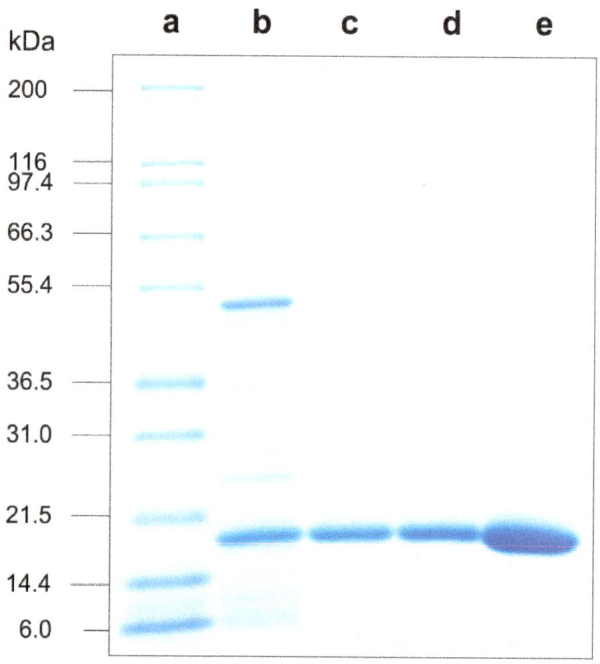

Figure 4: SDS-PAGE analysis of in-process controls.

(a) Mark12™ Standard; (b) Purification step 1 elution pool; (c) Purification step 2 elution pool; (d) Purification step 3 elution pool; (e) Drug substance, HCP content: 30 ppm.

Table 2: Comparison of identified HCPs with and without HCP affinity enrichment

			Direct analysis		**After HCP enrichment**	
ACC	**Identified *E. coli* protein**	**MW [kDa]**	**SC**	**COV [%]**	**SC**	**COV [%]**
P00634	Alkaline phosphatase	49.4	**458**	92	**251**	83
P0A6Y8	Chaperone protein dnaK	69.1	**250**	80	**278**	74
P23843	Periplasmic oligopeptide-binding protein	60.9	**214**	78	**155**	64
P0A6P1	Elongation factor Ts	30.4	**163**	76	**152**	67
P0A6P9	Enolase	45.6	**116**	69	**105**	63
P0A877	Tryptophan synthase alpha chain	28.7	**103**	87	**115**	76
P0AE08	Alkyl hydroperoxide reductase subunit C	20.7	**97**	84	**71**	84
P0AFM2	Glycine betaine-binding periplasmic protein	36.0	**92**	79	**53**	71
P0ABK5	Cysteine synthase A	34.5	**84**	76	**75**	64
P77395	Uncharacterized protein ybbN	31.8	**68**	58	**73**	72

P0A6P7	Probable GTP-binding protein engB	23.5	**65**	68	**78**	77
P0A799	Phosphoglycerate kinase	41.1	**64**	45	**90**	63
P39180	Antigen 43	106.8	**62**	21	**39**	16
P0A862	Thiol peroxidase	17.8	**60**	76	**53**	76
P69913	Carbon storage regulator	6.9	**56**	33	**<20**	33
	Total number of identified HCPs (score >20)		**76**		**84**	

Database query was conducted by analyzing LC-MS/MS CID spectra using Proteome Discoverer V1.3 and a false discovery rate FDR < 1% of purification step 1 elution pool samples. The Top 15 HCPs were sorted according to the score value of the direct analysis at purification step 1 level. ACC, accession number (http://www.uniprot.org/); SC, score; MW, theoretical molecular weight; COV, Sequence coverage.

Next, we employed the described approach to identify HCPs at the final drug substance level. A total of 12 bacterial proteins (with an identification score ≥ 20), not detected without affinity enrichment, were identified at final bulk level (Table 3). Eight proteins were already verified at purification step 1 elution pool level (including BAP and Alkyl hydroperoxide reductase subunit C). However, the Protein tolB, DNA protection during starvation protein, 2-amino-4-hydroxy-6-hydroxymethyldihydropteridine pyrophosphokinase, and N-acetylmuramoyl-L-alanine amidase AmiD were only detected at final drug substance level suggesting a relative enrichment of the protein through the purification process.

Table 3: Identified HCPs at drug substance level after HCP affinity enrichment

ACC	**Identified *E. coli* protein**	**MW [kDa]**	**SC**	**COV [%]**
P23843	Periplasmic oligopeptide-binding protein	60.9	**93**	60
P0A6Y8	Chaperone protein dnaK	69.1	77	40
P23847	Periplasmic dipeptide transport protein	60.3	77	46
P00634	Alkaline phosphatase	49.4	**48**	43
P0A855	Protein tolB	45.9	**42**	37
P0ABT2	DNA protection during starvation protein	18.7	**38**	60
P0A6F5	60 kDa chaperonin	57.3	**32**	22
P0AE08	Alkyl hydroperoxide reductase subunit C	20.7	**26**	47
P26281	2-amino-4-hydroxy-6-hydroxymethyldihydropteridine pyrophosphokinase	18.1	**26**	58
P69441	Adenylate kinase	23.6	**22**	36
P75820	N-acetylmuramoyl-L-alanine amidase AmiD	31.1	**21**	30
P0A910	Outer membrane protein A	37.2	**20**	26
	Total number of identified HCPs (score >20)		**12**	

Database query was conducted by analyzing LC-MS/MS CID spectra using Proteome Discoverer V1.3 and a false discovery rate FDR < 1%. ACC, accession number (http://www.uniprot.org/); SC, score; MW, theoretical molecular weight; COV, Sequence coverage.

In summary, the application of affinity chromatography combined with comprehensive LC-MS was adequate to identify low abundant HCPs at the final drug substance level.

Since BAP was identified as being the most abundant HCP at purification step 1 elution pool level and is still traceable at final drug substance level we developed two different assays for enzymatic and immunological BAP monitoring on a cobas INTEGRA® 400 plus and a cobas e 411 system, respectively[1]. The method validation results for both cobas® systems demonstrated acceptable analytical performance and are in accordance with the manufacturer's accuracy and imprecision criteria (Table 4). The cobas® analysis of all total purification step elution pools and the final drug substance material does demonstrate an almost complete BAP removal by the applied purification process (Table 5). At final drug substance level the detected immunological BAP activity of 0.1 U/mg was close to the quantification limit (0.12 U/mL) and the observed enzymatic BAP activity was below the detection limit of 0.2 mU/mL (see Table 4). As initially described, several batches with increased HCP levels were observed at final drug substance level by a process-specific ELISA system. To verify if BAP does contribute to the elevated total HCP levels the enzymatic and immunological BAP activity of various batches was analyzed at purification step 3 elution pool level. The results are summarized in Table 6 and demonstrate that no causal relationship between elevated total HCP levels and enzymatic and immunological BAP activity is verifiable.

Table 4: Analytical performance of the BAP ECLIA and BAP enzymatic activity assay

Instrument	cobas e 411	cobas INTEGRA® 400 plus
Assay	BAP ECLIA	BAP Enzymatic activity
Detection Limit [mU/mL]	40	0.2
Quantitation Limit [mU/mL]	120	1.0
Range [mU/mL]	120 - 15 000	1.0 - 1200
Accuracy: Recovery of spike [%]	90 - 118	72 - 105
Precision: Repeatability RSD [%]	< 10	1 - 12
Performance	100 samples/120 min	100 samples/35 min
Dilution of samples	Done by system	Done by system

BAP, Bacterial Alkaline Phosphatase; ECLIA, Electrochemiluminescence Immunoassay.

Table 5: Immunological and enzymatic BAP activities at different process levels

	Protein	HCP ELISA	BAP ECLIA	BAP Enzymatic activity
	[mg/mL]	*[ng/mg]*	*[U/mg]*	*[mU/mg]*
Purification Step 1	1.44	n.a.	8390	970
Purification Step 2	0.28	n.a.	38	0.7
Purification Step 3	6.44	264	9.0	0.4
Drug substance	1.74	16	0.1	<DL

BAP, Bacterial Alkaline Phosphatase; ECLIA, Electrochemiluminescence Immunoassay; n.a., not applicable; DL, Detection limit

Table 6: HCP content and BAP enzymatic and immunological activities of various drug substance batches

	Drug substance	Purification step 3		
	HCP ELISA	**Protein**	**BAP ECLIA**	**BAP Enzymatic activity**
	[ng/mg]	*[mg/mL]*	*[U/mg]*	*[mU/mg]*
Batch 3	15	6.61	25	0.3
Batch 4	32	5.78	17	0.3
Batch 5	22	5.70	19	0.3
Batch 6	30	6.13	20	0.2
Batch 7	19	6.23	18	0.2
Batch 8	20	6.56	13	< QL
Batch 9	19	6.40	18	0.2
Batch 10	32	7.57	27	0.4
Batch 11	36	7.42	18	0.3
Batch 12	8	6.78	22	0.2

BAP, Bacterial Alkaline Phosphatase; ECLIA, Electrochemiluminescence Immunoassay; QL, Quantification limit.

DISCUSSION

For the identification and quantification of HCPs in biotherapeutics, a test system employing HCP affinity enrichment, highly sensitive LC-MS, and high throughput immunoassay testing was developed. Direct LC-MS analysis was capable of identifying 76 HCPs at purification step 1 level but did not verify the presence of HCPs at the final drug substance level. In contrast, the application of affinity chromatography for HCP enrichment combined with LC-MS was adequate to identify 85 HCPs at purification step 1 level. In addition, the results achieved do not suggest, from a qualitative point of view, significant alterations of the HCP profile related to the affinity enrichment step. The described approach resulted in the confirmation of 12 low abundant HCPs in the final drug substance. All identified bacterial HCPs have the potential to trigger an immune response in human, although the respond will depend on composition and amount of bacterial proteins administered [2,3]. Moreover, five low abundant bacterial proteins with possible catalytic activity were verified.

Bacterial Alkaline Phosphatase (BAP) is a widely distributed non-specific phosphomonoesterase that also catalyzes phosphoryl transfer reaction to various alcohols [31,32]. *E. coli* Alkyl hydroperoxide reductase (AhpC) directly reduces organic hydroperoxides in its reduced dithiol form and might act as an antioxidant enzyme [33]. 2-amino-4-hydroxy-6-hydroxymethyldihydropteridine pyrophosphokinase, Adenylate kinase, and N-acetylmuramoyl-L-alanine amidase AmiD were also detected at the final drug substance level. The identified bacterial enzymes are involved in folic acid biosynthesis, nucleotide biosynthesis, and cell wall biogenesis/degradation [34–37]. The described catalytic activities do not suggest a negative impact on product stability. However, bacterial enzymes could theoretically also have enzymatic effects in humans, although, to the author's knowledge, reports to this risk have not been published [3]. BAP, AhpC, and Adenylate kinase were detected at purification step 1 and final drug substance level whereas 2-amino-4-hydroxy-6-hydroxymethyldihydropteridine pyrophosphokinase and N-acetylmuramoyl-L-alanine amidase AmiD were only detected at the final drug substance level. Thus, the data indicate a less effective removal or relative enrichment of both enzymes through the purification process.

Subsequently, we focused on developing test systems for high throughput monitoring of specific bacterial HCPs. Since BAP was identified as being the most abundant HCP at purification step 1 level, we firstly established two different assays for enzymatic and immunological BAP monitoring using the cobas® technology. The obtained results demonstrate an almost complete removal of BAP enzymatic and immunological activity by the applied purification process. However, since BAP enzymatic activity was verified until purification step 3 level BAP activity at the final drug substance level is most likely, although to a much lower extent. These results are in agreement with the data obtained by comprehensive LC-MS analysis, in which BAP at final bulk level was only found after enrichment by affinity chromatography. In addition, we assessed if BAP does contribute to the elevated total HCP levels of some drug substance batches. The results revealed that no causal relationship between elevated total HCP levels and enzymatic and immunological BAP activity is traceable. Currently, we are developing novel immunological and enzymatic cobas® test systems to assess AhpC, 2-amino-4-hydroxy-6-hydroxymethyldihydropteridine pyrophosphokinase, Adenylate kinase, and N-acetylmuramoyl-L-alanine amidase AmiD removal by the applied purification process and perhaps more importantly, their catalytic activity at the final drug substance level. Recently, the identification and quantification of HCPs in biotherapeutics by 2D–LC-MS was demonstrated [29,30]. The described approaches allow the simultaneous quantification of various low abundance HCPs. In the present study, the application of affinity chromatography combined with comprehensive LC-MS analysis and cobas® technology was adequate to identify low abundant HCPs at final drug substance level and to subsequently monitor the enzymatic and immunological activity of BAP at various purifications steps. Accordingly, the impact of fermentation, purification, and formulation conditions on HCP removal and biological activity can be conducted by monitoring process-specific HCPs in a GMP-compatible and high-throughput (> 1000 samples/day) manner.

MATERIALS AND METHODS

Reversed Phase Chromatography (RP-HPLC)

Reversed phase chromatography was performed on a Dionex Summit® HPLC system (Thermo Fisher Scientific, Bremen, Germany) with UV detection at 210 nm. The separation was carried out on a YMC-Pack ODS-AQ analytical column (3 x 150 mm, S-3μ, 200 Å, carbon content: 11.0-11.5 %, YMC, Tokyo, Japan) between 20°C and 25°C. A step gradient using 0.1% TFA, 30 % acetonitrile as solvent A and 0.1 % TFA, 80 % acetonitrile as solvent B at 0.4 mL/min was applied. For the chromatographic analysis 6 μg of total protein was injected. Fractions were collected manually.

Sodium dodecyl sulfate polyacrylamide gel electrophoresis (SDS-PAGE)

One-dimensional SDS-PAGE was performed with Novex® 18% Tris-Glycine gels in a XCell SureLock® Mini-Cell (Life Technologies Corporation, Darmstadt, Germany). Samples were reduced with NuPAGE® Sample Reducing Agent (catalogue number: NP0004) and gel electrophoresis was carried out according to the Novex® Tris-Glycine Midi Gels instruction (quick reference card, 25-0913 Version B; 12 May 2008). 5 μg of protein was loaded per lane. Low concentrated fractions from reverse phase chromatography were evaporated to dryness in a RVC 2-25 CD plus Rotational-Vacuum-Concentrator (Martin Christ Gefriertrocknungsanlagen GmbH, Osterode am Harz, Germany). The gels were stained with SimplyBlue™ SafeStain (Life Technologies Corporation) and destained in ultrapure water.

In-gel proteolytic digestion

In-gel digestion was carried out using OMX-S® devices (OMX GmbH, Martinsried, Germany) according to the OMX-S® pro Instruction Manual. Protein bands were washed and destained with 50% acetonitrile, 50% ammonium bicarbonate solution (50 mM, pH 8.0). The digest was performed in 20 μL freshly prepared trypsin solution (0.01 μg/μl) in 50 mM ammonium bicarbonate solution (pH 8.0) at 37°C for 45 min.

HCP identification by Nano ESI-MS/MS

For the Nano ESI-MS/MS analysis of the in-gel digests, peptides were desalted and concentrated with ZipTip® C18 Pipette Tips (Millipore Corporation, Billerica, USA) and eluted in 20 μL 1% formic acid, 50% acetonitrile. Nano ESI-MS/MS analyses were performed on a QTOF Ultima mass spectrometer (Waters, Manchester, U.K.) equipped with a TriVersa NanoMate (Advion, Inc., Ithaca, USA). Spectra were recorded in the positive ion mode. Sequencing was performed by low-energy collision-induced dissociation (CID) using argon as collision gas. The collision energy was set from 20 to 45 eV. Spectra were searched against the UniProt database of *Escherichia coli* using Protein Prospector (UCSF, University of California, San Francisco; http://prospector.ucsf.edu/prospector/mshome.htm) and MASCOT (Matrix Science Inc, Boston, USA; http://www.matrixscience.com/search_form_select.html).

In-solution digestion

For the proteolytic digestion, samples were denatured in 0.4 M Tris-HCl, 8 M guanidine hydrochloride, pH 8.5 by diluting 150 µg of protein in a total volume of 300 µL. For reduction, 10 µl of 0.1 g/mL dithiothreitol was added followed by incubation at 50°C for 1 hour. After alkylation of free cysteine by adding 10 µl of 0.33 g/mL iodoacetic acid and incubation at room temperature under exclusion of light for 30 min, the buffer was exchanged to digestion buffer (0.1 M Tris-HCl, pH 8.5) by application onto an illustra™ NAP™-5 gel filtration column (G-25, GE Healthcare, Buckinghamshire, UK). The NAP™-5 eluate (500 µL) was mixed with 30 µL of a solution of 0.1 mg/mL sequencing grade trypsin (Promega, Madison, USA) in 10 mM HCl and incubated at 37°C for 18 h.

HCP identification by LC-MS/MS

LC-MS/MS analysis of in solution digests were performed on a LTQ Orbitrap Velos mass spectrometer (Thermo Fisher Scientific, Bremen, Germany) coupled to an Acquity UPLC system (Waters, Manchester, UK). Peptides were separated on a BEH C18 column (1.7 µm 2.1x150 mm, Waters, Manchester, UK) using a binary gradient (solvent A: 0.1% formic acid, solvent B: 0.1% formic acid, 100% acetonitrile) from 1% to 45% B at a flow rate of 0.3 mL/min in 40 min. 5 µg of digested protein was loaded. Low concentrated digests were evaporated to 30 µL in a RVC 2 - 25 CD plus Rotational-Vacuum-Concentrator and completely injected. Data acquisition was controlled by XCalibure software (Thermo, Waltham, MA). For the top10 CID method, survey full scan MS spectra (from m/z 200 - 2000) were acquired by the Orbitrap system with a resolution of r = 30000. The ten most abundant peptide ions with charge states > +1 were sequentially isolated and fragmented with CID and a normalized collision energy of 40 V using helium as collision gas. The resulting fragment ions were detected by the ion trap. The automatic gain control (AGC) target values were set to $1*10^6$ for Full MS scans in the Orbitrap mass analyzer and $1*10^4$ for MS/MS scans in the ion trap mass analyzer.

LC-MS/MS Database Query

CID spectra were searched against an in-house *E. coli* database using Proteome Discoverer V1.3 (Thermo Fisher Scientific, Bremen, Germany). The custom protein database was compiled from 5,967 *E.coli* protein sequences (from actual Swiss Prot K12 database), the sequence of the therapeutic protein, and the sequence of porcine trypsin. The following SEQUEST® search parameters were applied: (1) trypsin with a maximum of one missed cleavage, (2) carboxymethylation of cysteines as fixed and (3) oxidation of methionine as variable modifications. Precursor mass tolerance was set to 10 ppm and the fragment mass tolerance was set to 0.8 Da. A False Discovery Rate (FDR) of 1% was calculated. Only proteins specified with a score value ≥ 20 and with high confidence unique peptides (FDR < 1%) were considered as positive hits. The mass spectrometry proteomics data for HCP identification at drug substance level have been deposited to the ProteomeXchange Consortium (http://proteomecentral.proteomexchange.org) via the PRIDE partner repository[38,39] with the dataset identifier PXD000509 and DOI 10.6019/PXD000509.

HCP Enrichment by Affinity Chromatography

For the preparation of the affinity resin, NHS activated sepharoseTM 4 fast flow (GE Healthcare, Buckinghamshire, UK) and anti-*E. coli* antibody (Dako Deutschland GmbH, Hamburg, Germany) were used. The antibody solution was dialyzed against coupling buffer (200 mM potassium phosphate, pH 8.4) and adjusted to a concentration of ca. 10 mg/mL. Coupling was performed with an adapted procedure derived from technical note 71 5000 14 AD (GE Healthcare, Buckinghamshire, UK). Unspecific binding sites of the resin were blocked by incubating with drug substance solution. The prepared affinity resin was filled into a Kronlab Eco glass column (10 x 250 mm, YMC Europe GmbH, Dinslaken, Germany) and regenerated by the following steps: (1) 0.5 M NaCl, 0.05 % Tween20, pH 7.5, 4 CV (column volumes); (2) 30 mM NaCl, 4 CV; (3) 1 M propionic acid, 2 CV; (4) 50 mM potassium phosphate, 150 mM NaCl pH 7.5, 2 CV. 2.2 mg of drug substance solution containing 80 µg HCP were loaded on the affinity resin. Column equilibration was performed with 10 mM potassium phosphate, 154 mM NaCl, 0.005 % NaN_3, 0.05 % Triton-x 100, 0.1 % BSA pH 7.0, 4 CV followed by washing step 1 with 10 mM potassium phosphate, 100 mM NaCl, 0.005 % NaN_3, 0.05 % Tween20, 0.5 mM EDTA, pH 6.5 (4 CV) and washing step 2 using 10 mM potassium phosphate, 30 mM NaCl, pH 7.5 (4 CV). HCPs were eluted with 3 CV of 1 M propionic acid. Flow rate was set to 0.15 ml/min. The eluate was collected as a single fraction in potassium phosphate (pH 7.5) and was adjusted to pH 7.5. To remove propionic acid the eluate was dialyzed against 10 mM potassium phosphate, 154 mM NaCl, pH 7.5.

Quantitative Determination of the Enzymatic Activity of Alkaline Phosphatase

The colorimetric assay was carried out on a cobas INTEGRA® 400 plus system using the ALP IFCC Gen.2 cassettes (Roche Diagnostics Ltd., Basel, Switzerland) according to the manufacturer's guidelines. Briefly, the principle of the assay is the cleavage of p-nitrophenyl phosphate by alkaline phosphatase into phosphate and p-nitrophenol. The p-nitrophenol released is directly proportional to the catalytic alkaline phosphatase activity. The activity is determined by measuring the increase in absorbance at 409 nm. The assay is performed at 37°C. A minimal sample volume of 250 µL was required. Calibration was done with Bacterial Alkaline Phosphatase (Life Technologies GmbH, Darmstadt, Germany, Catalogue number 18011-015).

Bacterial Alkaline Phosphatase (BAP) ECLIA

The immunological BAP content was determined by an electrochemiluminescence immunoassay (ECLIA) on a cobas e 411 analyzer (Roche Diagnostics Ltd., Basel, Switzerland) according to the manufacturer's guidelines. Briefly, the assay is based on a sandwich principle using a mouse monoclonal anti-BAP antibody (in-house development). First, 30 µl of sample, biotinylated anti-BAP capture antibody and ruthenium-labeled anti-BAP detection antibody were incubated for 9 min forming a ternary complex. In a second step after addition of streptavidin-coated microparticles, the complex is bound to the solid phase via interaction of biotin and streptavidin during 9 min of incubation. The reaction mixture is aspirated into the measuring cell where the microparticles are magnetically captured to the surface of the electrode. Voltage-induced chemiluminescence is measured by a photomultiplier. The concentration of BAP in the test sample is finally calculated from a BAP (Life Technologies GmbH, Darmstadt, Germany, Catalogue number 18011-015) standard curve of known concentration.

Supporting Information

Table S1. Repeatability of HCP identification results. Database query was conducted by analyzing LC-MS/MS CID spectra using Proteome Discoverer V1.3 and a false discovery rate FDR < 1% of three purification step 1 elution pool samples (three independent sample preparations). The Top 15 HCPs were sorted according to the score value of Analysis 1. Accession number, http://www.uniprot.org/; MW, theoretical molecular weight.

			Analysis 1		Analysis 2		Analysis 3	
Accession	Identified E. coli protein	MW [kDa]	Score	Coverage [%]	Score	Coverage [%]	Score	Coverage [%]
P00634	Alkaline phosphatase	49.4	458	92	450	92	561	87
P0A6Y8	Chaperone protein dnaK	69.1	250	80	247	77	357	72
P23843	Periplasmic oligopeptide-binding protein	60.9	214	78	219	75	176	69
P0A6P1	Elongation factor Ts	30.4	163	76	160	76	128	66
P0A6P9	Enolase	45.6	116	69	116	71	113	63
P0A877	Tryptophan synthase alpha chain	28.7	103	87	100	87	75	69
P0AE08	Alkyl hydroperoxide reductase subunit C	20.7	97	84	93	84	97	75
P0AFM2	Glycine betaine-binding periplasmic protein	36.0	92	79	96	78	94	70
P0ABK5	Cysteine synthase A	34.5	84	76	81	70	74	70
P77395	Uncharacterized protein ybbN	31.8	68	58	73	66	76	65
P0A6P7	Probable GTP-binding protein engB	23.5	65	68	71	81	78	66
P0A799	Phosphoglycerate kinase	41.1	64	45	75	61	54	45
P39180	Antigen 43	106.8	62	21	40	14	56	17
P0A862	Thiol peroxidase	17.8	60	76	66	76	69	76
P69913	Carbon storage regulator	6.9	56	33	67	43	88	33
	Total number of identified HCPs (score >20)		76		75		72	

ACKNOWLEDGMENTS

We are indebted to all members of the laboratories in Penzberg for valuable discussions and Prof. Dr. Oliver Eickelberg for manuscript proofreading. We thank Attila Csordas and the other members of the PRIDE team at the EMBL-EBI for their assistance in making the data used for this manuscript publicly accessible via the PRIDE repository. COBAS, COBAS E and COBAS INTEGRA are trademarks of Roche.

REFERENCES

1. Briggs J, Panfili PR (1991) Quantitation of DNA and protein impurities in biopharmaceuticals. Anal Chem 63: 850-859. doi:10.1021/ac00009a003. PubMed: 1858980.
2. Janeway CA, Travers P, Walport M, Shlomchik M (2005) Immunobiology: the immune system in health and disease. Garland Science Publishing, New York, USA p. S 6. pp. 90-91.
3. Wang X, Hunter AK, Mozier NM (2009) Host cell proteins in biologics development: Identification, quantitation and risk assessment. Biotechnol Bioeng 103: 446-458. doi:10.1002/bit.22304. PubMed: 19388135.
4. Gao SX, Zhang Y, Stansberry-Perkins K, Buko A, Bai S et al. (2011) Fragmentation of a highly purified monoclonal antibody attributed to residual CHO cell protease activity. Biotechnol Bioeng 108: 977-982. doi:10.1002/bit.22982. PubMed: 21404269.
5. ICH (1999) Guidance for industry Q6B specifications : Test procedures and acceptance criteria for biotechnological /biological products. Rockville, MD, U.S. Dept. of Health and Human Services, Food and Drug Administration, Center for Drug Evaluation and Research, Center for Biologics Evaluation and Research.
6. Leader B, Baca QJ, Golan DE (2008) Protein therapeutics: a summary and pharmacological classification. Nat Rev Drug Discov 7: 21-39. doi:10.1038/nrd2399. PubMed: 18097458.
7. Blattner FR, Plunkett G 3rd, Bloch CA, Perna NT, Burland V et al. (1997) The complete genome sequence of Escherichia coli K-12. Science 277: 1453-1462. doi:10.1126/science.277.5331.1453. PubMed: 9278503.
8. Gibbs RA, Weinstock GM, Metzker ML, Muzny DM, Sodergren EJ et al. (2004) Genome sequence of the Brown Norway rat yields insights into mammalian evolution. Nature 428: 493-521. doi:10.1038/nature02426. PubMed: 15057822.
9. Mouse Genome Sequencing Consortium, Waterston RH, Lindblad-Toh K, Birney E, Rogers J, et al. (2002) Initial sequencing and comparative analysis of the mouse genome. Nature 420: 520-562. doi:10.1038/nature01262. PubMed: 12466850.
10. Hart RA, Rinas U, Bailey JE (1990) Protein composition of Vitreoscilla hemoglobin inclusion bodies produced in Escherichia coli. J Biol Chem 265: 12728-12733. PubMed: 2197280.
11. Rinas U, Bailey JE (1992) Protein compositional analysis of inclusion bodies produced in recombinant Escherichia coli. Appl Microbiol Biotechnol 37: 609-614. PubMed: 1369400.
12. Rinas U, Boone TC, Bailey JE (1993) Characterization of inclusion bodies in recombinant Escherichia

coli producing high levels of porcine somatotropin. J Biotechnol 28: 313-320. doi:10.1016/0168-1656(93)90179-Q. PubMed: 7763564.

13. Veeraragavan K (1989) Studies on two major contaminating proteins of the cytoplasmic inclusion bodies in Escherichia coli. FEMS Microbiol Lett 52: 149-152. PubMed: 2689277.
14. Eaton LC (1995) Host cell contaminant protein assay development for recombinant biopharmaceuticals. J Chromatogr A 705: 105-114. doi:10.1016/0021-9673(94)01249-E. PubMed: 7620564.
15. Hoffman K (2000) Strategies for host cell protein analysis 13. Biopharm. pp. 38-45.
16. Rathore AS, Sobacke SE, Kocot TJ, Morgan DR, Dufield RL et al. (2003) Analysis for residual host cell proteins and DNA in process streams of a recombinant protein product expressed in Escherichia coli cells. J Pharm Biomed Anal 32: 1199-1211. doi:10.1016/S0731-7085(03)00157-2. PubMed: 12907264.
17. Savino E, Hu B, Sellers J, Sobjak A, Majewski N et al. (2011) Development of an in-house, process-specific ELISA for detecting HCP in a therapeutic antibody, Part 2. Bioprocess International 9: 68-75.
18. Wang X, Schomogy T, Wells K, Mozier NM (2010) Improved HCP quantitation by minimizing antibody cross-reactivity to target proteins. Bioprocess International 8: 18-24.
19. Hayduk EJ, Choe LH, Lee KH (2004) A two-dimensional electrophoresis map of Chinese hamster ovary cell proteins based on fluorescence staining. Electrophoresis 25: 2545-2556. doi:10.1002/elps.200406010. PubMed: 15300775.
20. Jin M, Szapiel N, Zhang J, Hickey J, Ghose S (2010) Profiling of host cell proteins by two-dimensional difference gel electrophoresis (2D-DIGE): Implications for downstream process development. Biotechnol Bioeng 105: 306-316. doi:10.1002/bit.22532. PubMed: 19739084.
21. Aebersold R, Mann M (2003) Mass spectrometry-based proteomics. Nature 422: 198-207. doi:10.1038/nature01511. PubMed: 12634793.
22. Domon B, Aebersold R (2006) Mass spectrometry and protein analysis. Science 312: 212-217. doi:10.1126/science.1124619. PubMed: 16614208.
23. Kaltashov IA, Bobst CE, Abzalimov RR, Wang G, Baykal B et al. (2012) Advances and challenges in analytical characterization of biotechnology products: mass spectrometry-based approaches to study properties and behavior of protein therapeutics. Biotechnol Adv 30: 210-222. doi:10.1016/j.biotechadv.2011.05.006. PubMed: 21619926.
24. Yates JR, Ruse CI, Nakorchevsky A (2009) Proteomics by mass spectrometry: approaches, advances, and applications. Annu Rev Biomed Eng 11: 49-79. doi:10.1146/annurev-bioeng-061008-124934. PubMed: 19400705.
25. Zhang Z, Pan H, Chen X (2009) Mass spectrometry for structural characterization of therapeutic antibodies. Mass Spectrom Rev 28: 147-176. doi:10.1002/mas.20190. PubMed: 18720354.
26. Issaq HJ, Chan KC, Janini GM, Conrads TP, Veenstra TD (2005) Multidimensional separation of peptides for effective proteomic analysis. J Chromatogr B Analyt Technol Biomed Life Sci 817: 35-47. doi:10.1016/j.jchromb.2004.07.042. PubMed: 15680787.
27. Motoyama A, Yates JR 3rd (2008) Multidimensional LC separations in shotgun proteomics. Anal Chem 80: 7187-7193. doi:10.1021/ac8013669. PubMed: 18826178.
28. Washburn MP, Wolters D, Yates JR 3rd (2001) Large-scale analysis of the yeast proteome by multidimensional protein identification technology. Nat Biotechnol 19: 242-247. doi:10.1038/85686. PubMed: 11231557.
29. Doneanu CE, Xenopoulos A, Fadgen K, Murphy J, Skilton SJ, et al. (2012) Analysis of host-cell proteins in biotherapeutic proteins by comprehensive online two-dimensional liquid chromatography/mass spectrometry. mAbs 4: 24-44.
30. Schenauer MR, Flynn GC, Goetze AM (2012) Identification and quantification of host cell protein impurities in biotherapeutics using mass spectrometry. Anal Biochem 428: 150-157. doi:10.1016/j.ab.2012.05.018. PubMed: 22640604.
31. Kim EE, Wyckoff HW (1991) Reaction mechanism of alkaline phosphatase based on crystal structures. Two-metal ion catalysis. J Mol Biol 218: 449-464. doi:10.1016/0022-2836(91)90724-K. PubMed: 2010919.
32. Sowadski JM, Handschumacher MD, Murthy HM, Foster BA, Wyckoff HW (1985) Refined structure of alkaline phosphatase from Escherichia coli at 2.8 A resolution. J Mol Biol 186: 417-433. doi:10.1016/0022-2836(85)90115-9. PubMed: 3910843.
33. Cha MK, Kim HK, Kim IH (1995) Thioredoxin-linked “thiol peroxidase” from periplasmic space of Escherichia coli. J Biol Chem 270: 28635-28641. doi:10.1074/jbc.270.48.28635. PubMed: 7499381.
34. Brune M, Schumann R, Wittinghofer F (1985) Cloning and sequencing of the adenylate kinase gene (adk) of Escherichia coli. Nucleic Acids Res 13: 7139-7151. doi:10.1093/nar/13.19.7139. PubMed: 2997739.
35. Kerff F, Petrella S, Mercier F, Sauvage E, Herman R et al. (2010) Specific structural features of the N-acetylmuramoyl-L-alanine amidase AmiD from Escherichia coli and mechanistic implications for enzymes of this family. J Mol Biol 397: 249-259. doi:10.1016/j.jmb.2009.12.038. PubMed: 20036252.
36. Reinstein J, Schlichting I, Wittinghofer A (1990) Structurally and catalytically important residues in the phosphate binding loop of adenylate kinase of Escherichia coli. Biochemistry 29: 7451-7459. doi:10.1021/bi00484a014. PubMed: 2223776.
37. Talarico TL, Dev IK, Dallas WS, Ferone R, Ray PH (1991) Purification and partial characterization of 7,8-dihydro-6-hydroxymethylpterin-pyrophosphokinase and 7,8-dihydropteroate synthase from Escherichia coli MC4100. J Bacteriol 173: 7029-7032. PubMed: 1657875.

38. Vizcaíno JA, Côté RG, Csordas A, Dianes JA, Fabregat A et al. (2013) The PRoteomics IDEntifications (PRIDE) database and associated tools: status in 2013. Nucleic Acids Res 41: D1063-D1069. doi:10.1093/nar/gks1262. PubMed: 23203882.

39. Wang R, Fabregat A, Ríos D, Ovelleiro D, Foster JM et al. (2012) PRIDE Inspector: a tool to visualize and validate MS proteomics data. Nat Biotechnol 30: 135-137. doi:10.1038/nbt.2112. PubMed: 22318026.

CHAPTER 11

AN IMMUNOHISTOLOGICAL STUDY IN MOUSE TISSUES

Jean-Marc Collombet, Mikael Elias, Guillaume Gotthard, Elise Four, Frédérique Renault, Aurélie Joffre, Dominique Baubichon, Daniel Rochu, Eric Chabrière

INTRODUCTION

DING proteins, named according to their four conserved N-terminal amino-acid residues, encompass a recently discovered protein family [1]. Intriguingly, eukaryotic DING genes are consistently missing from genomic databases although proteins belonging to this family seem to be ubiquitous in eukaryotes: they have been identified in animals (human, monkey, rat, turkey), plants (*Hypericum perforatum*, *Arabidopsis thaliana*, potato, tobacco) and fungi (*Candida albicans, Ganoderma lucidum*) [2], [3] mostly as a 40 kDa protein or higher molecular weight DING proteins [4]. Although no complete eukaryotic DING coding sequence is available in databases, few partial DNA sequences have been either cloned [3] or identified in non-annoted parts of genomes [2]. These few pieces of sequences show that DING proteins are strongly conserved [2]. DING proteins have also been isolated from several prokaryotes [5], [6], and their coding genes are in some cases available, such as the gene encoding PfluDING, the protein isolated from *P. fluorescens* [7], [8], [9]. The high sequence identity between known eukaryotic DING sequences and available prokaryotic DING sequences (>70% sequence identity) and the systematic absence of eukaryotic DING genes raised a controversy about their prokaryotic [10] or eukaryotic origins [11].

DING proteins have been mostly isolated by virtue of a biological function. One of the most striking examples as such, remains the search for a new HIV inhibitor in St John›s Wort that led to the characterization of a novel DING protein named p27^{SJ} [3]. In humans, several DING proteins have been identified from different tissues [2], [12], [13]. The human phosphate binding protein (HPBP) is a serendipitously discovered plasma apolipoprotein that binds phosphate and is isolated from human plasma [14], [15]. HPBP structure was solved [16] and its physiological function, i.e. its association with paraoxonase (HPON1), an enzyme involved in atherosclerosis [17], has been extensively studied [18], [19], [20]. The complete protein sequence of HPBP was recently determined by a tandem use of mass spectrometry and X-ray crystallography [21]. Such a sequence stands out as the single complete eukaryotic sequence of a DING representative, known to date. Three other human DING proteins involve the crystal adhesion inhibitor (CAI), the human synovial stimulatory protein (SSP), and the X-DING-CD4^{+}from human CD4^{+} T lymphocytes [22]. Comparison of sequenced N-terminal and internal HPBP, CAI SSP, and X-DING-CD4^{+} peptides strongly suggests these stem from 4 different genes, all lacking from the sequenced human genome. The CAI isolated from human kidney cells is assumed to prevent the growth of kidney stones [23]. The SSP, isolated from human synovial liquid, possesses auto-antigen activity, lymphocyte stimulatory activity and a putative role in the etiology of rheumatoid arthritis [24], [25]. The X-DING-CD4^{+} was isolated from CD4+ T cells that are resistant to HIV infection and was shown to block the HIV-1 LTR promoted expression and the replication of HIV-1 [22]. The involvement of DING proteins in a large spectrum of diseases enhances the potential therapeutic value of this specific protein family, and further raises the question of the molecular mechanisms involved in such biological properties.

Although the amount of data concerning this protein family has increased over the last few years, their physiological functions remain largely unknown, and their origin in

Citation: Collombet J-M, Elias M, Gotthard G, Four E, Renault F, Joffre A, et al. (2010) An Immunohistological Study in Mouse Tissues. PLoS ONE 5(2): e9099. doi:10.1371/journal.pone.0009099.

eukaryotes is still under debate. Hence, we performed a mapping of the DING localization in a murine model.

This study focused on several mouse tissues i.e. brain, liver, lung, heart, aorta, artery and skin. Findings revealed that eukaryotic DING proteins have an intracellular localization. It also provides an essential background for future investigations as regards the numerous biological roles of eukaryotic DING proteins.

MATERIAL AND METHODS

Animal Care and Sample Collection

Nine-week old adult male B6D2F1/j@rj mice (Janvier Laboratories - France) were housed in cages under standard conditions of temperature (24°C) and humidity (50–60%), with lights on between 07:00 and 19:00. Mice had free access to water and standard laboratory chow.

All the experiments in our study were reviewed and approved by the Institutional Animal Care and Research Advisory Committee in accordance with French law and leading international guidelines.

Pentobarbital (80 mg/kg) anaesthetized mice were sacrificed by intracardiac perfusion of saline with heparin (5 UI/ml) followed by a fixative solution of 4% formaldehyde and 3% acetic acid in saline. Brain, liver, lung, heart, aorta artery and skin were collected, post-fixed in 4% formaldehyde for 48 hours and then processed for paraffin embedding. For the brain tissue, coronal sections (6 μm thick) were serially cut with a microtome at +0.74 mm (ventricular and striatal areas) and –1.82 mm (hippocampus area) from the bregma, as shown in the Franklin and Paxinos stereotaxic mouse brain atlas [26]. For all other collected tissues (liver, lung, heart, aorta artery and skin), transverse sections were prepared.

Plasma was purified from wild-type and germ-free C57BL/6 mouse blood using standard protocols. Wild-type and germ-free C57BL/6 mouse plasma was kindly provided by the European Mouse Mutant Archive (EMMA; http://emmanet.org).

Histological Staining

Hemalun-phloxin (H&P) staining was performed on paraffin-embedded tissue sections as previously described by Lillie and Fullmer [27]. For skin and lung sections, a saffron staining step was added after the H&P staining (incubation of sections in 2% saffron solution in ethanol for 10 min).

Immunohistochemistry

HPBP was purified from human blood plasma as previously described [28]. Rabbit polyclonal and mouse monoclonal antibodies raised against HPBP were prepared by the Genecust Company (Dudelange, Luxembourg) using standard protocols. All polyclonal antibodies and some monoclonal antibodies raised against HPBP are able to recognize other eukaryotic DING proteins, because of the high sequence identity existing in this family.

For DING protein immunohistochemistry, sections from all tested tissues were deparaffinized, rehydrated and treated for 10 min in TBS containing 0.3% v/v H_2O_2. For brain tissue, a demasking step in boiling 1 mM EDTA pH 8.0 for 20 min was added. Sections were then successively incubated for 1 h at room temperature in TBS-BSA (TBS containing 1% w/v BSA) and overnight at +4°C in TBS-BSA containing primary antibodies. After 3 washes (15 min each) in TBS, secondary biotinylated IgG antibodies in TBS-BSA were applied to sections for 1 h at room temperature. Visualisation was performed using Vectastain ABC Elite kit (Vector) and diaminobenzidine (DAB; Sigma). Dilutions for primary and secondary antibodies were: as follows 1:1000 rabbit polyclonal anti-HPBP (antibody C); 1:50 mouse monoclonal anti-HPBP (antibody 1D3 targeting the N-terminal peptide of HPBP); 1:400 biotinylated anti-rabbit IgG (Vector) and 1:1000 biotinylated anti-mouse IgG (Vector). To ensure proper control processing, some sections from all tested tissues were similarly treated except for the fact that the incubation step in monoclonal or polyclonal HPBP primary antibodies was omitted. In addition, to assess the specificity of polyclonal HPBP antibody, a competition experiment was conducted by adding 0.4, 2, 10 or 40 μg of purified HPBP on brain section slides (3 brain sections per slide) in the primary antibody incubation step.

The following markers were considered for visualization of the main types of specific brain cells: GFAP for activated astroglia, *Griffonia simplifolia* lectin (GSA) for activated microglia and NeuN for mature neurons. Double-labeling detections were achieved on deparaffinized and hydrated sections by performing DAB-stained DING protein immunochemistry (brown staining) as described above, followed by GFAP or NeuN immunolabeling using SG vector dye (blue staining) for visualization [29]. For the detection of DING protein in activated microglia, GSA staining was carried out as previously described by Streit [30] with DAB-staining, followed by DING protein immunochemistry using SG vector as dye revelator.

In control mice, GFAP or GSA staining is very faint since activated astroglial and microglial cells are almost completely absent. Therefore, for the specific detection of DING protein in activated glial cells, brain sections from soman-intoxicated mice were used. Soman, an irreversible cholinesterase inhibitor, is a powerful warfare neurotoxicant triggering epileptic seizures leading to neuronal cell death and subsequent glial activation [29]. For this purpose, nine week old adult male B6D2F1/j@rj mice were subcutaneously injected with 110 μg/kg soman (200 μl in saline buffer; soman was provided by the "Centre d›Etudes du Bouchet" - France) followed 1 min. later by an intraperitoneal injection (200 μl in saline) of 5.0 mg/kg atropine methyl nitrate. Pentobarbital (80 mg/kg) anaesthetized mice were sacrificed on day 3 (pick of microglial cell activation) and day 8 (pick of astroglial cell activation) post-poisoning using intracardiac perfusion of formaldehyde and collected brains were processed for immunohistochemistry as described above for control mice.

Western Blots Assays

Anaesthetized mice were decapitated and tissues such as the whole brain without cerebellum, liver, lung, shaven skin and heart ventricle were immediately collected. Brain and liver were homogenized with a mini-potter in 5 volumes of cold

RIPA buffer containing 20 mM Tris-HCl pH 8.0, 150 mM NaCl, 1 mM EDTA, 1% v/v NP40, 0.5% w/v SDS, 0.5% w/v deoxycholic acid and 0.5% v/v protease inhibitor cocktail set III (Calbiochem - Merck). Lung, skin or heart were disrupted using a mixer mill (Retsch MM301) calibrated for two sessions of 2 min shaking each, at 30 Hz. For disruption, tissues were transferred in a 2 ml microfuge tube containing 5 volumes of cold RIPA buffer (see above) and two 3 mm tungsten carbide beads (Retsch). Subsequently, homogenates were centrifuged at 14000 g for 20 min at +4°C and supernatants were frozen at −20°C for further western blot analysis. Prior to freezing, protein concentrations were determined in the supernatants, using the Lowry method [31].

Western immunoblotting was achieved as previously described [32]. For each tissue homogenate or plasma sample, 20 µg of total protein per well were loaded onto a 10% SDS-PAGE gel. Gel electro-transfer was performed onto 0.2 µm nitrocellulose membrane using a specific transfer buffer (48 mM Tris; 39 mM glycine; 20% methanol; 1.3 mM SDS; pH 9.2). For DING proteins detection on tissues, membranes were incubated with 1:400 monoclonal HPBP antibody and 1:1000 biotinylated-IgG anti-mouse (Vector). Western blots on plasma samples were performed using 1:2000 polyclonal anti-DING antibodies and 1:2500 anti-rabbit antibodies (BioRad). The size of DING proteins bands was calculated according to the migration of Precision plus protein kaleidoscope standard (BioRad) on the same gel for all experiments, except for the western blot on plasma samples, where Prestained Protein Ladder was used (Fermentas life science).

RESULTS

Western Blot Analysis

Western blot analysis was performed on brain, shaven skin, lung, heart and liver prepared from B6D2F1 mouse samples. Anti-DING monoclonal antibody revealed several bands ranging from 41 to 140 kDa in all tested mouse tissues (Figure 1). The 41 kDa protein band corresponds to the size of eukaryotic DING proteins already described in the literature [1]. Intensities of 41 kDa bands were very similar in all tested mouse tissues except in shaven skin where the band intensity is weaker. Other bands between 52 and 140 kDa are more likely high molecular weight DING proteins (HMW-DING) comparable to the ones already observed in plants [4]. A similar band pattern was found in mouse lung, heart and liver with 4 major HMW-DING bands located at 140 kDa, 71 kDa (double band of HMW-DING), 62 kDa and 52 kDa. In the heart, the intensity of the double 71 kDa band is more important than the one detected in lung and liver. In the brain, the 3 HMW-DING bands at 140 kDa, 71 kDa (double band) and 62 kDa are revealed but the 52 kDa HMW-DING protein was not present. In the shaven skin, only one HMW-DING was identified with a very intense band located at 52 kDa (Figure 1).

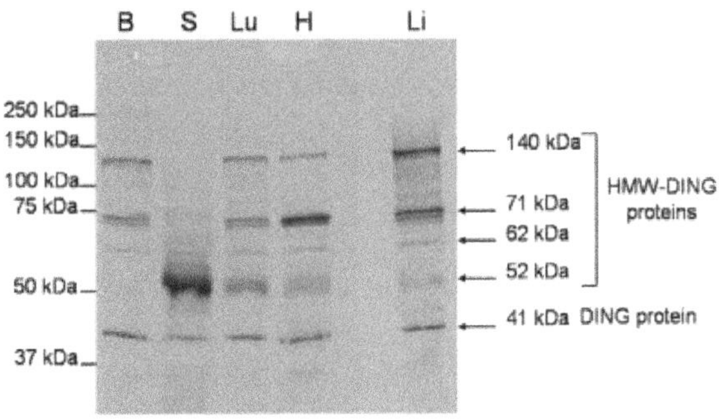

Figure 1: Characterization of DING proteins by western blot analysis.

Western blots were achieved with protein homogenates prepared from B6D2F1 mouse brain, shaven skin, lung, heart and liver (loading of 20 µg total proteins in each well). DING proteins were identified with mouse monoclonal anti-DING antibody. Diaminobenzidine was used for the band revelation. Abbreviations are: B = brain; S = shaven skin; Lu = lung; H = heart; Li = liver; HMW = high molecular weight.

Furthermore, western blot analysis was carried out on plasma purified from wild-type or germ-free C57BL/6 mice to determine whether or not the presence of DING proteins in rodent was due to a symbiotic or contaminating microbe. In both wild-type and germ-free C57BL/6 plasma, a similar pattern was observed (Figure 2). This indicates that plasma DING proteins do not originate from bacteria but are directly produced by eukaryotic cells and are subsequently secreted in the circulating blood. Anti-DING polyclonal antibody revealed several bands ranging from 35 to 130 kDa, with a slightly different pattern from that observed in mouse tissues. As a case in point, 2 bands of HMW-DING at 130 kDa and 100 kDa and a shorter DING protein of 35 kDa were specifically observed. On the other hand, 2 bands corresponding to HMW-DING at 52 kDa and 71 kDa were shared with other mouse tissues. The band at 71 kDa is very strong, suggesting that this isoform is widely predominant in mouse plasma.

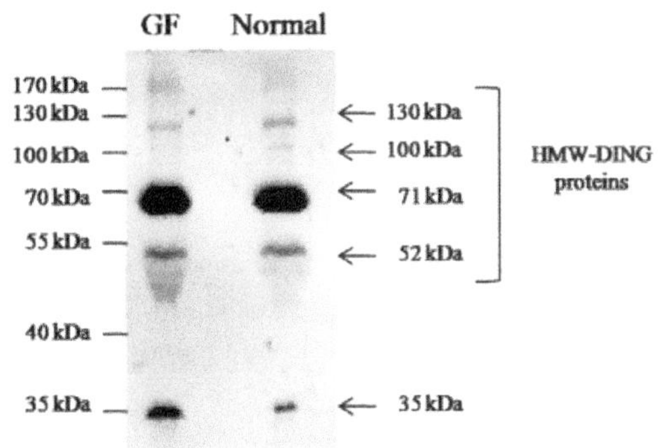

Figure 2: Western blot analysis on plasma samples from normal and germ-free mouse.

Western blot was achieved with plasma from wild type and germ-free C57BL/6 mice (loading of 20 µg total proteins in each well). Abbreviations are: normal = wild-type and GF = germ-free.

DING Protein Detection in the Mouse Brain

DING protein staining was detected in all cerebral regions of brain sections using polyclonal antibody. The specificity of the polyclonal antibody was verified in competition experiments where various quantities of purified HPBP (ranging from 0.4 to 10 µg per brain section) were added in the primary antibody incubation step (Figure 3). The addition of 0.4 µg HPBP (Figure 3B) is sufficient enough to induce a significant reduction of the intensity of DING immunolabeling previously observed in brain sections in absence of purified HPBP competitor (Figure 3A). An almost complete depletion of DING protein immunolabeling was obtained by the addition of either 2 or 10 µg of purified HPBP competitor (Figures 3C and 3D). This demonstrates the high specificity of polyclonal antibody raised against mouse DING proteins and HPBP.

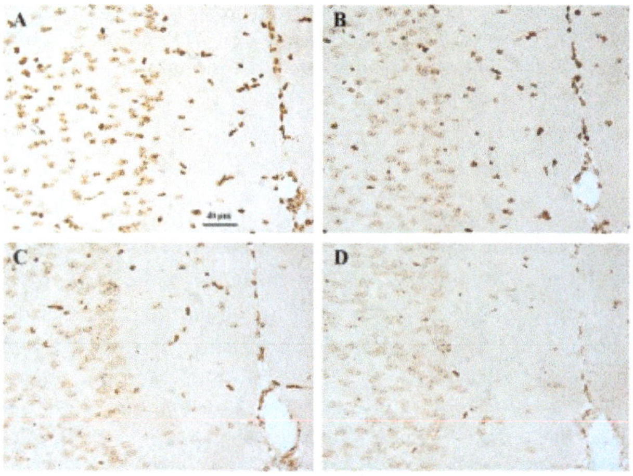

Figure 3: Competition assays to assess polyclonal antibody specificity.

Anti-DING immunohistochemistry was performed on brain sections from control mice (panel A). In a competition experiment, 0.4 µg (panel B), 2 µg (panel C) or 10 µg (panel D) of human purified HPBP protein was added in the primary antibody incubation step. In each panel, the same brain area (cingulate cortex area) was photographed with the same magnification (see scale bar on panel A).

In the brain, DING labeling was exclusively detected in cell nuclei but following two different staining patterns. In the first one, the whole nucleus is strongly labeled (Figure 4A). This labeling can be either evenly distributed throughout the nucleus or some more intensely stained patches can be spotted in the labeled nuclei. In the second pattern, detected DING proteins appeared as small patches scattered in a poorly labeled nucleus (Figure 4A). The relative proportion of strongly- or poorly-labeled nuclei is dependent on the considered cerebral regions. For example, strongly-labeled nuclei are almost entirely present in epithelial cells constituting blood vessels (Figure 4F) and are dominant in cells located in the subventricular zone and the cerebral cortex (Figures 4B and 4C). In contrast, the majority of "poorly"-labeled nuclei are found in the lateral septum, the striatum and the hippocampus (dentate gyrus and CA1, CA2 or CA3 hippocampal fields). Regardless of the strongly- or poorly- stained status of nuclei, the distribution of DING protein-positive cells is also dependent on the related brain areas. In a semi-qualitative study, the highest number of labeled cells was observed in the granular layer of the dentate gyrus (Figure 4E), the CA1, CA2 and CA3 fields of the hippocampus and the subventricular zone (Figure 4B). To a lesser extent, the density of DING protein-labeled cells is also important in the hypothalamus, the corpus callosum, the amygdala, the choroid plexus and all cortices including cingular, piriform and cerebral cortices (Figure 4C). The quantity of DING protein-positive cells was low in the thalamus (Figure 4D), the lateral septum, the striatum and some hippocampal areas deprived of pyramidal neurons such as the stratum radiatum, the lacunosum moleculare layer and the molecular layer of the dentate gyrus.

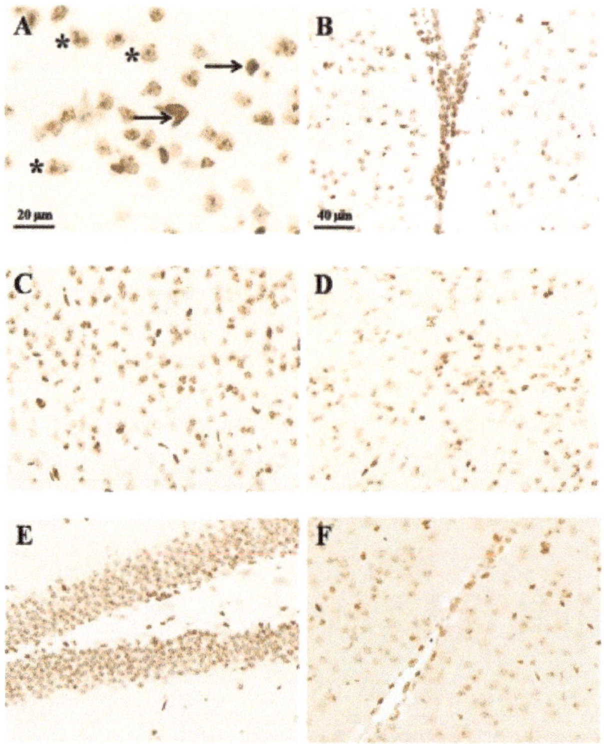

Figure 4: DING immunochemistry in the mouse brain.

Different brain areas were photographed on control mouse brain sections labeled by anti-DING immunochemistry, using diaminobenzidine as revelator dye. The different brain regions are: the cerebral cortex (panels A and C), the sub-ventricular zone or SVZ (panel B), the thalamus (panel D), the granular layer of the dentate gyrus (panel E) and epithelial cells from blood vessels (panel F). Scale bars represent 20 µm for panel A or 40 µm for panels B to F. In panel A, black arrows indicate brain cells with intense DING labeling throughout the whole nucleus while black asterisks refer to brain cells with small patches of DING labeling in poorly labeled nuclei.

Both H&P staining and DING protein immunochemistry were combined on same brain sections (co-labeling experiments) to ensure that all brain nuclei are positively labeled with anti-DING antibody (data not shown). In all checked cerebral regions, non-H&P-stained nuclei were deprived of DING protein labeling. Therefore, the density of DING protein labeling in a given brain area is directly correlated to the density of cell nuclei in the specific cerebral region.

The presence of large numbers of DING protein-positive cells in the hippocampal CA1 field or in the granular layer of the dentate gyrus undoubtedly means that these positively-stained cells are neurons since these brain areas involve pyramidal neurons for the most part. As assessed by DING protein/NeuN double labeling (Figures 5A and 5B), co-localization of NeuN and DING proteins was observed in many cell nuclei confirming the presence of DING protein in neurons throughout the brain.

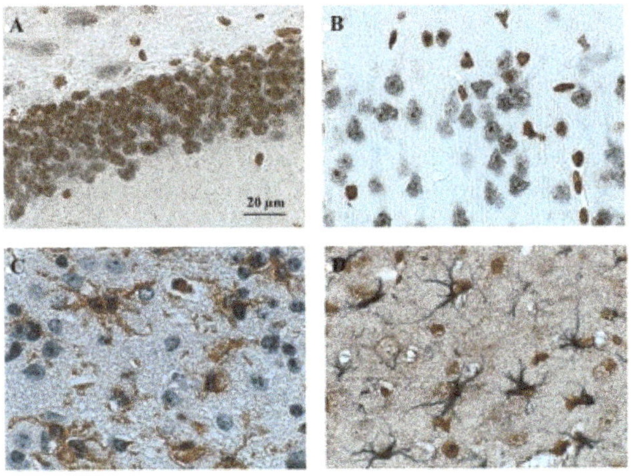

Figure 5: Characterization of DING-labeling in brain cells.

Anti-DING/anti-NeuN double staining was performed in brain sections of control mice to detect DING-expressing neurons (panel A: granular layer of the dentate gyrus; panel B: cerebral cortex). Diaminobenzidine (brown labeling) and SG vector dye (blue labeling) were used to view DING and NeuN, respectively. Activated microglia (panel C) and astroglia (panel D) expressing DING proteins were revealed in brain sections of soman-poisoned mice with anti-DING/GSA lectin or anti-DING/anti-GFAP double staining immunochemistry, respectively. Blue staining was obtained with SG vector (labeling of DING proteins in microglia and GFAP in astrocytes) while brown staining was achieved using diaminobenzidine (labeling of DING proteins in astroglia and GSA lectin in microglia).

To address the issue as to whether DING protein was also present in astroglial or microglial cells, DING protein/GFAP or DING protein/lectin GSA double staining were performed in the brain of soman-poisoned mice, respectively. Usually, resting glial cells are not easy to detect due to the thinness of their perinuclear cytoplasmic processes and the smallness of their nuclei. Therefore, a mouse model containing activated glial cells with prominent cytoplasmic branching processes and hypertrophied nuclei, namely the soman-intoxicated mouse, was chosen. The presence of DING protein was demonstrated in numerous activated microglial or astroglial cells after soman poisoning, as shown in Figures 5C and 5D, respectively.

DING Protein Detection in Other Mouse Tissues

In the skin, a massive DING protein-positive staining was observed in the *stratum corneum*, epidermis (including basal keratinocytes) and cutaneous underlying muscles (Figures 6A and 6B). In the dermis, only fibroblasts were strongly labeled with anti-DING antibody. However, a weak DING protein labeling was found in the dermis extracellular matrix mainly consisting of collagen fibers (Figures 6A and 6B).

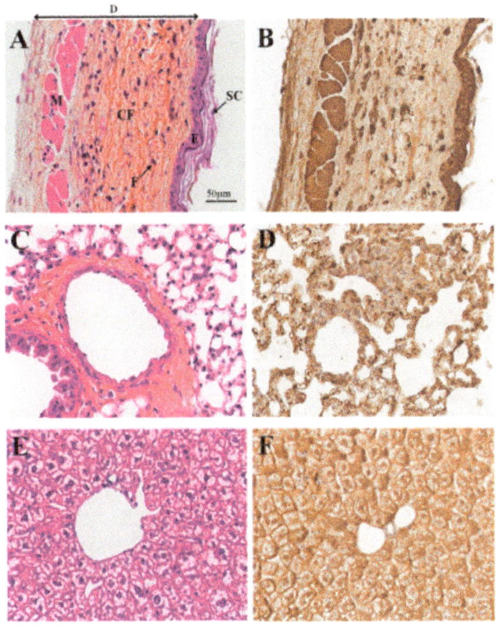

Figure 6: DING immunochemistry in different mouse tissues.

Skin (panels A and B), lung (panels C and D) and liver (panels E and F) were collected from control mice and processed for hemalun-phloxin-saffron staining (panels A, C and E) or anti-HPBP immunochemistry (panels B, D and F). The same magnification was used for all the photographs (see scale bar on panel A). Abbreviations are: SC = *stratum corneum*; E = epidermis; D = dermis; F = fibroblast; CF = collagen fibers and M = cutaneous underlying muscles.

In the heart, muscle fibers were mildly stained with anti-DING antibody in their entirety, including cardiomyocyte nuclei. DING protein was also detected in the nuclei of endothelial cells from blood vessels (data not shown).

The presence of a heterogeneous DING protein labeling was observed in the aortic media and adventitia. An intense labeling was evidenced in the myocyte and fibrocyte nuclei while a slighter labeling was displayed in the aortic amorphous ground substance enriched in chondroitin sulfate. We observed a lack of DING protein staining in elastic concentric membranes and collagen fibrils of the aorta (data not shown).

In the lung, a positive DING protein labeling was identified in cells of the pulmonary alveoli and bronchioles with folded mucous membranes (Figures 6C and 6D). DING protein labeling is mainly concentrated in cell nuclei. A positive staining is also present in cytoplasm but in a more diffuse pattern.

In the liver, all the hepatocytes are stained with anti-DING antibody. A strong staining was localized in the nucleus and plasma membrane of hepatocytes while a weaker staining was noticed in the cytoplasm (Figures 6E and 6F).

Altogether, these results clearly substantiate the presence of DING protein in all tested mouse tissues. At the cellular level, the strongest labeling was generally localized in nuclei and to a lesser extent in the cytoplasm of considered cells. Moreover, it is noteworthy that DING proteins were rarely spotted in the extracellular matrix. Indeed, DING proteins were only found in the aortic amorphous ground substance or in the skin epidermis.

DISCUSSION

Origin of Mice DING Proteins

The origin of DING proteins is prone to controversy [11]. Indeed, in the post-genomic era, their genes are still consistently missing from databases and the few partial nucleic sequences identified in non-annoted parts of genomes are highly similar to bacterial DING representatives, such as *Pseudomonas* DING proteins. In addition, their codon usage is similar to that of *Pseudomonas*, leading to the hypothesis of a bacterial origin [10]. Because of the numerous biological implications of DING proteins in eukaryotes, the hypothesis of *Pseudomonas*contamination has been discarded [11], [33], but the hypothesis of an unknown microbial symbiosis with eukaryotes remains a viable hypothesis [11]. In order to investigate the possibility of microbial symbiotic origin of DING proteins in eukaryotes, we analyzed wild-type and germ-free mouse plasma samples using western blot assays. The specificity of the used antibodies has been checked using competition assays (Figure 3). In addition, the experiment was performed using different kind of polyclonal antibodies, targeted against HPBP (Figure 2), and targeted against the very conserved N-terminal peptide of DING proteins. The similar patterns obtained in both experiments evidence the specificity of antibodies against DING proteins. The DING protein profiles were compared in both wild-type and germ-free C56BL/6 mouse plasma. The present study shows a similar distribution of DING proteins in either wild-type or germ-free C57BL/6 mouse plasma. This indicates that the presence of DING proteins in eukaryotes is likely not to be related to microbial symbiosis nor to contaminations. Therefore, regarding data provided in this study, the more likely hypothesis concerning the origin of eukaryotic DING proteins is a synthesis by eukaryotic cells themselves.

In addition, the presence of mouse plasma DING protein is consistent with the recent purification of a human DING representative HPBP in the blood as published by Morales et al. [16]. The existence of DING proteins in mammalian plasma suggests therefore that these proteins are synthesized by eukaryotic cells and are subsequently secreted in the circulating blood. To date, the secretion route of DING proteins remains unidentified. The sequence of DING protein genes or the full sequencing of HMW-DING proteins is likely to shed light on the understanding of mechanisms involved in the secretion of these proteins.

Omnipresence of DING Proteins in Mouse Tissues

As assessed by western blot analysis, DING proteins were detected in all explored mouse tissues, namely: brain, skin, heart, aorta, lung and liver. Our present results provide substantial evidence that the omnipresence of DING proteins in various mouse tissues is consistent with data previously published in other mammalian models. Indeed, the 40 kDa cotinine receptor, a member of the DING protein family, was purified from rat brains and sequenced [34]. More recently, the 38 kDa apolipoprotein HPBP has been isolated from human blood and its structure was solved using X-ray crystallography [16], [35]. HPBP being a apolipoprotein [16], it could be produced by hepatocytes and could be subsequently secreted in the circulating blood. Therefore, it is not surprising to detect DING proteins in both the mouse liver and plasma, in keeping with substantiated evidence from our experiments.

As mentioned above, only the 41 kDa DING protein was present in mouse liver, heart, brain, skin or lung. Further, the quantity of this protein was more or less similar in all investigated tissues. However, the distribution pattern of HMW-DING proteins was different depending on the nature of the related tissue. A total of four major HMW-DING at 140 kDa, 71 kDa (double bands), 62 kDa and 52 kDa were revealed in tissues, and two others at 130 kDa and 100 kDa were revealed in plasma samples. For example, the 52 kDa HMW-DING was predominant in the skin while the quantities of 140 and 71 kDa HMW-DING were more important in the liver as compared to the other tested mouse tissues. The diversity of HMW-DING proteins possibly results in different physiological involvements. The various forms of DING proteins detected in these assays, different than the classical 41 kDa form, might correspond to higher molecular weight DING protein precursors and truncated or maturated DING proteins. Because of the high sequence conservation within the DING protein family, these bands might also correspond to uncharacterized mouse DING proteins.

Intracellular Localization of Mouse DING Proteins

DING proteins are mainly localized in the nucleus of every cell types present in all investigated mouse tissues. Generally, nuclear stainings are very intense, except in the brain where neuronal nuclei exhibit either strong or reduced labeling. However, as regards other cerebral cells such as microglia or astroglia, all nuclei are deeply stained with anti-DING antibody. Since we investigated the cellular localization of DING proteins with antibodies that recognizes various DING protein forms, the observed signal could be derived from any of these forms. The presence of DING proteins in cell nucleus is consistent with biological activities identified for some of these proteins. For example, bacterial PfluDING protein isolated from *Pseudomonas fluorescens* is competent to stimulate the proliferation of cultured human fibroblasts as assessed by ^{3}H-thymidine incorporation experiment [7]. Another DING protein, p27^{SJ}, suppresses expression of HIV-1 genome [36]. This suppression of expression is mediated by the physical and functional association of p27^{SJ} with human C/EBPβ transcription factor and viral Tat transactivator. C/EBPβ is a factor stimulating HIV-1 gene transcription and regulating the expression of several genes involved in mammalian cell proliferation or differentiation [3], [36], [37]. Tat transactivator is a viral protein triggering the transcription of HIV-1 viral genes. Moreover, p27SJ possess a phosphatase activity inducing a dysregulation at S and G2/M phases in cell cycles related to alteration of Erk1/2 phosphorylation state [38]. In addition, the X-DING-CD4^{+} seems to interact with transcription factors in the nucleus, and is believed to be involved in the resistance to HIV infection of non-progressive patients [22], [39]. Since DING proteins are clearly involved in cell cycle regulation and cell proliferation which are complex processes within the nucleus, it may implies a nuclear localization of these proteins for an optimal activity. Our present investigation provides substantial evidence of the nuclear localization of DING proteins.

The nuclear localization of DING proteins raises the issue of the pathways for these proteins to the nucleus after synthesis in the cytoplasm. The import of proteins into the nucleus is tightly regulated and specific nuclear localization signals (NLS) are required for the transport process [40], [41]. Concerning DING proteins, none of the available protein sequences indicate the presence of such a NLS. However, despite being mostly isolated, sequenced and characterized as 38–41 kDa proteins, DING proteins exist also as higher molecular weight proteins [4]. Our study provides evidence to that effect. Then, it could be assumed that NLS might be present in HMW-DING proteins rather than in mature DING proteins. The sequencing of these HMW-DING proteins would be useful to address this issue. DING proteins are also detected in the cytoplasm of liver, lung, skin and aortic cells. Nevertheless, the quantity of DING proteins in cytoplasm is much lower than the quantity revealed in nucleus. DING proteins are completely absent in the cytoplasm of cerebral cells, including neurons, microglia and astroglia. Moreover, the liver is the only tested tissue of our study for which DING proteins was massively localized in the plasma membrane, reinforcing the hypothesis of a possible secretion of these proteins from liver cells to the circulating blood, via a secretion of the DING protein through cell plasma membrane. Since our study demonstrates that 52 kDa and 71 kDa-DING proteins are both intracellular and secreted, this could argue in favor of an unconventional route for DING proteins secretion rather than a secretion pathway via N-terminal secretion signal peptides.

CONCLUSION

Our study hereby, provides extensive data as regards intracellular DING protein localization in several mouse tissues. DING proteins seem to be ubiquitous in all tested tissues (i.e. brain, skin, heart, aorta, liver and lung) and exists as different isoforms, since we identified, in addition to the common 41 kDa-DING protein, High Molecular Weight DING proteins in all tested mice tissues. The localization of DING proteins is tissue-dependant: such proteins exhibit an intracellular localization in the brain while these proteins are detected either in the nucleus or cytoplasm of other investigated tissues. As for liver, DING proteins were also recovered in the plasma membrane, findings back up therefore the hypothesis of a possible secretion of DING proteins from liver to circulating blood, as evidenced by the presence of DING proteins both in intracellular and in plasma. Finally, the comparison of western blot profiles performed on blood plasma purified from wild-type and germ-free mice further evidenced the assumption that DING proteins are likely to be produced by eukaryotic cells.

REFERENCES

1. Berna A, Bernier F, Scott K, Stuhlmuller B (2002) Ring up the curtain on DING proteins. FEBS Lett 524: 6–10.
2. Berna A, Bernier F, Chabriere E, Perera T, Scott K (2008) DING proteins; novel members of a prokaryotic phosphate-binding protein superfamily which extends into the eukaryotic kingdom. Int J Biochem Cell Biol 40: 170–175.
3. Darbinian-Sarkissian N, Darbinyan A, Otte J, Radhakrishnan S, Sawaya BE, et al. (2006) p27(SJ), a novel protein in St John's Wort, that suppresses expression of HIV-1 genome. Gene Ther 13: 288–295.
4. Perera T, Berna A, Scott K, Lemaitre-Guillier C, Bernier F (2008) Proteins related to St. John's Wort p27SJ, a suppressor of HIV-1 expression, are ubiquitous in plants. Phytochemistry 69: 865–872.
5. Scott K, Wu L (2005) Functional properties of a recombinant bacterial DING protein: comparison with a homologous human protein. Biochim Biophys Acta 1744: 234–244.
6. Pantazaki AA, Tsolkas GP, Kyriakidis DA (2007) A DING phosphatase in Thermus thermophilus. Amino Acids.
7. Ahn S, Moniot S, Elias M, Chabriere E, Kim D, et al. (2007) Structure-function relationships in a bacterial DING protein. FEBS Lett 581: 3455–3460.
8. Moniot S, Elias M, Kim D, Scott K, Chabriere E (2007) Crystallization, diffraction data collection and preliminary crystallographic analysis of DING protein from Pseudomonas fluorescens. Acta Crystallograph Sect F Struct Biol Cryst Commun 63: 590–592.
9. Liebschner D, Elias M, Moniot S, Fournier B, Scott K, et al. (2009) Elucidation of the Phosphate Binding Mode of DING Proteins Revealed by Subangstrom X-ray Crystallography. J Am Chem Soc 131: 7879–7886.
10. Lewis AP, Crowther D (2005) DING proteins are from Pseudomonas. FEMS Microbiol Lett 252: 215–222.
11. Berna A, Scott K, Chabriere E, Bernier F (2009) The DING family of proteins: ubiquitous in eukaryotes, but where are the genes? Bioessays 31: 570–580.
12. Belenky M, Prasain J, Kim H, Barnes S (2003) DING, a genistein target in human breast cancer: a protein without a gene. J Nutr 133: 2497S–2501S.
13. Adams L, Davey S, Scott K (2002) The DING protein: an autocrine growth-stimulatory protein related to the human synovial stimulatory protein. Biochim Biophys Acta 1586: 254–264.
14. Contreras-Martel C, Carpentier P, Morales R, Renault F, Chesne-Seck ML, et al. (2006) Crystallization and preliminary X-ray diffraction analysis of human phosphate-binding protein. Acta Crystallograph Sect F Struct Biol Cryst Commun 62: 67–69.
15. Fokine A, Morales R, Contreras-Martel C, Carpentier P, Renault F, et al. (2003) Direct phasing at low resolution of a protein copurified with human paraoxonase (PON1). Acta Crystallogr D Biol Crystallogr 59: 2083–2087.
16. Morales R, Berna A, Carpentier P, Contreras-Martel C, Renault F, et al. (2006) Serendipitous discovery and X-ray structure of a human phosphate binding apolipoprotein. Structure 14: 601–609.
17. Shih DM, Gu L, Xia YR, Navab M, Li WF, et al. (1998) Mice lacking serum paraoxonase are susceptible to organophosphate toxicity and atherosclerosis. Nature 394: 284–287.
18. Rochu D, Renault F, Elias M, Hanne S, Cléry-Barraud C, et al. (2007) Functional states, storage and thermal

stability of human paraoxonase: Drawbacks, advantages and potential. Toxicology 142:

19. Rochu D, Chabriere E, Renault F, Elias M, Clery-Barraud C, et al. (2007) Stabilization of the active form(s) of human paraoxonase by human phosphate-binding protein. Biochem Soc Trans 35: 1616–1620.
20. Rochu D, Chabriere E, Elias M, Renault F, Clery-Barraud C, et al. (2008) Stabilisation of Active Form of Natural Human PON1 Requires HPBP in The Paraoxonases: Their Role in Disease Development and Xenobiotic Metabolism Springer Netherlands: 171–183.
21. Diemer H, Elias M, Renault F, Rochu D, Contreras-Martel C, et al. (2008) Tandem use of X-ray crystallography and mass spectrometry to obtain ab initio the complete and exact amino acids sequence of HPBP, a human 38-kDa apolipoprotein. Proteins 71: 1708–1720.
22. Lesner A, Shilpi R, Ivanova A, Gawinowicz MA, Lesniak J, et al. (2009) Identification of X-DING-CD4, a new member of human DING protein family that is secreted by HIV-1 resistant CD4+ T cells and has antiviral activity. Biochem Biophys Res Commun.
23. Kumar V, Yu S, Farell G, Toback FG, Lieske JC (2004) Renal epithelial cells constitutively produce a protein that blocks adhesion of crystals to their surface. Am J Physiol Renal Physiol 287: F373–383.
24. Hain N, Alsalameh S, Bertling WM, Kalden JR, Burmester GR (1990) Stimulation of rheumatoid synovial and blood T cells and lines by synovial fluid and interleukin-2: characterization of clones and recognition of a co-stimulatory effect. Rheumatol Int 10: 203–210.
25. Hain NA, Stuhlmuller B, Hahn GR, Kalden JR, Deutzmann R, et al. (1996) Biochemical characterization and microsequencing of a 205-kDa synovial protein stimulatory for T cells and reactive with rheumatoid factor containing sera. J Immunol 157: 1773–1780.
26. Franklin KBJ, Paxinos G (1997) The mouse brain in stereotaxic coordinates. Academic Press, San Diego
27. Lillie RD, Fullmer HM (1976) Histopathologic technique and practice. McGraw-Hill, New-York 208–209.
28. Renault F, Chabriere E, Andrieu JP, Dublet B, Masson P, et al. (2006) Tandem purification of two HDL-associated partner proteins in human plasma, paraoxonase (PON1) and phosphate binding protein (HPBP) using hydroxyapatite chromatography. J Chromatogr B Analyt Technol Biomed Life Sci 836: 15–21.
29. Collombet JM, Four E, Bernabe D, Masqueliez C, Burckhart MF, et al. (2005) Soman poisoning increases neural progenitor proliferation and induces long-term glial activation in mouse brain. Toxicology 208: 319–334.
30. Streit WJ (1990) An improved staining method for rat microglial cells using the lectin from Griffonia Simplicifolia (GSA I-B4). J Histochem Cytochem 38: 1683–1686.
31. Lowry OH, Rosebrough NJ, Farr AL, Randall RJ (1951) Protein measurement with the Folin phenol reagent. J Biol Chem 193: 265–275.
32. Collombet JM, Masqueliez C, Four E, Burckhart MF, Bernabe D, et al. (2006) Early reduction of NeuN antigenicity induced by soman poisoning in mice can be used to predict delayed neuronal degeneration in the hippocampus. Neurosci Lett 398: 337–342.
33. Berna A, Bernier F, Chabriere E, Elias M, Scott K, et al. (2009) For whom the bell tolls? DING proteins in health and disease. Cell Mol Life Sci.
34. Riah O, Dousset JC, Bofill-Cardona E, Courriere P (2000) Isolation and microsequencing of a novel cotinine receptor. Cell Mol Neurobiol 20: 653–664.
35. Morales R, Berna A, Carpentier P, Contreras-Martel C, Renault F, et al. (2007) Discovery and crystallographic structure of human apolipoprotein. Ann Pharm Fr 65: 98–107.
36. Darbinian N, Popov Y, Khalili K, Amini S (2008) Creation of a bi-directional protein transduction system for suppression of HIV-1 expression by p27SJ. Antiviral Res 79: 136–141.
37. Mukerjee R, Deshmane SL, Darbinian N, Czernik M, Khalili K, et al. (2008) St. John's Wort protein, p27(SJ), regulates the MCP-1 promoter. Mol Immunol 45: 4028–4035.
38. Darbinian N, Czernik M, Darbinyan A, Elias M, Chabriere E, et al. (2009) Evidence for phosphatase activity of p27SJ and its impact on the cell cycle. J Cell Biochem 107: 400–407.
39. Lesner A, Li Y, Nitkiewicz J, Li G, Kartvelishvili A, et al. (2005) A soluble factor secreted by an HIV-1-resistant cell line blocks transcription through inactivating the DNA-binding capacity of the NF-kappa B p65/p50 dimer. J Immunol 175: 2548–2554.
40. Kalderon D, Roberts BL, Richardson WD, Smith AE (1984) A short amino acid sequence able to specify nuclear location. Cell 39: 499–509.
41. Dingwall C, Robbins J, Dilworth SM, Roberts B, Richardson WD (1988) The nucleoplasmin nuclear location sequence is larger and more complex than that of SV-40 large T antigen. J Cell Biol 107: 841–849.

CHAPTER 12

IN SITU PROTEIN DETECTION FOR COMPANION DIAGNOSTICS

Gabriela Gremel, Karin Grannas, Lesley Ann Sutton, Fredrik Pontén and Agata Zieba

Keywords: Companion diagnostics, immunohistochemistry, Her2, alternative binders, proximity ligation assays

INTRODUCTION

Throughout recent decades, our understanding of the molecular basis of cancer development has dramatically improved. This is reflected in the growing number of targeted cancer therapies and significantly affects today's standard of care in oncology. Nevertheless, a prerequisite for an effective, targeted cancer treatment concerns the selection of patient, which creates a growing demand for reliable companion diagnostic devices. The rationale behind such developments is to ensure that treatment is not withheld from patients whom it may benefit while at the same time protecting them from overtreatment, the risk of unnecessary side effects and, most importantly, a delay in receiving treatment with a more suitable agent.

Companion diagnostics also play an important role during the pre-clinical stages of drug testing. A potent effect observed in a small patient population may be missed by the absence of a reliable companion diagnostic test. Conversely, a novel subset of patients may be found to benefit from treatment or no difference in efficiency may be detected, regardless of biomarker positivity. These issues pose a challenge to the parallel development of drug and companion diagnostic tests and consequently, the latter should be fully validated before the initiation of clinical trials and the trial design adjusted accordingly (1). Despite much advances, the corresponding regulatory framework is still incomplete and while the US Food and Drug Administration (FDA) dictates a stringent premarket approval procedure for all companion diagnostic devices, similar legislation is still under review in Europe (1). Currently, only 19 companion diagnostic devices have been approved by the FDA, 10 of which are intended for the detection of the human epidermal growth factor receptor 2 (ERBB2, also referred to as HER2)[1].

Most companion diagnostic tests used in a clinical setting are based on immunohistochemistry (IHC), real-time reverse transcription PCR (qRT-PCR), or *in situ* hybridization (ISH). With regard to ISH, assay systems based on either fluorescent (FISH) or colorimetric (CISH) signal detection have been established and each testing modality is associated with a number of advantages and disadvantages (Table 1).

Citation: Gremel G, Grannas K, Sutton LA, Pontén F and Zieba A (2013) In situ protein detection for companion diagnostics. Front. Oncol. 3:271. doi: 10.3389/fonc.2013.00271

Table 1: Advantages and disadvantages of currently used companion diagnostic techniques

Technique	Advantage	Disadvantage
IHC	Routinely performed; low technological requirements; time and cost effective; preservation of histological information; suitable for small tumor samples	Semi-quantitative; subjective interpretation of results; variability dependent on fixation procedure, staining protocol, and antibody selection
qRT-PCR	Quantitative; large dynamic range	No histological information retained; contamination of test results by stromal/normal tissue possible; increased technological requirements; increased time and cost requirements; variability dependent on tissue quality, RNA extraction/processing procedures and primer/probe selection
ISH	Quantitative for genetic alterations; higher reproducibility	Increased technological requirements (especially for FISH); increased time and cost requirements; added expertise in result interpretation necessary

IHC, immunohistochemistry; qRT-PCR, quantitative real-time PCR; ISH, in situ hybridization; FISH, fluorescent in situ hybridization; CISH, colorimetric in situ hybridization.

While the scope of companion diagnostics is broad, with this review we will focus on techniques designed to detect proteins in formalin-fixed, paraffin-embedded (FFPE) tissue. We will discuss currently applied companion diagnostic tests which use IHC and also novel developments regarding mutation-specific antibodies, *in situ* proximity ligation assays (PLA), and alternative protein binders.

APPLICATION OF IMMUNOHISTOCHEMISTRY IN CLINICALLY USED COMPANION DIAGNOSTICS

Estrogen Receptor

The introduction of tamoxifen, a selective estrogen receptor (ER) modulator, over 30 years ago has revolutionized the clinical management of breast cancer. However, since significant treatment benefits were only observed in ER-positive patients (2, 3), companion diagnostic testing became imperative. Originally, various ligand binding assays (LBAs) were used to quantify the expression of ER, however, they required homogenization of fresh frozen tumor material and were thus laborious in their execution. With the development of monoclonal antibodies targeting the ER and antigen retrieval methods for the use of FFPE tissue, LBAs were soon replaced and IHC became the standard diagnostic tool. Several grading systems were subsequently introduced to describe IHC-based ER expression levels, including (1) Allred score (range: 0–8) (4), (2) Quick score (range: 0–7) (5) (both of which are based on the sum of fraction and intensity units of the stained cells), (3) *J*-score (range: 0–3, based on the fraction of stained cells) (6) and (4) H-score (range: 0–300, based on the product of fraction and the intensity unit of stained cells) (7). Differences between positive/negative definitions together with variations regarding antibody clones, tissue fixation, antigen retrieval, and detection protocols, all contributed to a significant rate of variability in ER detection (8–10). For instance, a study headed by the UK National External Quality Assessment Scheme for Immunocytochemistry (NEQAS-ICC) reported false negativity rates ranging from 30 to 60% following the testing of a standardized sample with low ER expression by 200 laboratories throughout 26 countries (8).

Due to the historic nature of ER testing, there are currently no FDA-approved companion diagnostic devices available. To minimize inter-laboratory variation, the American Society of Clinical Oncology and the College of American Pathologists (ASCO/CAP) have recently published a document outlining their recommendations for the immunohistochemical testing of ER in breast cancer (11). The optimal testing conditions and tissue handling requirements were defined together with guidelines for both the internal and external quality assurance procedure. The same guidelines were also applicable to the detection of the progesterone receptor (PR) via IHC. PR is located downstream of ER and a positive PR test result may be indicative of an intact estrogen signaling cascade (12). This line of thinking was corroborated by the finding that patients with PR positive tumors had a better prognosis than patients with ER-positive/PR negative breast cancers (13). Alternative methods for the detection of ER and PR are continuously under investigation and Oncotype DX is one such example. This is a qRT-PCR-based assay system designed to estimate the probability of distant tumor recurrence in tamoxifen-treated, node-negative breast cancers (14) and measures the expression PR and ER, together with 19 other genes, in mRNA extracted from FFPE tissue. Proof-of-concept studies on the applicability of Oncotype DX as a companion diagnostic tool for tamoxifen treatment reported varying conclusions. In a study supported by Genomic Health Inc., Badve and colleagues reasoned that ER/PR determination using Oncotype DX performed comparably well to IHC-based detection systems (15). This was in contrast to an independent evaluation by Kraus et al. who concluded that IHC was superior to the Oncotype DX qRT-PCR-based test, not only due to higher sensitivity but also the lower cost, the ease of application and the preservation of morphological information (16).

Human Epidermal Growth Factor Receptor 2

Overexpression of the HER2 protein and/or amplification of the HER2-encoding gene have been associated with an unfavorable prognosis in several types of cancer, including breast, gastric, and pancreatic cancer (17–19). Trastuzumab (Herceptin), an antibody-based inhibitor, was the first HER2-targeted drug to be approved for the treatment of breast cancer and has since been shown to significantly improve survival in a metastatic and adjuvant setting (20, 21). Numerous studies support the close relationship between HER2 positivity and trastuzumab responsiveness (20, 22) and bearing in mind that a HER2-amplification rate of approximately 25% occurs in breast cancer, initial clinical trials may not have yielded significant data had no pre-selection of patients according to HER2 status taken place (23). Since gene-amplification is the primary cause of HER2 overexpression (24), both FISH- (or CISH-) and IHC-based companion diagnostic devices have been approved by the FDA. Nevertheless, the initial evaluation of HER2 status is usually performed using an IHC-based method and only ambiguous (or equivocal) cases are subjected to FISH reflex testing. Substantial inter-laboratory variations in test results are an inherent problem when considering IHC-based tests. Similar to the guidelines established for ER, ASCO/CAP has produced recommendations for HER2 testing in breast cancer (25, 26). In contrast to the instructions for the commonly used FDA-approved HercepTest (Dako), which states that a finding of more than 10% of cells with strong, uniform membrane staining qualifies as a positive result, the ASCO/CAP guidelines require complete intense membrane staining in >30% of cells in order to qualify as a positive test result following IHC testing. In addition, unlike the FDA-approved cut-off ratio of 2.0 for HER2/Chromosome 17 centromere (CEP17) testing via FISH (or four HER2 copies in assays without internal CEP17 probes), ASCO/CAP considered the range of ratios between 1.8 and 2.2 (or four to six HER2 copies) as equivocal and stated that only cases with HER2/CEP17 ratios >2.2 (or more than six copies of HER2) could be deemed to be positive based on FISH analysis. The aim of the new ASCO/CAP guidelines was to reduce the number of inconclusive cases and although some groups were positive to these new definitions (27, 28), others saw no added benefit (29). While high concordance between IHC- and FISH-based HER2 testing was demonstrated by several studies, thus justifying the use of routine IHC as an initial test (30), critics are keen to highlight the technical superiority of FISH over IHC and consequently advocate FISH as the gold standard for HER2 testing (31). Hence, it is evident that more conclusive studies on the clinical significance of both testing modality are required.

Epidermal Growth Factor Receptor

The epidermal growth factor receptor (EGFR) is a prominent therapeutic target in both colorectal and non-small cell lung cancer (NSCLC). In colorectal cancer, it is primarily targeted by the monoclonal antibody-based drugs cetuximab and panitumumab. These drugs target the extracellular domain of the EGFR and block down-stream signaling. Clinical trials for both agents initially required the pre-selection of patients based on positive expression of the EGFR protein, as determined by IHC, however, it soon became evident that IHC-based protein expression levels did not correlate with therapy outcome (32, 33) and that even patients with EGFR-negative tumors may benefit from EGFR-targeted therapy (34, 35). The causes for this discrepancy may be of a technical nature and connected to the variability/sensitivity of immunohistochemical techniques, or they may be a direct consequence of biological determinants. For instance, metastatic tumors may have lost the expression of EGFR, rendering them unresponsive to therapy (36). In addition, Chung and co-workers reasoned that antibodies used within IHC-based detection systems were unable to discriminate between high- and low-affinity EGFRs. Consequently, the relative distribution of such high- and low-affinity EGFRs within colorectal cancer tissue may be crucial in determining the response to therapy (34). Furthermore, it has been noted that therapeutic antibodies that target EGFR may induce antibody-dependent, cell-mediated cytotoxicity, resulting in an indirect beneficial effect owing to the recruitment of cytotoxic immune cells such as monocytes and natural killer cells to the tumor (34).

While the immunohistochemical detection of EGFR expression did not prove to be decisive in determining the clinical response, promising data has been generated in support of using the EGFR gene copy number as a predictive biomarker for EGFR-targeted therapy (37). Nevertheless, in order to achieve definitive proof and to facilitate the development of standardized testing modalities further investigation is required. In NSCLC, EGFR is targeted primarily using the small molecule inhibitors gefitinib and erlotinib. In contrast to colorectal cancer, mutations within the EGFR in NSCLC are common and mutational testing is recommended for all NSCLC cases (38). The application of mutation-specific antibodies for this purpose is discussed below. A further distinguishing feature regarding the testing of EGFR in colorectal cancer and NSCLC is that in the latter, IHC positivity or high EGFR gene copy numbers showed no conclusive correlation with treatment response (38).

V-kit Hardy-Zuckerman 4 Feline Sarcoma Viral Oncogene Homolog

Immunohistochemistry provides an excellent tool for the differential diagnosis of gastrointestinal stromal tumors (GIST). This is largely due to the fact that greater than 85% of GIST test positive for v-kit Hardy-Zuckerman 4 feline sarcoma viral oncogene homolog (KIT), in contrast to the negative result generated by most other mesenchymal tumors (39, 40). Imatinib mesylate (Gleevec, Novartis, Basel, Switzerland) is a specific tyrosine kinase inhibitor that exhibits high therapeutic activity in patients with chronic myeloid leukemia by targeting the fusion protein BCR-ABL (41). Additional targets of imatinib mesylate include the platelet-derived growth factor receptor (PDGFR) and KIT. For patients with unresectable or metastatic GIST, a positive immunohistochemical staining for KIT was initially required as an entry criteria into clinical trials investigating the efficacy of imatinib mesylate (42, 43). Significant clinical responses were recorded and this revolutionized the management of advanced GIST, a malignancy that had previously failed to respond to conventional chemotherapy. Activating mutations within the KIT gene and, to a lesser degree, PDGFR, are commonly found in patients with GIST and depending on their location within the coding region of the respective gene, they are highly correlated with the likelihood of a response to imatinib mesylate treatment (44, 45). That notwithstanding, since a small percentage of patients with GIST do not express detectable levels of KIT or do not harbor mutations within KIT/PDGFR (44–46) IHC or mutational analysis should not be used to deny treatment with imatinib mesylate since these patients may still be sensitive to this therapy.

Anaplastic Lymphoma Kinase Rearrangements

In addition to EGFR, the anaplastic lymphoma kinase (ALK) represents a second therapeutic target in NSCLC. Chromosomal rearrangements involving the associated gene have been detected in approximately 5% of cases, most frequently resulting in the fusion to echinoderm microtubule-associated protein-like 4 (EML4) and the constitutive expression of a chimeric tyrosine kinase protein (47, 48). Second-line treatment of NSCLC patients with confirmed ALK rearrangements, using the small molecule inhibitor crizotinib, has recently been shown to significantly prolong progression-free survival compared to standard chemotherapy (49). The current "gold standard" for ALK rearrangement testing is dual-color break-apart FISH. However, interpretation of test results may be challenging since EML4 and ALK are located on the same chromosome, resulting in limited separation of the 5′ and 3′ probes. To define a positive test result, only signals separated by more than two signal diameters and/or single 3′ signals (correlating to the ALK kinase domain) should be counted. In addition, at least 50 cells should be reviewed with a positive signal detectable in at least 15% (50). The immunohistochemical detection of ALK has been considered as an attractive addition to routine FISH testing. Since ALK is not expressed in lung tissue unless driven by promoter rearrangement, a good correlation between IHC and FISH results and low IHC background staining have been reported. In addition, a number of studies confirm that IHC-negative cases are almost exclusively negative in FISH analysis and therefore indicate that IHC could be applicable as a quick and cost-effective screening tool for ALK rearrangements (51–54). FISH reflex testing for all IHC positive cases has been proposed, somewhat similar to the evaluation strategy for HER2 (55). Interestingly, the percentage of ALK rearrangement positive cells during FISH evaluation did not significantly correlate with the response to crizotinib (56). Nonetheless, comprehensive data on the correlation between the intensity of ALK staining as determined by IHC and treatment response is still lacking.

MUTATION-SPECIFIC ANTIBODIES

The selection of patients for a targeted cancer treatment frequently relies on the detection of specific gene mutations. The routinely applied techniques are generally based on the isolation of chromosomal DNA from fresh, frozen or FFPE material and analysis can involve various techniques such as mutation-specific real-time PCR, direct sequencing, mass spectrometry, mismatch ligation assays, high-resolution melting curve assays, or denaturating high-performance liquid chromatography, among others. A common drawback relates to the fact that information on tissue morphology is lost and also that "contamination" of tumor material with normal cells may hamper detection or obscure the results. In addition, increased demands on sample size and quality and extra requirements regarding technology and expertise, associated with higher cost and expenditure of time, frequently apply. The development of mutation-specific antibodies and their application in routine IHC may provide a convenient addition to DNA-based profiling techniques.

BRAF V600E

The v-raf murine sarcoma viral oncogene homolog B1 (BRAF) represents an outstanding target for the development of a mutation-specific antibody. Mutations of the associated gene occur in a range of human malignancies including cutaneous melanoma, colorectal cancer, NSCLC, papillary thyroid cancer, and hairy-cell leukemia (57–59). By far, the most common BRAF mutation results in the substitution of valine for glutamic acid at position 600 (V600E), leading to the constitutive activation of the protein's kinase domain. In human cutaneous melanoma, mutated BRAF has been detected in 40–50% of cases, with up 90% of these alterations concerning the V-E substitution at codon 600 (60). Vemurafenib and dabrafenib are two potent small molecule inhibitor drugs that specifically target BRAF V600E and have demonstrated remarkable response rates in metastatic melanoma patients (61, 62). Mutational testing of the patient tumor material is required before commencement of treatment and is to date commonly based on the detection of genomic alterations. As an addition to DNA testing, Capper et al. recently proposed a mutation-specific antibody for the detection of BRAF V600E in FFPE tissue specimens by means of IHC (Figure 1) (63). The results obtained from using this antibody to determine the BRAF mutational status in melanoma and thyroid cancer samples were identical to those achieved following DNA sequencing-based profiling. These results have since been substantiated by numerous studies with similarly high levels of specificity and sensitivity (up to 100%, respectively) (64–68).

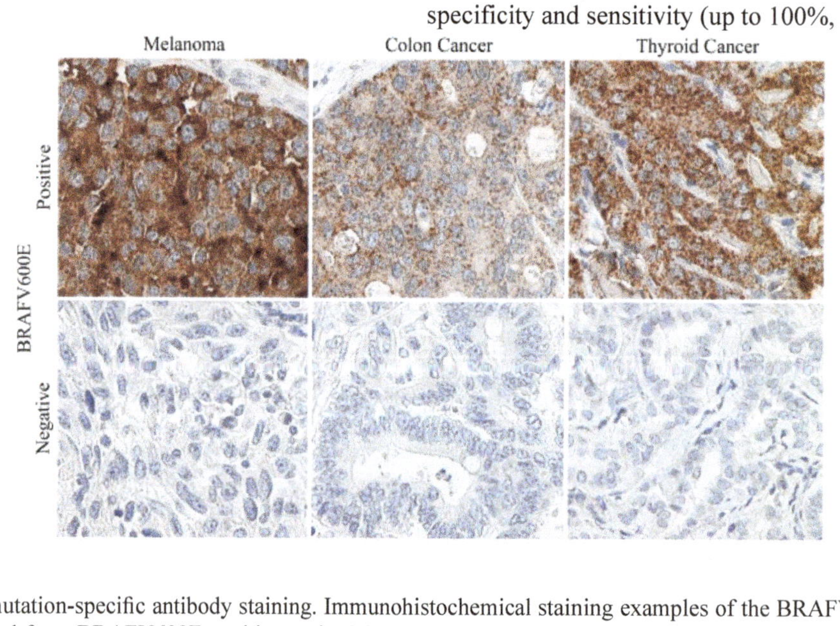

Figure 1: BRAFV600E mutation-specific antibody staining. Immunohistochemical staining examples of the BRAFV600E mutation-specific antibody VE1 are presented for a BRAFV600E-positive and a BRAFV600E-negative case of melanoma, colon cancer, and thyroid cancer,

respectively. BRAFV600E-positive staining is generally detected as a granular, cytoplasmic signal that can easily be distinguished from BRAFV600E-negative cases. In the presented example images, 3,3′-Diaminobenzidine (DAB) was used as a chromogen.

In samples where the number of tumor cells is low, IHC-based BRAF testing was suggested to be more sensitive than direct DNA sequencing or high-resolution melting curve analysis (64, 65). In addition, IHC-based staining results showed low inter-observer variability (68). Nevertheless, despite the benefits of using IHC-based methods for determining the presence/absence of mutations within the BRAF gene, the presence of (non-specific) strong, nuclear staining may complicate the assessment of staining results. In addition, false-negative IHC results may occur due to unsuitable or incomplete tissue fixation, the presence of necrotic or pre-necrotic tissue areas or low levels of total protein expression (63, 64). The latter may be controlled for through the use of an additional antibody capable of detecting total BRAF protein expression. With regard to the intra-tumor heterogeneity of BRAF V600E, only few cases with non-homogenous expression have been observed following immunohistochemical detection (67, 69). These results are in direct contrast to previous reports describing significant variability of BRAF mutational status among individual cells within a tumor and warrant further investigation (70, 71). Regarding the possible relationship between BRAF V600E protein expression and clinical outcome, no significant correlation was seen between the percentage of BRAF V600E positive tumor cells and the response to treatment with either dabrafenib or vemurafenib (72). Similarly, the total intensity of mutation-specific antibody staining did not significantly correlate with patient outcome.

EGFR L858R and E746_A750del

Epidermal growth factor receptor mutations have been detected in 2–17% of NSCLC patients from Europe and the United States, however, the mutational frequency increases to 30% when analyzing cases from East Asia (73–75). Specific mutations, in particular those affecting the EGFR kinase domain, have been associated with response to gefitinib and erlotinib treatment (76, 77). The two most common types of EGFR mutations are in-frame deletions of exon 19 and a leucine to arginine substitution at codon 858 (L858R) in exon 21. Taken together, alterations at these sites account for up to 90% of all EGFR mutations (78). Exon 19 deletions may affect a varying number of nucleotides. For example, E746_A750del results in a five amino acid deletion in the corresponding protein and is the most common deletion detected, occurring in approximately 70% of cases (79). The application of mutation-specific antibodies designed to target L858R and the E746_A750del modification, have yielded varying levels of detection specificity and sensitivity. For L858R, several studies reported sensitivity values in the range of 70–100% and specificities exceeding 95% (79–83). While these results were promising, sensitivities as low as 36 and 40% have also been described for the same antibody clone (84, 85). Similarly, regarding the E746_A750del-specific antibody, the same studies published sensitivity and specificity values of 40–100% and 95–100%, respectively. The possible sources of variation are numerous and include the application of different scoring systems, discrepancy between the definitions of positivity/negativity, different DNA-based reference techniques, different tissue fixation methods, and the types of specimens analyzed. While initial attempts to determine optimal tissue preparation and staining evaluation have been presented (86), additional steps toward a standardized protocol for the detection of EGFR mutations using IHC should be undertaken.

The overall high levels of specificity associated with IHC-based EGFR-mutational testing imply that IHC may be suitable as a pre-screening tool for the identification of NSCLC patients that are eligible for EGFR-inhibitor treatment. Since a number of mutations are not currently detectable by antibody-based profiling, the additional testing of IHC-negative cases using direct DNA sequencing or similar assays is necessary (79, 81). The applicability of IHC in predicting response to EGFR-targeted therapy remains controversial. Confirming the importance of EGFR-mutational status for treatment response, positive IHC staining has been associated with longer progression-free survival compared to IHC-negative or -equivocal cases (83, 87). In addition, high mutant EGFR expression (as defined by the sum of scores for fraction and intensity) was significantly related to elevated progression-free survival but not overall survival (88) and a fraction of positive tumor cells exceeding 50% of all cells predicted better response to EGFR inhibition treatment in univariate but not multivariate analysis (89). Despite the aforementioned results, a study by Kato and co-workers could not detect a significant correlation between IHC staining and treatment response or survival (82). Shortcomings in the significance of IHC-based detection methods in predicting survival benefit, in particular when compared to DNA-based techniques, may occur due to the limited mutation spectrum detected via IHC. Furthermore, EGFR-mutation-specific antibodies have been shown to occasionally detect mutations associated with EGFR-inhibitor resistance via mechanisms that are not yet fully understood (84).

Alternative Protein Binders

In situ affinity-based detection of proteins remains one of the best sources of information about either the healthy status of an individual tissue or potential pathological changes, and is thus applicable within several medical settings. Molecular imaging allows for the early detection and classification of many human diseases and, when specific, permits improved, target-directed therapies. Molecules generated through immunization such as polyclonal, monospecific polyclonal, and monoclonal antibodies continue to be the best established and most widely used binders in diagnostics (90, 91). Methods for the detection of proteins based on antibody recognition often encounter problems due to poor selectivity and/or sensitivity (92). Poorly characterized antibodies and/or insufficient quality control often render them as unsuitable for demanding applications such as companion diagnostics (93). Commercially available antibodies frequently perform very differently within various laboratories and often do not perform as advertised, thus raising doubts regarding their reliability when incorporated into assays requiring high specificity (94). Antibodies can be biochemically and physiologically modified and use of their derivatives, such as single chain variable fragments (scFv) or Fab fragments, may result in the improved detection of a wide range of target molecules (Figure 2) (95). Currently only a few antibodies and recombinant proteins are used within clinical settings, largely due to the reasons outlined above. Recombinant binders that are generated in immune-free, *in vitro*-based approaches, hold the potential of taking priority over conventional antibodies (96). Stability, specificity, ease of manipulation, low cost, high throughput, and reproducibility of production are some of the advantages that make novel scaffold molecules highly desirable (97). Alternative binders are promising molecules for novel approaches in individualized medicine (Figure 2). They can serve as personalized molecular imaging tools for *in vivo*, live diagnostics of the changes occurring in the expression of markers following treatment (95).

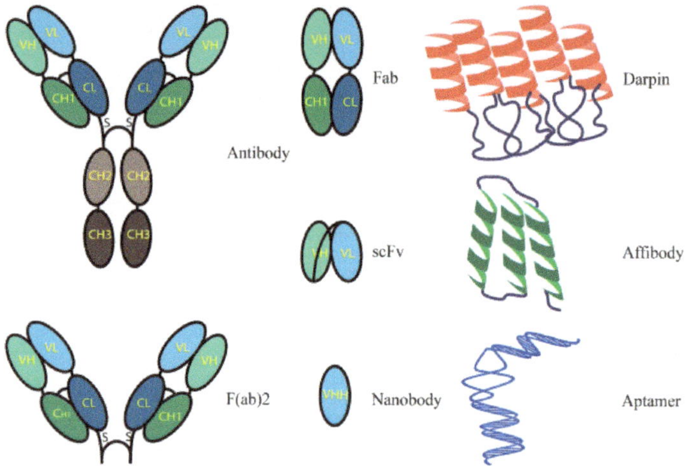

Figure 2: Schematic representation of binder formats.

Recombinant Antibody Fragments

Antibody fragments are generated in order to obtain binders with improved characteristics, compared to conventional antibodies, but similar functional and recognition properties. Fab and $F(ab)_2$ fragments are antigen-binding fragments generated after proteolysis of full length antibodies. Single chain variable fragments (scFvs) are smaller than Fab fragments and are composed of genetically linked light and heavy chains containing variable regions. These molecules can also exist as dimers (98). Another class of antibody-derived antigen-binding molecules, termed nanobodies, are small, single-domain polypeptides derived from the variable part of the heavy chain (VHH) of light-chain deficient antibodies that were originally discovered in camelids (camels, llamas) (99, 100). Their reduced size, greater stability and solubility, and antibody-like binding characteristics make nanobodies ideal for use in the targeting and imaging of antigens in live cells, protein precipitation *in vivo*, and targeted enzymes modulations (101–103). As a result of their smaller size (only 15 kDa), nanobodies can bind to epitopes that are hidden or shielded and reach affinities within the range of nanomolar to picomolar. Nanobodies are highly specific for their targets and have no known cross-reactivity to structurally related proteins, which makes them excellent tools for targeting kinases and tyrosine phosphatases. In addition, nanobodies have technological advantages that render them superior to conventional antibodies. They are easily modified to avoid chemically reactive groups such a primary amines or to alter the primary amine number to allow more selective and controlled chemical conjugation. The selection of binders for certain applications is usually based on their performance in experimental settings and depends on their preference for particular epitopes and the accessibility of binding sites.

Affibody Molecules

Affibody molecules are small (~7 kDa), alpha-helical *Z*-domain of Staphylococcal protein A, immune-independent affinity molecules that target a wide range of proteins (104, 105). They can be produced in functional form both via recombinant expression in *Escherichia coli* or peptide synthesis. They possess picomolar affinities, are highly soluble and stable. In addition, they are cysteine-free which prevents non-specific binding events when applied to tissues. Furthermore, the lack of cysteine provides an opportunity for site-specific labeling through the introduction of unique cysteine molecules. High affinity affibodies were engineered against targets such as the IL2 receptor, Alzheimer's amyloid-beta peptide or EGFR (106–108). They have been used in various types of experiments and are intended for both *in vivo* and *in vitro* imaging and also therapeutic applications including the detection of HER2 within different experimental settings (109, 110).

Designed Ankyrin Repeat Proteins

Designed ankyrin repeat proteins (DARPins) are potent alternatives to conventional antibodies. They detect antigens with high specificity and picomolar affinity, are independent of target immunogenicity and possess attractive molecular properties such as small size and high stability (111). They are synthetic, non-immunoglobulin binding proteins that form scaffolds containing tandem repeats of an elementary, structural motif, typically composed of 33 amino acid residues folded into a β-turn followed by two antiparallel α-helices. A single protein may contain up to 29 repeats of this motif. The production of DARPins does not require the use of animals at any step, therefore permitting the large scale, parallel production of variable binders. DARPins are correctly folded in both prokaryotes and eukaryotes, due to the absence of disulfide bonds, which enables their use in a variety of functional assays (112). They can easily be genetically modified to form fusion proteins and site-specifically targeted for chemical conjugation. DARPins against a wide range of protein targets, including extracellular, intracellular, and membrane proteins, were generated with high yield from synthetic libraries and successfully used as replacements for conventional antibodies. One such example is the DARPins generated against HER2; these displayed higher specificity and similar sensitivity when compared to FDA-approved antibodies for the *in situ* identification of HER2 expression status in FFPE breast cancer tissue (113). DARPins can easily be made functional for use in various biomedical applications through the introduction of site-specific, clickable modifications. Such alterations do not affect their physical properties (114).

Aptamers

Aptamers are a class of small, synthetic, self-folding, and single-stranded RNA or DNA molecules that form secondary and tertiary structures and specifically bind to proteins, small molecules, or other cellular targets such as nucleic acids (115, 116). They are comparable to antibodies in terms of their target recognition capabilities, their binding affinities, and the diversity of applications that they can be used in; however, they possess numerous significant characteristics that render them advantageous over their protein equivalents. Aptamers are highly specific, non-immunogenic, redox-insensitive, and temperature- and pH-tolerant. In addition, they do not have hydrophobic cores which are usual in proteins and, therefore, they do not aggregate. In order to select aptamers, information on protein conformation is not required, a feature which can be useful for screening for unidentified disease biomarkers. Aptamers can be generated through cell-based aptamer selection that utilizes differences between the molecular signatures of any two different cell types. The selected aptamers selectively bind to an unknown protein within one cell type only, are cross-linked to their targets and once the complex is purified the targets can be analyzed by mass spectrometry (117). Therefore, the cell-based selection of aptamer molecules has great potential for the development of specific probes suitable for biomarker discovery and companion diagnostics development. Since chemical synthesis is a process that is well defined and highly reproducible, the production of aptamers can easily be scaled up. They can be synthesized with specific, custom tailored functional groups attached to 5′ or 3′ termini which creates an easy approach to conjugation and multiplexing *in situ* assays. Furthermore, aptamer conjugations do not generally alter their binding affinity. With advances in imaging techniques, aptamers are already considered as prospective reagents for *in situ* targeting. To date, several aptamers have been developed against important clinical targets such as PDGF, von Willebrand factor (vWF), E-selectin, vascular endothelial growth factor (VEGF), and prostate specific membrane antigen (PSMA) and their applicability within a clinical setting is currently being investigated (118–121).

IN SITU PROXIMITY LIGATION ASSAY

Using traditional IHC techniques, the level of protein expression can easily be determined. However, the functional status of a cell cannot be evaluated by the level of expressed protein alone. The activity of signaling pathways, as assessed by the analysis of post-translation modifications (PTMs) and protein interactions, needs to be determined and taken into consideration (122). Cancer does not consist of a homologous mass of cells but of complex, heterogeneous cell populations that are affected by interactions with each other and the surrounding environment. Therefore, the analysis of cancer tissue at single cell resolution provides a much better understanding of the differences in signaling status and activity (123). *In situ* PLA enables a localized and specific detection by utilizing oligonucleotide-conjugated antibodies to determine the proximity between one or more targeted epitopes. This makes it a suitable method for detecting molecular events in cells and tissue, for example the status of a signaling pathway. The use of two independent binders and the additional requirement of proximity for reporting enable the specific detection of proteins, protein–protein interactions, and PTMs (124). Proximity ligation converts the recognition of a protein, protein complex, or PTM by two or more antibodies into an amplifiable, circular DNA molecule (Figure 3). Upon proximal binding of a pair of oligonucleotide-conjugated antibodies (PLA probes), the oligonucleotides guide the formation of a circle after applying two additional, single-stranded DNA molecules. This circular DNA molecule is then ligated and amplified by phi29 polymerase within a rolling-circle amplification (RCA) reaction, resulting in a localized, concatameric product. The latter is visualized by hybridization of detection oligonucleotides labeled with fluorophores or horse radish peroxidase (Figure 3) (125). Due to the environment of fixed cells and tissue the amplification product will collapse into a bundle with a diameter of approximately 1 μM (126) that can then be visualized as a bright dot that is quantifiable and easily distinguished from the background (127).

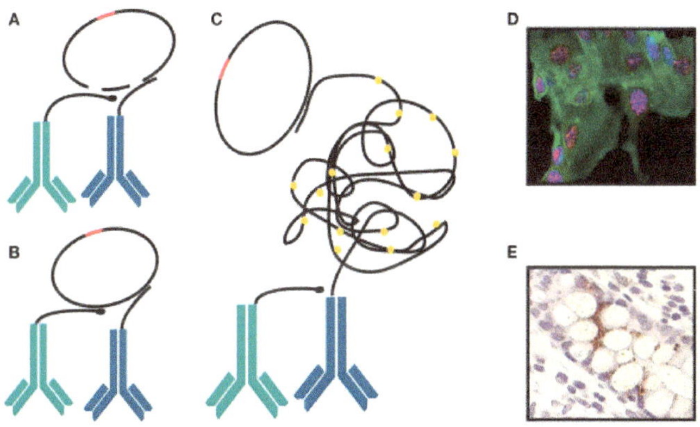

Figure 3: Proximity ligation assay. (A) Two probes stay in close proximity by binding to a protein or two proteins present in one complex. **(B)** They are joined and circularized by DNA ligation upon introduction of linear connector oligonucleotides. After ligation, rolling-circle amplification (RCA) is initiated. One of the proximity probes is used as a primer. **(C)** The single-stranded RCA products are hybridized with labeled detection oligonucleotide complementary to a multiplied motif in the sequence of the RCA product. The detection oligonucleotide can be labeled with fluorophore **(D)** or a horse radish peroxidase **(E)**.

Heterogeneity within a sample increases the demands on the dynamic range of a method in order to allow for the detection of both abundant and scarce targets within the same sample. *In situ* PLA uses an amplifiable DNA circle as a reporter molecule and by using reagents that give rise to three variants of the reporter DNA circles and adding them at decreasing concentrations the dynamic range of the PLA is increased. By labeling the circles with different fluorophores, the readout can be adjusted to the fluorophore whose concentration gives rise to quantifiable and easily distinguishable signals. In a heterogeneous sample, different readout fluorophores can be used for different parts of the sample, enabling the detection of a target that varies greatly within the sample without the risk of signal saturation. As the size of a patient sample is often limited, this approach reduces the need to optimize the binder concentration and enables the evaluation of patient samples where knowledge on the expected results is limited (128).

Multiplex *in situ* PLA permits the parallel analyses of multiple protein complexes involved in signaling pathways directly in tissue and cells thus making it possible to compare levels of protein complexes between individual cells and also providing information regarding the spatial distributions of these complexes. A tag-specific sequence within the PLA probe targeting a protein gives rise to a DNA circular molecule that carries information on the identity of the target protein. The amplified tags in the RCA products can then be visualized using oligonucleotides labeled with different fluorophores, to uniquely recognize the tag sequences corresponding to a certain target (129). *In situ* PLA has been shown to provide valuable information about the status of signaling pathways by detecting molecular events such as dimerizations, the formation of protein complexes and PTMs. It enables the detection of activity at different levels within a signaling pathway, thereby enabling specific aberrations to be pinpointed. *In situ* PLA has been utilized in studies investigating both EGFR dimerization and receptor activation, which has been proposed to play a crucial role during tumor progression, and also the development of drug resistance. Dimerization and aberrant activity has been shown to be independent of EGFR expression, explaining why the deregulated expression of the EGFR in several types of human malignancies was shown to have limited value as a prognostic or diagnostic marker. Receptor dimerization events detected by mutation-specific PLA appeared to be more suitable for the selection of patients for EGFR-targeted treatment (130).

Similarly, the overexpression of human epidermal growth factor receptors (HERs) has been linked to poor prognosis in patients with early breast cancer. Dimers containing the HER2 isoform were shown to be more stable and have prolonged active signaling compared to HER2 deficient dimers. Elevated levels of HER2-HER2 and HER2-HER3 complexes detected by PLA showed a significant association with decreased recurrent-free survival and a reduction in overall survival of breast cancer patients, proving that PLA and the detection of cellular signaling processes can be successfully implemented in studies on prognostic markers in clinical specimens (131). Through the application of *in situ* PLA, it is now possible to screen for the effects of a drug treatment on intracellular signaling, providing information on the specific level of signaling pathways. Being able to study primary cell lines and patient tissue sample gives valuable information of the signaling status within a specific tumor and allows to predict the response to a certain therapy (132). PLA technologies have been used to address a variety of biomedical problems and demonstrated the potential to address some difficulties, both concerning the validation of biomarkers and the applicability for clinical diagnostics. Implementing PLA techniques as an alternative to IHC in everyday laboratory practice allows for a more precise and quantitative evaluation of antibody performance characteristics and their suitability for an anticipated analytical use. Application of the PLA technique provides an opportunity to develop a high-quality procedure for *in situ* detection of proteins and signaling pathways in companion diagnostics. This will offer the medical industry powerful, universally applicable tools for clinical research and routine diagnostics.

CONCLUSION

Affinity proteomics for the analysis of proteins as companion diagnostics requires access to reagents that can be used in specific detection reactions. The comprehensive validation and improvement of existing and newly generated antibodies to obtain well characterized, high-quality, and well-controlled resources as tools for large scale studies of the human proteome in health and disease is a widely acknowledged demand. In many routine clinical, diagnostic, and life science applications, antibodies have proven to be the reagents of choice. IHC is routinely performed in the majority of clinical laboratories and widely acknowledged as superior to other analysis techniques regarding time- and cost-effective application. In selected cases, IHC and mutation-specific antibodies may even provide an attractive alternative to DNA-based testing methods. As a highly valuable resource documenting the availability and identification of novel biomarker candidates, the Human Protein Atlas[2] project has generated antibodies targeting proteins from over 15,000 genes, corresponding to about 75% of all human protein-coding genes (133, 134). All antibodies are routinely subjected to a series of validation steps, including protein arrays, western blots, and immunofluorescence and used to assess protein expression patterns in a broad spectrum of normal and cancer tissues through application of IHC. Nevertheless, efforts to detect proteins when high specificity is required often fail. Hence, there is a strong need for better methods and reagents for assessing protein expression in tissues as means of companion diagnostics and alternative binders or PLA in combination with existing antibodies represent promising candidate alternatives.

Conflict of Interest Statement

The authors declare that the research was conducted in the absence of any commercial or financial relationships that could be construed as a potential conflict of interest.

ACKNOWLEDGMENTS

This work was supported by grants from the Knut and Alice Wallenberg Foundation, from the Swedish Cancer Society and from the European Union Seventh Framework Program under grant agreement 241481 (Affinomics).

REFERENCES

1. Jorgensen JT. Companion diagnostics in oncology – current status and future aspects. *Oncology* (2013) 85:59–68. doi: 10.1159/000353454
2. Fisher B, Redmond C, Brown A, Wolmark N, Wittliff J, Fisher ER, et al. Treatment of primary breast cancer with chemotherapy and tamoxifen. *N Engl J Med* (1981) 305:1–6. doi:10.1056/NEJM198107023050101
3. Fisher B, Redmond C, Brown A, Wickerham DL, Wolmark N, Allegra J, et al. Influence of tumor estrogen and progesterone receptor levels on the response to tamoxifen and chemotherapy in primary breast cancer. *J Clin Oncol* (1983) 1:227–41.
4. Allred DC, Harvey JM, Berardo M, Clark GM. Prognostic and predictive factors in breast cancer by immunohistochemical analysis. *Mod Pathol* (1998) 11:155–68.
5. Barnes DM, Harris WH, Smith P, Millis RR, Rubens RD. Immunohistochemical determination of oestrogen receptor: comparison of different methods of assessment of staining and correlation with clinical outcome of breast cancer patients. *Br J Cancer* (1996) 74:1445–51. doi:10.1038/bjc.1996.563
6. Umemura S, Kurosumi M, Moriya T, Oyama T, Arihiro K, Yamashita H, et al. Immunohistochemical evaluation for hormone receptors in breast cancer: a practically useful evaluation system and handling protocol. *Breast Cancer* (2006) 13:232–5. doi:10.2325/jbcs.13.232
7. Kinsel LB, Szabo E, Greene GL, Konrath J, Leight GS, McCarty KS Jr. Immunocytochemical analysis of estrogen receptors as a predictor of prognosis in breast cancer patients: comparison with quantitative biochemical methods. *Cancer Res* (1989) 49:1052–6.
8. Rhodes A, Jasani B, Barnes DM, Bobrow LG, Miller KD. Reliability of immunohistochemical demonstration of oestrogen receptors in routine practice: interlaboratory variance in the sensitivity of detection and evaluation of scoring systems. *J Clin Pathol* (2000) 53:125–30. doi:10.1136/jcp.53.2.125
9. Rhodes A, Jasani B, Balaton AJ, Barnes DM, Miller KD. Frequency of oestrogen and progesterone receptor positivity by immunohistochemical analysis in 7016 breast carcinomas: correlation with patient age, assay sensitivity, threshold value, and mammographic screening. *J Clin Pathol*(2000) 53:688–96. doi:10.1136/jcp.53.9.688
10. Francis GD, Dimech M, Giles L, Hopkins A. Frequency and reliability of oestrogen receptor, progesterone receptor and HER2 in breast carcinoma determined by immunohistochemistry in Australasia: results of the RCPA Quality Assurance Program. *J Clin Pathol* (2007) 60:1277–83. doi:10.1136/jcp.2006.044701
11. Hammond ME, Hayes DF, Dowsett M, Allred DC, Hagerty KL, Badve S, et al. American Society of Clinical Oncology/College of American Pathologists guideline recommendations for immunohistochemical testing of estrogen and progesterone receptors in breast cancer (unabridged version). *Arch Pathol Lab Med* (2010) 134:e48–72. doi:10.1043/1543-2165-134.7.e48
12. Horwitz KB, McGuire WL. Predicting response to endocrine therapy in human breast cancer: a hypothesis. *Science* (1975) 189:726–7. doi:10.1126/science.168640
13. Clark GM, McGuire WL, Hubay CA, Pearson OH, Marshall JS. Progesterone receptors as a prognostic factor in Stage II breast cancer. *N Engl J Med* (1983) 309:1343–7. doi:10.1056/NEJM198312013092240
14. Paik S, Shak S, Tang G, Kim C, Baker J, Cronin M, et al. A multigene assay to predict recurrence of tamoxifen-treated, node-negative breast cancer. *N Engl J Med* (2004) 351:2817–26. doi:10.1056/NEJMoa041588
15. Badve SS, Baehner FL, Gray RP, Childs BH, Maddala T, Liu ML, et al. Estrogen- and progesterone-receptor status in ECOG 2197: comparison of immunohistochemistry by local and central laboratories and quantitative reverse transcription polymerase chain reaction by central laboratory. *J Clin Oncol* (2008) 26:2473–81. doi:10.1200/JCO.2007.13.6424
16. Kraus JA, Dabbs DJ, Beriwal S, Bhargava R. Semi-quantitative immunohistochemical assay versus oncotype DX(R) qRT-PCR assay for estrogen and progesterone receptors: an independent quality assurance study. *Mod Pathol* (2012) 25:869–76. doi:10.1038/modpathol.2011.219
17. Press MF, Bernstein L, Thomas PA, Meisner LF, Zhou JY, Ma Y, et al. HER-2/neu gene amplification characterized by fluorescence in situ hybridization: poor prognosis in node-negative breast carcinomas. *J Clin Oncol* (1997) 15:2894–904.
18. Lei S, Appert HE, Nakata B, Domenico DR, Kim K, Howard JM. Overexpression of HER2/neu oncogene in pancreatic cancer correlates with shortened survival. *Int J Pancreatol* (1995) 17:15–21.
19. Nakajima M, Sawada H, Yamada Y, Watanabe A, Tatsumi M, Yamashita J, et al. The prognostic significance of amplification and overexpression of c-met and c-erb B-2 in human gastric carcinomas. *Cancer* (1999) 85:1894–902. doi:10.1002/(SICI)1097-0142(19990501)85:93.0.CO;2-J
20. Slamon DJ, Leyland-Jones B, Shak S, Fuchs H, Paton V, Bajamonde A, et al. Use of chemotherapy plus a monoclonal antibody against HER2 for metastatic breast cancer that overexpresses HER2. *N Engl J Med* (2001) 344:783–92. doi:10.1056/NEJM200103153441101
21. Joensuu H, Kellokumpu-Lehtinen PL, Bono P, Alanko T, Kataja V, Asola R, et al. Adjuvant docetaxel or vinorelbine with or without trastuzumab for breast cancer. *N Engl J Med* (2006) 354:809–20. doi:10.1056/NEJMoa053028
22. Mass RD, Press MF, Anderson S, Cobleigh MA, Vogel CL, Dybdal N, et al. Evaluation of clinical outcomes according to HER2 detection by fluorescence in situ hybridization in women with metastatic breast cancer treated with trastuzumab. *Clin Breast Cancer* (2005) 6:240–6. doi:10.3816/CBC.2005.n.026
23. Maitland ML, Schilsky RL. Clinical trials in the era of

personalized oncology. *CA Cancer J Clin* (2011) 61:365–81. doi:10.3322/caac.20135

24. Slamon DJ, Godolphin W, Jones LA, Holt JA, Wong SG, Keith DE, et al. Studies of the HER-2/neu proto-oncogene in human breast and ovarian cancer. *Science* (1989) 244:707–12. doi:10.1126/science.2470152

25. Wolff AC, Hammond ME, Schwartz JN, Hagerty KL, Allred DC, Cote RJ, et al. American Society of Clinical Oncology/College of American Pathologists guideline recommendations for human epidermal growth factor receptor 2 testing in breast cancer. *Arch Pathol Lab Med* (2007) 131:18–43. doi:10.1043/1543-2165(2007)131

26. Hammond ME, Hayes DF, Wolff AC. Clinical Notice for American Society of Clinical Oncology-College of American Pathologists guideline recommendations on ER/PgR and HER2 testing in breast cancer. *J Clin Oncol* (2011) 29:e458. doi:10.1200/JCO.2011.35.2245

27. Middleton LP, Price KM, Puig P, Heydon LJ, Tarco E, Sneige N, et al. Implementation of American Society of Clinical Oncology/College of American Pathologists HER2 Guideline Recommendations in a tertiary care facility increases HER2 immunohistochemistry and fluorescence in situ hybridization concordance and decreases the number of inconclusive cases. *Arch Pathol Lab Med* (2009) 133:775–80. doi:10.1043/1543-2165-133.5.775

28. Shah SS, Ketterling RP, Goetz MP, Ingle JN, Reynolds CA, Perez EA, et al. Impact of American Society of Clinical Oncology/College of American Pathologists guideline recommendations on HER2 interpretation in breast cancer. *Hum Pathol* (2010) 41:103–6. doi:10.1016/j.humpath.2009.07.001

29. Vergara-LluriME,MoatamedNA,HongE,AppleSK.High concordance between HercepTest immunohistochemistry and ERBB2 fluorescence in situ hybridization before and after implementation of American Society of Clinical Oncology/College of American Pathology 2007 guidelines. *Mod Pathol* (2012) 25:1326–32. doi:10.1038/modpathol.2012.93

30. Jorgensen JT, Moller S, Rasmussen BB, Winther H, Schonau A, Knoop A. High concordance between two companion diagnostics tests: a concordance study between the HercepTest and the HER2 FISH pharmDx kit. *Am J Clin Pathol* (2011) 136:145–51. doi:10.1309/AJCPJPJ8ZWGDTTWC

31. Sauter G, Lee J, Bartlett JM, Slamon DJ, Press MF. Guidelines for human epidermal growth factor receptor 2 testing: biologic and methodologic considerations. *J Clin Oncol* (2009) 27:1323–33. doi:10.1200/JCO.2007.14.8197

32. Van Cutsem E, Peeters M, Siena S, Humblet Y, Hendlisz A, Neyns B, et al. Open-label phase III trial of panitumumab plus best supportive care compared with best supportive care alone in patients with chemotherapy-refractory metastatic colorectal cancer. *J Clin Oncol* (2007) 25:1658–64. doi:10.1200/JCO.2006.08.1620

33. Cunningham D, Humblet Y, Siena S, Khayat D, Bleiberg H, Santoro A, et al. Cetuximab monotherapy and cetuximab plus irinotecan in irinotecan-refractory metastatic colorectal cancer. *N Engl J Med* (2004) 351:337–45. doi:10.1056/NEJMoa033025

34. Chung KY, Shia J, Kemeny NE, Shah M, Schwartz GK, Tse A, et al. Cetuximab shows activity in colorectal cancer patients with tumors that do not express the epidermal growth factor receptor by immunohistochemistry. *J Clin Oncol* (2005) 23:1803–10. doi:10.1200/JCO.2005.08.037

35. Lenz HJ, Van Cutsem E, Khambata-Ford S, Mayer RJ, Gold P, Stella P, et al. Multicenter phase II and translational study of cetuximab in metastatic colorectal carcinoma refractory to irinotecan, oxaliplatin, and fluoropyrimidines. *J Clin Oncol* (2006) 24:4914–21. doi:10.1200/JCO.2006.06.7595

36. Scartozzi M, Bearzi I, Berardi R, Mandolesi A, Fabris G, Cascinu S. Epidermal growth factor receptor (EGFR) status in primary colorectal tumors does not correlate with EGFR expression in related metastatic sites: implications for treatment with EGFR-targeted monoclonal antibodies. *J Clin Oncol* (2004) 22:4772–8. doi:10.1200/JCO.2004.00.117

37. Custodio A, Feliu J. Prognostic and predictive biomarkers for epidermal growth factor receptor-targeted therapy in colorectal cancer: beyond KRAS mutations. *Crit Rev Oncol Hematol* (2013) 85:45–81. doi:10.1016/j.critrevonc.2012.05.001

38. Ellis PM, Blais N, Soulieres D, Ionescu DN, Kashyap M, Liu G, et al. A systematic review and Canadian consensus recommendations on the use of biomarkers in the treatment of non-small cell lung cancer. *J Thorac Oncol* (2011) 6:1379–91. doi:10.1097/JTO.0b013e318220cb8e

39. Sarlomo-Rikala M, Kovatich AJ, Barusevicius A, Miettinen M. CD117: a sensitive marker for gastrointestinal stromal tumors that is more specific than CD34. *Mod Pathol* (1998) 11:728–34.

40. Hirota S, Isozaki K, Moriyama Y, Hashimoto K, Nishida T, Ishiguro S, et al. Gain-of-function mutations of c-kit in human gastrointestinal stromal tumors. *Science* (1998) 279:577–80. doi:10.1126/science.279.5350.577

41. Goldman JM, Melo JV. Chronic myeloid leukemia – advances in biology and new approaches to treatment. *N Engl J Med* (2003) 349:1451–64. doi:10.1056/NEJMra020777

42. van Oosterom AT, Judson I, Verweij J, Stroobants S, Donatodi Paola E, Dimitrijevic S, et al. Safety 740 and efficacy of imatinib (STI571) in metastatic gastrointestinal stromal tumours: a 741 phase I study. *Lancet* (2001) 358:1421–3. doi:10.1016/S0140-6736(01)06535-7

43. Demetri GD, von Mehren M, Blanke CD, Van den Abbeele AD, Eisenberg B, Roberts PJ, et al. Efficacy and safety of imatinib mesylate in advanced gastrointestinal stromal tumors. *N Engl J Med* (2002) 347:472–80. doi:10.1056/NEJMoa020461

44. Debiec-Rychter M, Dumez H, Judson I, Wasag B, Verweij J, Brown M, et al. Use of c-KIT/PDGFRA mutational analysis to predict the clinical response to imatinib in patients with advanced gastrointestinal stromal tumours entered on phase I and II studies of the EORTC Soft Tissue and Bone Sarcoma Group. *Eur J Cancer* (2004) 40:689–95. doi:10.1016/j.ejca.2003.11.025
45. Heinrich MC, Corless CL, Demetri GD, Blanke CD, von Mehren M, Joensuu H, et al. Kinase mutations and imatinib response in patients with metastatic gastrointestinal stromal tumor. *J Clin Oncol* (2003) 21:4342–9. doi:10.1200/JCO.2003.04.190
46. Medeiros F, Corless CL, Duensing A, Hornick JL, Oliveira AM, Heinrich MC, et al. KIT-negative gastrointestinal stromal tumors: proof of concept and therapeutic implications. *Am J Surg Pathol* (2004) 28:889–94. doi:10.1097/00000478-200407000-00007
47. Soda M, Choi YL, Enomoto M, Takada S, Yamashita Y, Ishikawa S, et al. Identification of the transforming EML4-ALK fusion gene in non-small-cell lung cancer. *Nature* (2007) 448:561–6. doi:10.1038/nature05945
48. Rodig SJ, Mino-Kenudson M, Dacic S, Yeap BY, Shaw A, Barletta JA, et al. Unique clinicopathologic features characterize ALK-rearranged lung adenocarcinoma in the western population. *Clin Cancer Res* (2009) 15:5216–23. doi:10.1158/1078-0432.CCR-09-0802
49. Shaw AT, Kim DW, Nakagawa K, Seto T, Crino L, Ahn MJ, et al. Crizotinib versus chemotherapy in advanced ALK-positive lung cancer. *N Engl J Med* (2013) 368:2385–94. doi:10.1056/NEJMoa1214886
50. Thunnissen E, Bubendorf L, Dietel M, Elmberger G, Kerr K, Lopez-Rios F, et al. EML4-ALK testing in non-small cell carcinomas of the lung: a review with recommendations. *Virchows Arch* (2012) 461:245–57. doi:10.1007/s00428-012-1281-4
51. Park HS, Lee JK, Kim DW, Kulig K, Kim TM, Lee SH, et al. Immunohistochemical screening for anaplastic lymphoma kinase (ALK) rearrangement in advanced non-small cell lung cancer patients. *Lung Cancer* (2012) 77:288–92. doi:10.1016/j.lungcan.2012.03.004
52. Yi ES, Boland JM, Maleszewski JJ, Roden AC, Oliveira AM, Aubry MC, et al. Correlation of IHC and FISH for ALK gene rearrangement in non-small cell lung carcinoma: IHC score algorithm for FISH. *J Thorac Oncol* (2011) 6:459–65. doi:10.1097/JTO.0b013e318209edb9
53. Paik JH, Choe G, Kim H, Choe JY, Lee HJ, Lee CT, et al. Screening of anaplastic lymphoma kinase rearrangement by immunohistochemistry in non-small cell lung cancer: correlation with fluorescence in situ hybridization. *J Thorac Oncol* (2011) 6:466–72. doi:10.1097/JTO.0b013e31820b82e8
54. Selinger CI, Rogers TM, Russell PA, O'Toole S, Yip P, Wright GM, et al. Testing for ALK rearrangement in lung adenocarcinoma: a multicenter comparison of immunohistochemistry and fluorescent in situ hybridization. *Mod Pathol* (2013). doi:10.1038/modpathol.2013.87
55. Rothschild SI, Gautschi O. Crizotinib in the treatment of non-small-cell lung cancer. *Clin Lung Cancer* (2013) 14:473–80. doi:10.1016/j.cllc.2013.04.006
56. Camidge DR, Theodoro M, Maxson DA, Skokan M, O'Brien T, Lu X, et al. Correlations between the percentage of tumor cells showing an anaplastic lymphoma kinase (ALK) gene rearrangement, ALK signal copy number, and response to crizotinib therapy in ALK fluorescence in situ hybridization-positive nonsmall cell lung cancer. *Cancer* (2012) 118:4486–94. doi:10.1002/cncr.27411
57. Davies H, Bignell GR, Cox C, Stephens P, Edkins S, Clegg S, et al. Mutations of the BRAF gene in human cancer. *Nature* (2002) 417:949–54. doi:10.1038/nature00766
58. Nikiforov YE, Nikiforova MN. Molecular genetics and diagnosis of thyroid cancer. *Nat Rev Endocrinol* (2011) 7:569–80. doi:10.1038/nrendo.2011.142
59. Tiacci E, Trifonov V, Schiavoni G, Holmes A, Kern W, Martelli MP, et al. BRAF mutations in hairy-cell leukemia. *N Engl J Med* (2011) 364:2305–15. doi:10.1056/NEJMoa1014209
60. Platz A, Egyhazi S, Ringborg U, Hansson J. Human cutaneous melanoma; a review of NRAS and BRAF mutation frequencies in relation to histogenetic subclass and body site. *Mol Oncol* (2008) 1:395–405. doi:10.1016/j.molonc.2007.12.003
61. Flaherty KT, Puzanov I, Kim KB, Ribas A, McArthur GA, Sosman JA, et al. Inhibition of mutated, activated BRAF in metastatic melanoma. *N Engl J Med* (2010) 363:809–19. doi:10.1056/NEJMoa1002011
62. Hauschild A, Grob JJ, Demidov LV, Jouary T, Gutzmer R, Millward M, et al. Dabrafenib in BRAF-mutated metastatic melanoma: a multicentre, open-label, phase 3 randomised controlled trial. *Lancet* (2012) 380:358–65. doi:10.1016/S0140-6736(12)60868-X
63. Capper D, Preusser M, Habel A, Sahm F, Ackermann U, Schindler G, et al. Assessment of BRAF V600E mutation status by immunohistochemistry with a mutation-specific monoclonal antibody. *Acta Neuropathol* (2011) 122:11–9. doi:10.1007/s00401-011-0841-z
64. Capper D, Berghoff AS, Magerle M, Ilhan A, Wohrer A, Hackl M, et al. Immunohistochemical testing of BRAF V600E status in 1,120 tumor tissue samples of patients with brain metastases. *Acta Neuropathol* (2012) 123:223–33. doi:10.1007/s00401-011-0887-y
65. Long GV, Wilmott JS, Capper D, Preusser M, Zhang YE, Thompson JF, et al. Immunohistochemistry is highly sensitive and specific for the detection of V600E BRAF mutation in melanoma. *Am J Surg Pathol* (2013) 37:61–5. doi:10.1097/PAS.0b013e31826485c0
66. Colomba E, Helias-Rodzewicz Z, Von Deimling A, Marin C, Terrones N, Pechaud D, et al. Detection of BRAF p.V600E mutations in melanomas: comparison of four methods argues for sequential use of immunohistochemistry and pyrosequencing. *J*

Mol Diagn (2013) 15:94–100. doi:10.1016/j.jmoldx.2012.09.001

67. Busam KJ, Hedvat C, Pulitzer M, von Deimling A, Jungbluth AA. Immunohistochemical analysis of BRAF(V600E) expression of primary and metastatic melanoma and comparison with mutation status and melanocyte differentiation antigens of metastatic lesions. *Am J Surg Pathol*(2013) 37:413–20. doi:10.1097/PAS.0b013e318271249e
68. Marin C, Beauchet A, Capper D, Zimmermann U, Julie C, Ilie M, et al. Detection of BRAF p.V600E mutations in melanoma by immunohistochemistry has a good interobserver reproducibility. *Arch Pathol Lab Med* (2013). doi:10.5858/arpa.2013-0031-OA
69. Yeh I, von Deimling A, Bastian BC. Clonal BRAF mutations in melanocytic nevi and initiating role of BRAF in melanocytic neoplasia. *J Natl Cancer Inst* (2013) 105:917–9. doi:10.1093/jnci/djt119
70. Yancovitz M, Litterman A, Yoon J, Ng E, Shapiro RL, Berman RS, et al. Intra- and inter-tumor heterogeneity of BRAF(V600E) mutations in primary and metastatic melanoma. *PLoS ONE* (2012) 7:e29336. doi:10.1371/journal.pone.0029336
71. Lin J, Goto Y, Murata H, Sakaizawa K, Uchiyama A, Saida T, et al. Polyclonality of BRAF mutations in primary melanoma and the selection of mutant alleles during progression. *Br J Cancer* (2011) 104:464–8. doi:10.1038/sj.bjc.6606072
72. Wilmott JS, Menzies AM, Haydu LE, Capper D, Preusser M, Zhang YE, et al. (V600E) protein expression and outcome from BRAF inhibitor treatment in BRAF(V600E) metastatic melanoma. *Br J Cancer* (2013) 108:924–31. doi:10.1038/bjc.2013.29
73. Rosell R, Moran T, Queralt C, Porta R, Cardenal F, Camps C, et al. Screening for epidermal growth factor receptor mutations in lung cancer. *N Engl J Med* (2009) 361:958–67. doi:10.1056/NEJMoa0904554
74. Paez JG, Janne PA, Lee JC, Tracy S, Greulich H, Gabriel S, et al. EGFR mutations in lung cancer: correlation with clinical response to gefitinib therapy. *Science* (2004) 304:1497–500. doi:10.1126/science.1099314
75. Tanaka T, Matsuoka M, Sutani A, Gemma A, Maemondo M, Inoue A, et al. Frequency of and variables associated with the EGFR mutation and its subtypes. *Int J Cancer* (2010) 126:651–5. doi:10.1002/ijc.24746
76. Lynch TJ, Bell DW, Sordella R, Gurubhagavatula S, Okimoto RA, Brannigan BW, et al. Activating mutations in the epidermal growth factor receptor underlying responsiveness of non-small-cell lung cancer to gefitinib. *N Engl J Med* (2004) 350:2129–39. doi:10.1056/NEJMoa040938
77. Eberhard DA, Johnson BE, Amler LC, Goddard AD, Heldens SL, Herbst RS, et al. Mutations in the epidermal growth factor receptor and in KRAS are predictive and prognostic indicators in patients with non-small-cell lung cancer treated with chemotherapy alone and in combination with erlotinib. *J Clin Oncol* (2005) 23:5900–9. doi:10.1200/JCO.2005.02.857
78. Sharma SV, Bell DW, Settleman J, Haber DA. Epidermal growth factor receptor mutations in lung cancer. *Nat Rev Cancer* (2007) 7:169–81. doi:10.1038/nrc2088
79. Brevet M, Arcila M, Ladanyi M. Assessment of EGFR mutation status in lung adenocarcinoma by immunohistochemistry using antibodies specific to the two major forms of mutant EGFR. *J Mol Diagn* (2010) 12:169–76. doi:10.2353/jmoldx.2010.090140
80. Fan X, Liu B, Xu H, Yu B, Shi S, Zhang J, et al. Immunostaining with EGFR mutation-specific antibodies: a reliable screening method for lung adenocarcinomas harboring EGFR mutation in biopsy and resection samples. *Hum Pathol* (2013) 44:1499–507. doi:10.1016/j.humpath.2012.12.002
81. Ho HL, Chang FP, Ma HH, Liao LR, Chuang YT, Chang-Chien YC, et al. Molecular diagnostic algorithm for epidermal growth factor receptor mutation detection in Asian lung adenocarcinomas: comprehensive analyses of 445 Taiwanese cases with immunohistochemistry, PCR-direct sequencing and Scorpion/ARMS methods. *Respirology* (2013). doi:10.1111/resp.12148
82. Kato Y, Peled N, Wynes MW, Yoshida K, Pardo M, Mascaux C, et al. Novel epidermal growth factor receptor mutation-specific antibodies for non-small cell lung cancer: immunohistochemistry as a possible screening method for epidermal growth factor receptor mutations. *J Thorac Oncol* (2010) 5:1551–8. doi:10.1097/JTO.0b013e3181e9da60
83. Wu SG, Chang YL, Lin JW, Wu CT, Chen HY, Tsai MF, et al. Including total EGFR staining in scoring improves EGFR mutations detection by mutation-specific antibodies and EGFR TKIs response prediction. *PLoS ONE* (2011) 6:e23303. doi:10.1371/journal.pone.0023303
84. Kitamura A, Hosoda W, Sasaki E, Mitsudomi T, Yatabe Y. Immunohistochemical detection of EGFR mutation using mutation-specific antibodies in lung cancer. *Clin Cancer Res* (2010) 16:3349–55. doi:10.1158/1078-0432.CCR-10-0129
85. Angulo B, Conde E, Suarez-Gauthier A, Plaza C, Martinez R, Redondo P, et al. A comparison of EGFR mutation testing methods in lung carcinoma: direct sequencing, real-time PCR and immunohistochemistry. *PLoS ONE* (2012) 7:e43842. doi:10.1371/journal.pone.0043842
86. Xiong Y, Bai Y, Leong N, Laughlin TS, Rothberg PG, Xu H, et al. Immunohistochemical detection of mutations in the epidermal growth factor receptor gene in lung adenocarcinomas using mutation-specific antibodies. *Diagn Pathol* (2013) 8:27. doi:10.1186/1746-1596-8-27
87. Kawahara A, Taira T, Azuma K, Tominaga M, Hattori S, Kawahara M, et al. A diagnostic algorithm using EGFR mutation-specific antibodies for rapid response EGFR-TKI treatment in patients with non-small cell lung cancer. *Lung Cancer* (2012) 78:39–44. doi:10.1016/j.lungcan.2012.07.002
88. Azuma K, Okamoto I, Kawahara A, Taira T, Nakashima

K, Hattori S, et al. Association of the expression of mutant epidermal growth factor receptor protein as determined with mutation-specific antibodies in non-small cell lung cancer with progression-free survival after gefitinib treatment. *J Thorac Oncol* (2012) 7:122–7. doi:10.1097/JTO.0b013e31822eeba2

89. Kozu Y, Tsuta K, Kohno T, Sekine I, Yoshida A, Watanabe S, et al. The usefulness of mutation-specific antibodies in detecting epidermal growth factor receptor mutations and in predicting response to tyrosine kinase inhibitor therapy in lung adenocarcinoma. *Lung Cancer* (2011) 73:45–50. doi:10.1016/j.lungcan.2010.11.003

90. Wootla B, Denic A, Rodriguez M. Polyclonal and monoclonal antibodies in clinic. *Methods Mol Biol* (2014) 1060:79–110. doi:10.1007/978-1-62703-586-6_5

91. Saito M, Sakurai S, Motegi A, Saito K, Sano T, Nakajima T. Comparative study using rabbit-derived polyclonal, mouse-derived monoclonal, and rabbit-derived monoclonal antibodies for KIT immunostaining in GIST and other tumors. *Pathol Int* (2007) 57:200–4. doi:10.1111/j.1440-1827.2007.02081.x

92. Michel MC, Wieland T, Tsujimoto G. How reliable are G-protein-coupled receptor antibodies? *Naunyn Schmiedebergs Arch Pharmacol*(2009) 379:385–8. doi:10.1007/s00210-009-0395-y

93. Skliris GP, Parkes AT, Limer JL, Burdall SE, Carder PJ, Speirs V. Evaluation of seven oestrogen receptor beta antibodies for immunohistochemistry, western blotting, and flow cytometry in human breast tissue. *J Pathol* (2002) 197:155–62. doi:10.1002/path.1077

94. Bordeaux J, Welsh A, Agarwal S, Killiam E, Baquero M, Hanna J, et al. Antibody validation. *Biotechniques* (2010) 48:197–209. doi:10.2144/000113382

95. Romer T, Leonhardt H, Rothbauer U. Engineering antibodies and proteins for molecular in vivo imaging. *Curr Opin Biotechnol* (2011) 22:882–7. doi:10.1016/j.copbio.2011.06.007

96. Lofblom J, Frejd FY, Stahl S. Non-immunoglobulin based protein scaffolds. *Curr Opin Biotechnol* (2011) 22:843–8. doi:10.1016/j.copbio.2011.06.002

97. Wurch T, Lowe P, Beck A, Corvaia N. Protein scaffolds as alternatives to whole antibodies: from discovery research to clinical development. *Med Sci (Paris)* (2009) 25:1169–72. doi:10.1051/medsci/200925121169

98. Holliger P, Hudson PJ. Engineered antibody fragments and the rise of single domains. *Nat Biotechnol* (2005) 23:1126–36. doi:10.1038/nbt1142

99. Hamers-Casterman C, Atarhouch T, Muyldermans S, Robinson G, Hamers C, Songa EB, et al. Naturally occurring antibodies devoid of light chains. *Nature* (1993) 363:446–8. doi:10.1038/363446a0

100. Arbabi Ghahroudi M, Desmyter A, Wyns L, Hamers R, Muyldermans S. Selection and identification of single domain antibody fragments from camel heavy-chain antibodies. *FEBS Lett* (1997) 414:521–6. doi:10.1016/S0014-5793(97)01062-4

101. Jobling SA, Jarman C, Teh MM, Holmberg N, Blake C, Verhoeyen ME. Immunomodulation of enzyme function in plants by single-domain antibody fragments. *Nat Biotechnol* (2003) 21:77–80. doi:10.1038/nbt772

102. Rothbauer U, Zolghadr K, Tillib S, Nowak D, Schermelleh L, Gahl A, et al. Targeting and tracing antigens in live cells with fluorescent nanobodies. *Nat Methods* (2006) 3:887–9. doi:10.1038/nmeth953

103. Muyldermans S. Single domain camel antibodies: current status. *J Biotechnol* (2001) 74:277–302. doi:10.1016/S1389-0352(01)00021-6

104. Nilsson FY, Tolmachev V. Affibody molecules: new protein domains for molecular imaging and targeted tumor therapy. *Curr Opin Drug Discov Devel* (2007) 10:167–75.

105. Lofblom J, Feldwisch J, Tolmachev V, Carlsson J, Stahl S, Frejd FY. Affibody molecules: engineered proteins for therapeutic, diagnostic and biotechnological applications. *FEBS Lett* (2010) 584:2670–80. doi:10.1016/j.febslet.2010.04.014

106. Friedman M, Nordberg E, Hoiden-Guthenberg I, Brismar H, Adams GP, Nilsson FY, et al. Phage display selection of Affibody molecules with specific binding to the extracellular domain of the epidermal growth factor receptor. *Protein Eng Des Sel* (2007) 20:189–99. doi:10.1093/protein/gzm011

107. Hoyer W, Gronwall C, Jonsson A, Stahl S, Hard T. Stabilization of a beta-hairpin in monomeric Alzheimer's amyloid-beta peptide inhibits amyloid formation. *Proc Natl Acad Sci U S A* (2008) 105:5099–104. doi:10.1073/pnas.0711731105

108. Gronwall C, Snelders E, Palm AJ, Eriksson F, Herne N, Stahl S. Generation of Affibody ligands binding interleukin-2 receptor alpha/CD25. *Biotechnol Appl Biochem* (2008) 50:97–112. doi:10.1042/BA20070261

109. Kramer-Marek G, Kiesewetter DO, Martiniova L, Jagoda E, Lee SB, Capala J. [18F]FBEM-Z(HER2:342)-Affibody molecule-a new molecular tracer for in vivo monitoring of HER2 expression by positron emission tomography. *Eur J Nucl Med Mol Imaging* (2008) 35:1008–18. doi:10.1007/s00259-007-0658-0

110. Tran T, Orlova A, Sivaev I, Sandstrom M, Tolmachev V. Comparison of benzoate- and dodecaborate-based linkers for attachment of radioiodine to HER2-targeting Affibody ligand. *Int J Mol Med* (2007) 19:485–93.

111. Stumpp MT, Amstutz P. DARPins: a true alternative to antibodies. *Curr Opin Drug Discov Devel* (2007) 10:153–9.

112. Boersma YL, Pluckthun A. DARPins and other repeat protein scaffolds: advances in engineering and applications. *Curr Opin Biotechnol* (2011) 22:849–57. doi:10.1016/j.copbio.2011.06.004

113. Theurillat JP, Dreier B, Nagy-Davidescu G, Seifert B, Behnke S, Zurrer-Hardi U, et al. Designed ankyrin repeat proteins: a novel tool for testing epidermal growth factor receptor 2 expression in breast cancer. *Mod Pathol* (2010) 23:1289–97. doi:10.1038/modpathol.2010.103

114. Simon M, Zangemeister-Wittke U, Pluckthun A. Facile double-functionalization of designed ankyrin repeat proteins using click and thiol chemistries. *Bioconjug Chem* (2012) 23:279–86. doi:10.1021/bc200591x

115. Ni X, Castanares M, Mukherjee A, Lupold SE. Nucleic acid aptamers: clinical applications and promising new horizons. *Curr Med Chem*(2011) 18:4206–14. doi:10.2174/092986711797189600

116. Hu M, Zhang K. The application of aptamers in cancer research: an up-to-date review. *Future Oncol* (2013) 9:369–76. doi:10.2217/fon.12.201

117. Shangguan D, Li Y, Tang Z, Cao ZC, Chen HW, Mallikaratchy P, et al. Aptamers evolved from live cells as effective molecular probes for cancer study. *Proc Natl Acad Sci U S A* (2006) 103:11838–43. doi:10.1073/pnas.0602615103

118. Gilbert JC, DeFeo-Fraulini T, Hutabarat RM, Horvath CJ, Merlino PG, Marsh HN, et al. First-in-human evaluation of anti von Willebrand factor therapeutic aptamer ARC1779 in healthy volunteers. *Circulation* (2007) 116:2678–86. doi:10.1161/CIRCULATIONAHA.107.724864

119. Green LS, Jellinek D, Bell C, Beebe LA, Feistner BD, Gill SC, et al. Nuclease-resistant nucleic acid ligands to vascular permeability factor/vascular endothelial growth factor. *Chem Biol* (1995) 2:683–95. doi:10.1016/1074-5521(95)90032-2

120. Green LS, Jellinek D, Jenison R, Ostman A, Heldin CH, Janjic N. Inhibitory DNA ligands to platelet-derived growth factor B-chain. *Biochemistry* (1996) 35:14413–24. doi:10.1021/bi961544+

121. Lupold SE, Hicke BJ, Lin Y, Coffey DS. Identification and characterization of nuclease-stabilized RNA molecules that bind human prostate cancer cells via the prostate-specific membrane antigen. *Cancer Res* (2002) 62:4029–33.

122. Casado P, Alcolea MP, Iorio F, Rodriguez-Prados JC, Vanhaesebroeck B, Saez-Rodriguez J, et al. Phosphoproteomics data classify hematological cancer cell lines according to tumor type and sensitivity to kinase inhibitors. *Genome Biol* (2013) 14:R37. doi:10.1186/gb-2013-14-4-r37

123. Hanahan D, Weinberg RA. Hallmarks of cancer: the next generation. *Cell* (2011) 144:646–74. doi:10.1016/j.cell.2011.02.013

124. Soderberg O, Leuchowius KJ, Gullberg M, Jarvius M, Weibrecht I, Larsson LG, et al. Characterizing proteins and their interactions in cells and tissues using the in situ proximity ligation assay. *Methods* (2008) 45:227–32. doi:10.1016/j.ymeth.2008.06.014

125. Soderberg O, Gullberg M, Jarvius M, Ridderstrale K, Leuchowius KJ, Jarvius J, et al. Direct observation of individual endogenous protein complexes in situ by proximity ligation. *Nat Methods* (2006) 3:995–1000. doi:10.1038/nmeth947

126. Fredriksson S, Gullberg M, Jarvius J, Olsson C, Pietras K, Gustafsdottir SM, et al. Protein detection using proximity-dependent DNA ligation assays. *Nat Biotechnol* (2002) 20:473–7. doi:10.1038/nbt0502-473

127. Zieba A, Wahlby C, Hjelm F, Jordan L, Berg J, Landegren U, et al. Bright-field microscopy visualization of proteins and protein complexes by in situ proximity ligation with peroxidase detection. *Clin Chem* (2010) 56:99–110. doi:10.1373/clinchem.2009.134452

128. Clausson CM, Allalou A, Weibrecht I, Mahmoudi S, Farnebo M, Landegren U, et al. Increasing the dynamic range of in situ PLA. *Nat Methods*(2011) 8:892–3. doi:10.1038/nmeth.1743

129. Leuchowius KJ, Clausson CM, Grannas K, Erbilgin Y, Botling J, Zieba A, et al. Parallel visualization of multiple protein complexes in individual cells in tumor tissue. *Mol Cell Proteomics* (2013) 12:1563–71. doi:10.1074/mcp.O112.023374

130. Gajadhar AS, Bogdanovic E, Munoz DM, Guha A. In situ analysis of mutant EGFRs prevalent in glioblastoma multiforme reveals aberrant dimerization, activation, and differential response to anti-EGFR targeted therapy. *Mol Cancer Res* (2012) 10:428–40. doi:10.1158/1541-7786.MCR-11-0531

131. Spears M, Taylor KJ, Munro AF, Cunningham CA, Mallon EA, Twelves CJ, et al. In situ detection of HER2:HER2 and HER2:HER3 protein-protein interactions demonstrates prognostic significance in early breast cancer. *Breast Cancer Res Treat* (2012) 132:463–70. doi:10.1007/s10549-011-1606-z

132. Leuchowius KJ, Jarvius M, Wickstrom M, Rickardson L, Landegren U, Larsson R, et al. High content screening for inhibitors of protein interactions and post-translational modifications in primary cells by proximity ligation. *Mol Cell Proteomics* (2010) 9:178–83. doi:10.1074/mcp.M900331-MCP200

133. Uhlen M, Oksvold P, Fagerberg L, Lundberg E, Jonasson K, Forsberg M, et al. Towards a knowledge-based Human Protein Atlas. *Nat Biotechnol* (2010) 28:1248–50. doi:10.1038/nbt1210-1248

134. Ponten F, Schwenk JM, Asplund A, Edqvist PH. The Human Protein Atlas as a proteomic resource for biomarker discovery. *J Intern Med*(2011) 270:428–46. doi:10.1111/j.1365-2796.2011.02427.x

CHAPTER 13

SUBCELLULAR LOCALIZATION OF GALLOYLATED CATECHINS IN TEA PLANTS [CAMELLIA SINENSIS (L.) O. KUNTZE] ASSESSED VIA IMMUNOHISTOCHEMISTRY

Huanhuan Xu, Ya Wang, Yana Chen, Pan Zhang, Yi Zhao, Yewei Huang, Xuanjun Wang and Jun Sheng

Keywords: Camellia sinensis, catechins, galloylated catechins, subcellular localization, immunohistochemistry, HPLC

INTRODUCTION

Tea is one of the most consumed beverages globally for centuries (Huang et al., 2014), second only to water. It is produced from tea plants [*Camellia sinensis* (L.) O. Kuntze] buds (Kim et al., 2013b; Schramm, 2013; Sonoda et al., 2014). Tea infusion contains abundant nutrients and functional ingredients, which are beneficial to the human health (El-Shahawi et al., 2012); specifically, the tea plant polyphenols have many important physiological functions (Liu et al., 2012). Catechins, consisting the most important flavonoid group, account for approximately 80% of all the polyphenols, which in turn constitute approximately 18–36% of the dry leaf weight. The main catechins are (-)-epicatechin (EC), (-)-epigallocatechin (EGC), (-)-epicatechin-3-gallate (ECG), and (-)-epigallocatechin-3-gallate (EGCG; Liu et al., 2009; Roman, 2013; Lu et al., 2014). It is notable that galloylated catechins account for approximately 76% of all catechins, of which EGCG is the most abundant, active, and thoroughly investigated, followed by ECG. Their mechanism of action indicates that the polyphenolic structure of galloylated catechins makes them good donors for hydrogen bonding, which increases the water solubility of galloylated catechins and contributes to their high affinity to proteins and nucleic acids (Yang et al., 2007).

Galloylated catechins have stronger health effects as compared to the non-galloylated catechins, with respect to the product quality in tea processing and pharmacological efficacy in humans (Bigelow and Cardelli, 2006; Tsutsumi et al., 2011). Galloylated catechins possess antioxidant, antibacterial, and anti-inflammatory effects and alleviate cardiovascular diseases (Braicu et al., 2011; Jin et al., 2013; Kim et al., 2013a; Moravcova et al., 2014); however, their subcellular localization have not been fully addressed (Suzuki et al., 2003; Liu et al., 2009, 2012). Previous studies have demonstrated that catechins were mainly located in the chloroplasts or vacuoles at the subcellular level (Suzuki et al., 2003; Liu et al., 2009). These finding were largely attributable to the methodologies applied, each having a unique set of advantages and limitations. Although, the classical histochemical localization staining reagents, including vanillin-HCl, diazotized amines, 4-dimethylaminocinnamaldehyde (DMACA), and potassium permanganate (Feucht et al., 1992; Liu et al., 2009; Bhattacharya et al., 2015), are extensively used to determine the subcellular localization of polyphenols, they do not specifically detect the galloylated catechins. It is well known that immunohistochemistry could be used to localize small molecules specifically. Moreover, this method has been successfully used to localize some secondary metabolites in plant. Immunohistochemical localization with primary anti-caffeine antibodies and conjugated secondary antibodies on tea leaf sections proved at the tissue level that caffeine was localized and accumulated within vascular bundles, mainly the precursor phloem (van Breda et al., 2013). Similarly, delta 9-tetrahydrocannabinol (THC) localization in glandular trichomes and bracteal tissues of *Cannabis* was examined with a mAb, which can specifically recognize THC (Kim and Mahlberg, 1997). Therefore, the subcellular localization of galloylated catechins in the tea plant by mAb as a rapid and sensitive method is necessary.

Precise information regarding the subcellular localization of galloylated catechins in the tea plant would be helpful for

Citation: Xu H, Wang Y, Chen Y, Zhang P, Zhao Y, Huang Y, Wang X and Sheng J (2016) Subcellular Localization of Galloylated Catechins in Tea Plants [Camellia sinensis (L.) O. Kuntze] Assessed via Immunohistochemistry. Front. Plant Sci. 7:728. doi: 10.3389/fpls.2016.00728.

understanding how their biosynthesis is controlled, thereby providing additional insights into the related metabolic pathways. Advances in the high specificity of immunohistochemistry have prompted us to probe the subcellular localization of galloylated catechins in the tea plant. In this content, the anti-galloylated catechin mAb was generated. The high galloylated catechin content tissues were subsequently assessed via high-performance liquid chromatography (HPLC), and the determination of the subcellular localization of galloylated catechins was determined using immunohistochemistry.

This study reports production of a anti-galloylated catechin mAb which can recognize the galloylated catechins with high specificities and affinities. The high quality mAbs which exhibited excellent binding capability to galloylated catechins were further used to localize them in the tea plant. Our findings demonstrated that vacuoles were the primary sites of localization of galloylated catechins at the subcellular level, which is intuitive for their underlying mechanisms of biosynthesis, transport, storage, and physiological functions. Moreover, the subcellular localization of galloylated catechins in the tea plant assessed via immunohistochemistry may contribute toward a theoretical reference for the assessment of the subcellular localization of secondary metabolites in plants.

MATERIALS AND METHODS

Chemicals and Reagents

Epigallocatechin-3-gallate, ECG, EGC, EC, gallic acid (GA), and resveratrol (RSV) were of high purity grade (≥98%) and purchased from Aladdin (Shanghai, China). Culture media and serum were obtained from Thermo Fisher Scientific (Waltham, MA, USA) and Biological Industries Israel Beit Haemek Ltd., respectively. Optimal Cutting Temperature (OCT) Compound was purchased from Sakura Finetek, USA. Formalin was obtained from Jinan Biological Technology Co., Ltd. Paraformaldehyde (PFA) was obtained from the Tianjin Branch of Chemical Reagent Co., Ltd (Tianjin, China). The ABC high-HRP immunostaining kit was manufactured by Vectastain Co., Ltd. The haematoxylin stain was of high purity grade and was purchased from Sigma-Aldrich (St Louis, MO, USA). Normal mouse IgG (sc-2025) was obtained from Santa Cruz Biotechnologies (Santa Cruz, CA, USA). The HRP-DAB Chromogenic Substrate Kit was obtained from Tiangen Biotech (Beijing, China) Co., Ltd. Neutral red was obtained from Shanghai Yuanye Biological Technology Co., Ltd (Shanghai, China). Acetonitrile and trifluoroacetic acid used in the mobile phases were of HPLC grade and procured from Tedia Co., Inc. (Fairfield, OH, USA) and Merck KGaA (Darmstadt, Germany), respectively.

Plant Materials

Tea plant [*C. sinensis* (L.) O. Kuntze] samples were obtained from the Yunnan Agricultural University, Kunming, China. Each sample included bud, first leaf, second leaf, third leaf, and tender stem, which were separated from the tea plant. The samples were maintained at 4°C to inhibit air contact prior to analysis.

Animals

Healthy male BALB/c mice (6–8 weeks old) were purchased from Nanjing Peng-sheng Biotechnology Co., Ltd, China. All mice were housed in polypropylene cages with sterile paddy husk; the animals were maintained under ambient conditions of temperature and humidity with a 12 h light/dark cycle. Food and water were provided *ad libitum*. All mice experiments were performed in the animal facility according to the institutional guidelines and were approved by the Institutional Animal Care and Use Committee of Yunnan Agricultural University. The physical condition of the animals was monitored daily, and any adverse events were not observed. The animals were anesthetized prior to immunization, and spleen cells were obtained from the immunized mice, which were euthanized via cervical dislocation following CO_2 anesthesia.

Production of Monoclonal Antibodies

Two BALB/c mice were immunized with oxidized tea polyphenols (OTP), which contains EGCG as the major group (Huang et al., 2014). Briefly, each mouse was vaccinated five times with 40 μg of OTP at a 2-week interval. The first immunization was performed using Freund's complete adjuvant; the incomplete adjuvant was used for the subsequent immunizations. Following the immunization procedure, spleen cells from the immunized mice were mixed with myeloma SP2/0 cells at a ratio of 5:1. The mixture was washed twice with pre-warmed RPMI-1640 (37°C) and pre-warmed 50% polyethylene glycol (PEG) 1500 (Sigma–Aldrich, Germany) was used for fusion. A HAT selective medium (Sigma–Aldrich, Germany) was consecutively used for the selection of hybridoma cells. Direct Enzyme-linked immunosorbent assay (ELISA) was performed to screen the EGCG positive hybridoma cells, with the plates coated with EGCG during the cloning of EGCG hybridomas. One hybridoma clone, P6C2, was selected from 326 clones raised against EGCG. Positive hybridomas were cultured for 2 weeks. The anti-galloylated catechin antibody was purified from the culture supernatants via affinity chromatography using a Pierce™ protein A/G column (Bayat et al., 2013). The eluted antibody was dialyzed against phosphate buffered saline (PBS) at pH = 7.2. SDS-PAGE analysis was performed following the Laemmli method, with a 12.0% separating gel to assess the purity and molecular weight of the mAb. The gel was stained with 0.25% Coomassie Brilliant Blue G-250.

Amino Acid Sequence of the Light Chain Variable Region Gene in the P6C2 Monoclonal Antibody

RNA was extracted from P6C2 hybridoma cells by RNeasy (Qiagen, Inc.). Reverse transcription was performed using Superscript™ III (Invitrogen, Inc.). cDNA fragments of the P6C2 light chain variable region gene were amplified via PCR using Fast-Pfu (Transgene, Beijing, China) with universal primers (Wang et al., 2000) as follows:

F-Kc: 5′-ACAAATGCCTATGCAGAYATTGTGMTSAC-MCARWCTMCA-3′, R-Kc: 5′-GGATACAGTTGGTG-CAGCATC-3′.

The amplified PCR fragment was cloned into the pBR322 vector with an infusion kit (Clontech Inc., Mountain View, CA, USA) according to the manufacturer's protocol. The DNA insert was sequenced by Invitrogen (Shanghai, China), and the primary structure of the kappa chain variable region was deduced.

Antibody Specificity Analysis

Epicatechin, EGC, ECG, and EGCG have a basic 2-phenylchromone structure (Figure 1), and non-galloylated catechins (EC and EGC) and GA are the precursor substances of galloylated catechins (ECG and EGCG). These compounds and RSV were used to evaluate the mAb's specificity. Direct ELISA was performed on 96-well immunoplate (Nunc Polysorp; Thermo Fisher Scientific), which were coated with EGCG, ECG, EGC, EC, GA, and RSV (at the same concentration, 50 µg mL^{-1}) overnight at 4°C and then blocked by incubation with 1% bovine serum albumin (BSA). The mAbs were applied to duplicate wells, followed by HRP-conjugated goat anti-mouse IgG (Thermo Fisher Scientific, Waltham, MA, USA) as the secondary antibody. Tetramethylbenzidine (TMB) high sensitivity substrate solution (BioLegend, San Diego, CA, USA) was added subsequently and the absorbance was recorded at 450 nm using an ELISA reader (Thermo Fisher Scientific, Waltham, MA, USA).

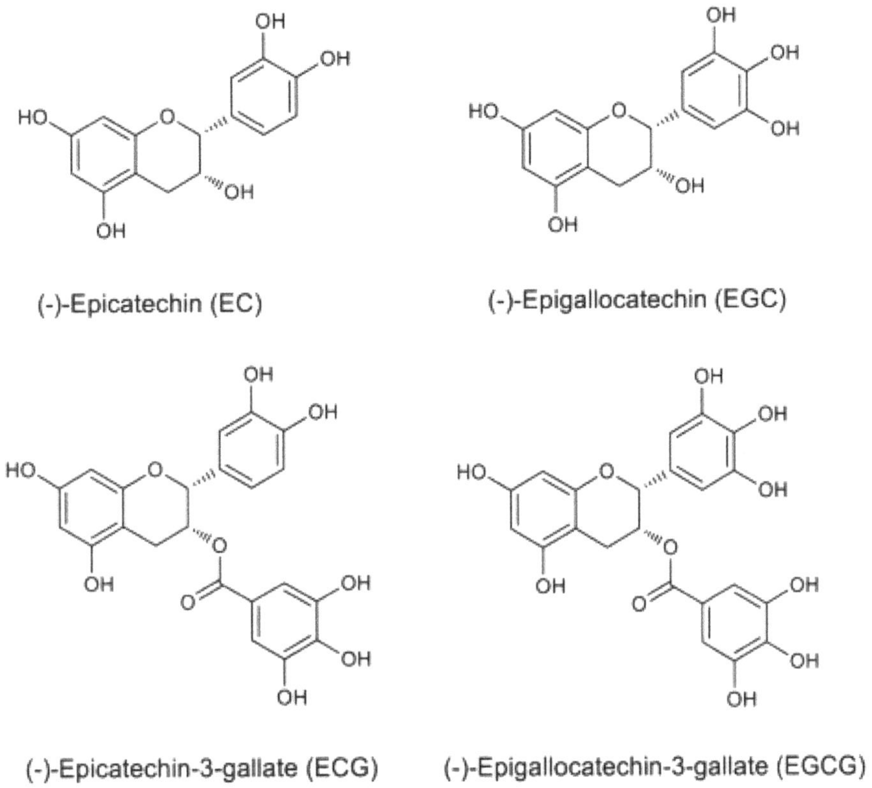

Figure 1: Structures of selected catechins.

Furthermore, the interactions between the anti-galloylated catechin antibody and EGCG, ECG, EGC, EC, and GA, were determined using Super Streptavidin (SSA) biosensors in an Octet Red 96 instrument (ForteBio Inc., Menlo Park, CA, USA). Interactions were assessed at 30°C in PBS (pH = 6.5) unless otherwise stated. Briefly, the antibody was biotinylated at a 1:1 stoichiometry for 1-h at room temperature (RT). The biotinylated antibody was subsequently desalinated by a PD SpinTrap™ G-25 column (GE Healthcare, UK). SSA tips were pre-wet for 10 min in buffer immediately prior to use, and the 96-well black plates utilized in the Octet were filled with 200 µL of sample or buffer per well and agitated at 1000 rpm. The antibody was loaded to the SSA biosensors, which were washed with the buffer for 120 s and transferred to the wells that contained the compounds.

Antibody Binding Affinity Determined by Octet

The binding affinity of anti-galloylated catechin antibody with EGCG or ECG was determined using SSA biosensors in the Octet Red 96 instrument. The biotinylated antibody and EGCG or ECG at different concentrations were prepared in the assay buffer (PBS, pH = 6.5) as described above. We measured EGCG and ECG association and dissociation for 10 min, respectively. The kinetic parameters and affinities were calculated from a non-linear global fit of the data between the galloylated catechins and the antibody, using Octet Data Analysis software version 7.0 (ForteBio Inc., Menlo Park, CA, USA).

HPLC Analysis

The required sample amounts were crushed under liquid N_2 to increase the extraction yield. An 80% methanol–water mixture was used as the extraction solvent (El-Shahawi et al., 2012; Otles and Yalcin, 2012). HPLC analysis was performed using a linear gradient system with mobile phase A (100% acetonitrile) and mobile phase B (0.03% trifluoroacetic acid), which were filtered through a 0.45 µm filter. The mobile phase A was increased from 10 to 60% in 36 min (Ning et al., 2009).

A 10 μL sample was analyzed using an auto sampler (G1329B, 1260ALS, Agilent, USA), an ultraviolet detector (G1314F, 1260VWD, Agilent, USA) at 280 nm, and a HPLC pump (G1311B, 1260Quat Pump, Agilent, USA) at 1.0 mL min^{-1} flow at 40°C (G1316A, 1260TCC, Agilent, USA) through a C_{18} ODS column (ZORBAX SB-C_{18} 4.6 mm × 250 mm, 5 microns, Agilent, USA).

Tissue Slicing and Immunohistochemistry

Fixation, embedding, sectioning, and staining of tea tissues were performed using the standard methods. Briefly, the tea tissues were fixed for 24 h at RT in 10% neutral buffered formalin. The OCT embedded tissues were cut into 20 μm sections using a Cryostat Microtome (Leica, Germany). The slides were fixed with 4% PFA for 10 min at 4°C and blocked with Blocking Solution (SP-6000, Vector Laboratories, Inc.) for 20 min at 37°C. After blocking for 30 min at 37°C with normal serum, histological sections of the tea tissues were incubated overnight at 4°C with the anti-galloylated catechin antibody. The sections were then sequentially incubated with biotinylated antibody and the ABC reagent for 30 min at 37°C. The reaction was visualized with DAB, and counterstaining was conducted with haematoxylin for 5 min. The sections were subsequently analyzed via fluorescence microscopy (Leica). Images of the tea tissue sections were acquired before and after staining.

Statistical Analyses

All values were presented as mean ± standard errors of the mean (SEM). All analyses were performed using SPSS 17.0 (Chicago, IL, USA), Graphpad Prism 5 (Graphpad Software, Inc., La Jolla, CA, USA) and Octet Data Analysis software version 7.0 (ForteBio Inc., Menlo Park, CA, USA).

RESULTS

Antibody Expression

The anti-galloylated catechin antibody was expressed in hybridoma cells and purified by affinity chromatography using a Pierce™ protein A/G column. The SDS-PAGE analysis of the purified mAb demonstrated the whole protein in the non-reducing conditions (~150 kDa) and 50 and 25 kDa heavy and light chains, respectively, in the reducing conditions (Figure 2).

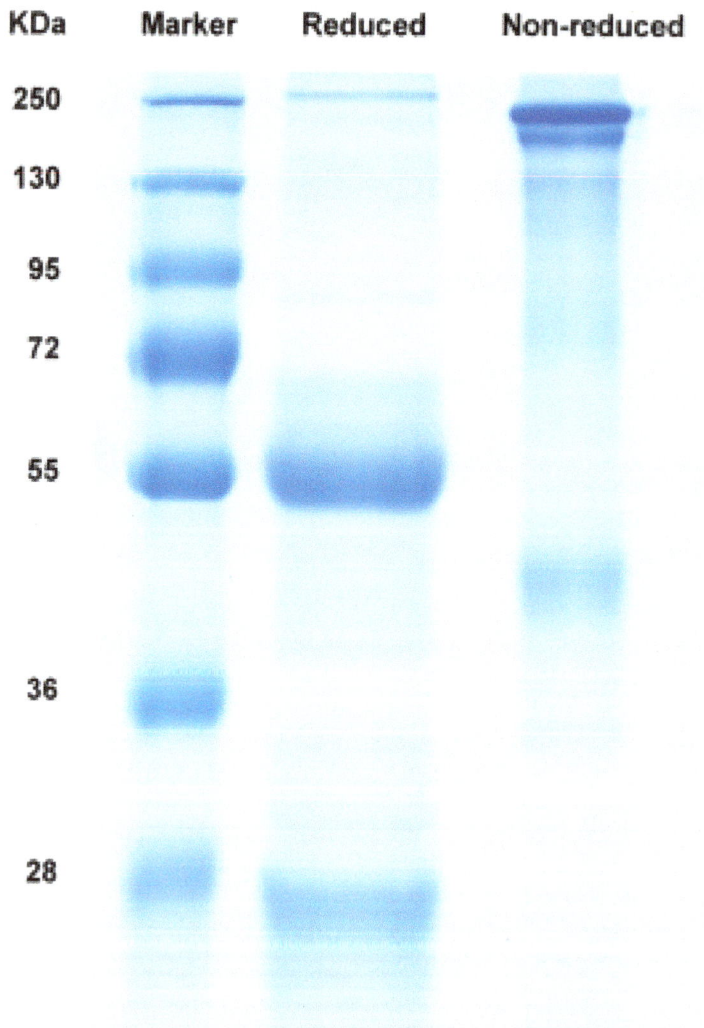

Figure 2: SDS-PAGE analysis of the purified mAb following Coomassie blue staining.

Amino Acid Sequence of the Kappa Chain Variable Region of the mAb

The sequence of the P6C2 kappa chain variable region was deduced from the sequence of DNA cloned into the pBR322 vector, as shown in Supplementary Figure S1. According to NCBI-blast, it was closely associated with the kappa chain variable region of the immunoglobulin raised under chloramphenicol selection.

Specificity of Antibody

The specificity of the purified mAb was assessed by direct ELISA on EGCG, ECG, EGC, EC, GA (tea polyphenols), and RSV (non-tea polyphenol; Figure 3). Our finding showed that the mAb specifically recognized EGCG and ECG, rather than EGC, EC, GA, and RSV. Besides, the specificity of the mAb was identified by Bio-Layer Interferometry (BLI) technique. The real-time interactions between the mAb and precursor substances of galloylated catechins, including the main non-galloylated catechins (EC and EGC) and GA, were determined using the ForteBio Octet system (ForteBio Inc., Menlo Park, CA, USA; Figure 4). The curves correspond to the phases of association and dissociation. In the association steps, as anticipated, EGCG and ECG could significantly bind to the anti-galloylated catechin antibody (Figures 4A,B), the binding signal values were gradually increased and finally achieved 0.40 and 0.28 nm, respectively. Whereas there were scarcely any signals in the interactions between the mAb and EGC, EC, and GA (Figures 4C–E), which means that the mAb could not recognize them. In consideration of catechin structures, EGCG and ECG contain a GA moiety at position 3 on the C ring, whereas other compounds (EGC, EC, and GA) do not contain this functional group (Figure 1), that may be the reason why the binding curves for EGCG and ECG are so different from the binding curves for EGC, EC, and GA. It indicates that the GA moiety functional group is necessary for anti-galloylated catechin antibody binding. The results above showed that the mAbs were capable of recognizing galloylated catechins with high specificity.

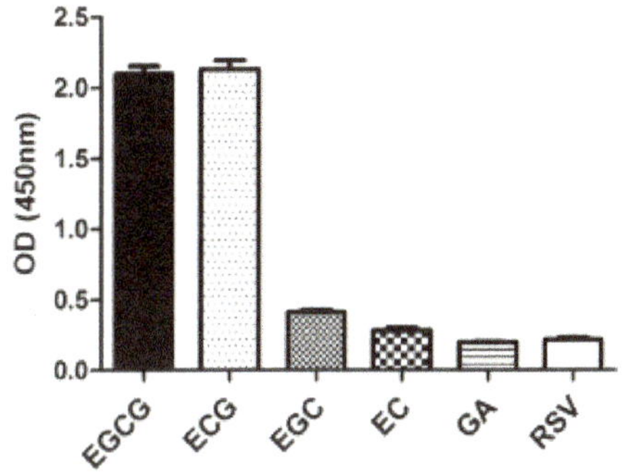

Figure 3: Determination of specificity of the anti-galloylated catechin mAb by direct ELISA. The anti-galloylated catechin mAb was tested against epigallocatechin-3-gallate (EGCG), epicatechin-3-gallate (ECG), epigallocatechin (EGC), epicatechin (EC), GA (gallic acid), and resveratrol (RSV) at the same concentration (50 μg mL^{-1}). Data were presented as mean ± SEM of three independent experiments.

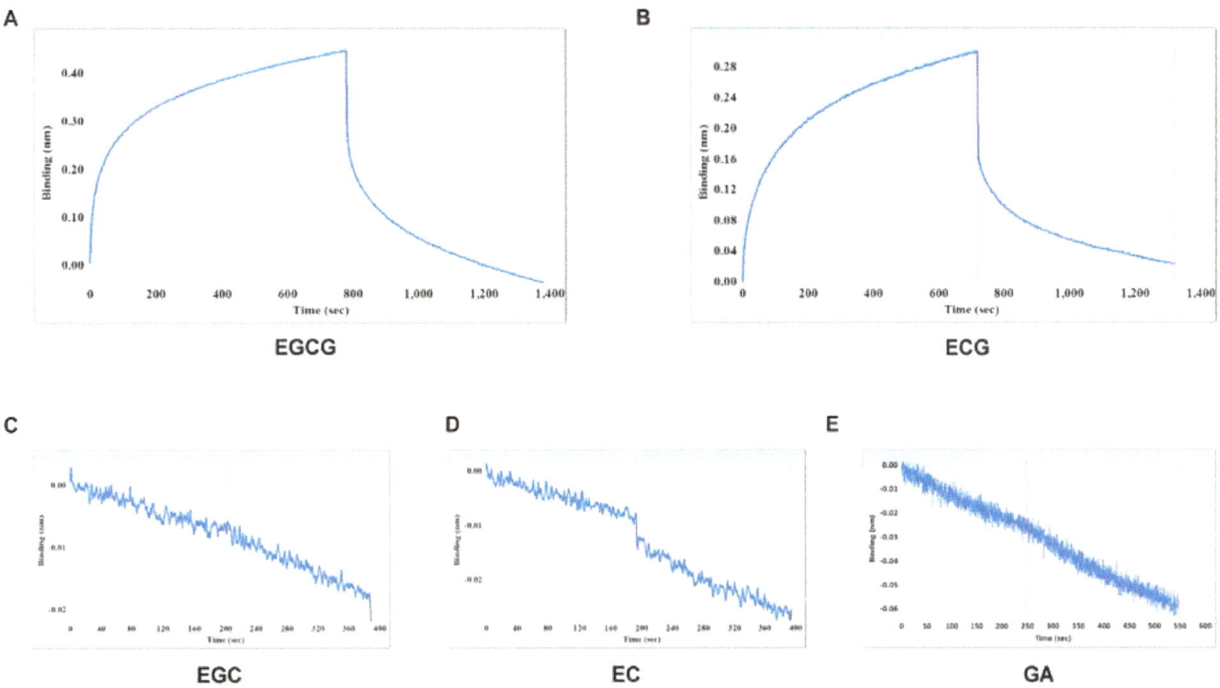

Figure 4: Interactions between the main compounds and anti-galloylated catechin antibody assessed via the label-free ForteBio Octet Red 96 System assay. **(A)** EGCG; **(B)** ECG; **(C)** EGC; **(D)** EC; **(E)** GA. Concentration, 50 μM. Curves correspond to the phases of association and dissociation.

Evaluation of Binding Affinity of mAbs

Furthermore, kinetic studies were performed to determine the binding affinities of the anti-galloylated catechin mAbs to serially diluted galloylated catechins from 32 to 1 µM (Figure 5; Table 1). The on-rate kinetic (K_{on}) values were displayed by EGCG at $2.27E + 02$ Ms^{-1} and ECG at $2.65E + 03$ Ms^{-1}, respectively; and the off-rate kinetic (K_{off}) values were displayed by EGCG at $2.10E - 03$ s^{-1} and ECG at $5.14E - 04$ s^{-1}, respectively. To understand the binding affinity value, the equilibrium dissociation constant (K_D) was calculated by K_{off}/K_{on}. This showed that the mAb had strong affinity to EGCG and ECG, with the K_D values of $9.25E - 06$ and $1.97E - 07$ M, respectively. The results indicated that the galloylated catechins had strong binding abilities with the anti-galloylated catechin antibody.

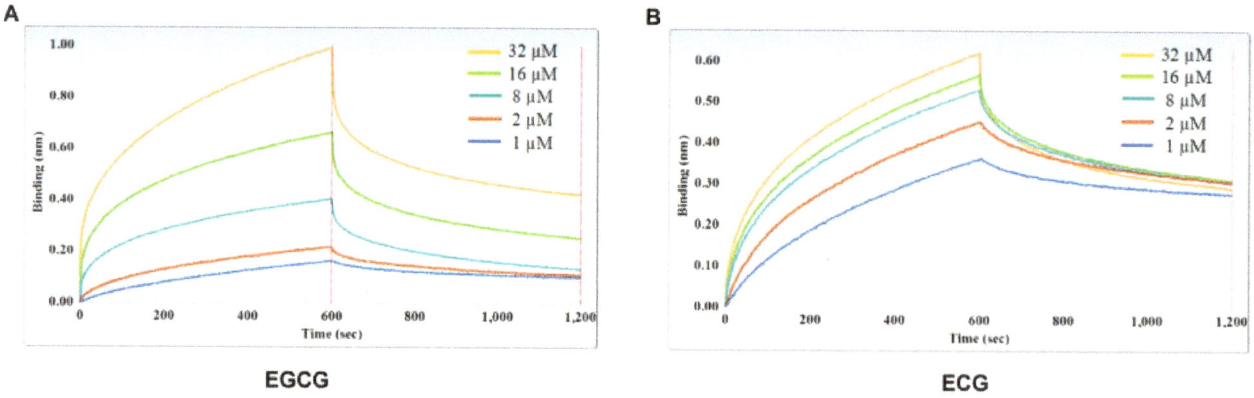

Figure 5: Binding affinity measurements of anti-galloylated catechin antibody with galloylated catechins assessed via the ForteBio system. **(A)** EGCG; **(B)** ECG. Curves correspond to the phases of association and dissociation of galloylated catechins at various concentrations on the monoclonal antibody anchored to the sensor chip. These curves may be used to determine the K_D, K_{on}, and K_{off}.

Table 1: Binding kinetics of the anti-galloylated catechin antibody to EGCG and ECG using the ForteBio system.

Variant	K_D (M)	K_{on} (1/Ms)	K_{off} (1/s)	R^2
EGCG	9.25 – 06	2.27E + 02	2.10E – 03	0.893
ECG	1.97E – 07	2.65E + 03	5.14E – 04	0.694

*Off-rate kinetics (K_{off}) were measured by saturating the SSA with the anti-galloylated catechin antibody and monitoring the dissociation after switching to buffer. The on-rate kinetics (K_{on}) were measured using different concentrations of EGCG or ECG. K_D, the equilibrium dissociation constant, was calculated as K_{off}/K_{on}. EGCG, ECG (**Figure 5**).*

Identification of High Galloylated Catechin Content Tissues

To identify the optimal tissue for the assessment of the subcellular localization of galloylated catechins via immunohistochemistry, high galloylated catechin content tissues were ascertained using HPLC. Peaks were identified by retention time compared with EGCG and ECG standards, and calibration curves were performed using serially diluted standards (Supplementary Figure S2). The total galloylated catechin amounts were highest in the first tea leaf, followed by the tea bud, second leaf, and third leaf, with only small quantities of galloylated catechins in the tender stem (Supplementary Figure S3; Table 2). The EGCG content was higher as compared to the ECG, which is consistent with previous studies. Furthermore, the galloylated catechins were mainly distributed in the tea plant's tender shoots.

Table 2: Galloylated catechin content (percentage of dry weight) of different tea tissues[a]

Tissue	EGCG	ECG	SUM
First leaf	14.17 ± 0.15	8.80 ± 0.16	22.97 ± 0.31
Bud	11.78 ± 0.17	8.86 ± 0.19	20.64 ± 0.36
Second leaf	7.38 ± 0.15	3.62 ± 0.02	11.00 ± 0.17
Third leaf	2.88 ± 0.05	1.68 ± 0.02	4.56 ± 0.07
Tender stem	0.72 ± 0.00	0.45 ± 0.01	1.17 ± 0.01

[a]*Data were presented as mean ± SEM of three independent experiments.*

Subcellular Localization of Galloylated Catechins via Immunohistochemistry

The observation that anti-galloylated catechin antibody specifically recognized galloylated catechins prompted us to probe the subcellular localization of these compounds in the tea plant. The tea bud is a galloylated catechin-rich tissue and is suitable for frozen section preparation. Thus, it was selected for neutral red staining and immunohistochemistry. Using both the methods, sharp microphotographs were acquired (Figure 6). Vacuole localization was typically examined by neutral red staining since it specifically reacted with the plant vacuoles to yield a red complex. Following neutral red staining, the red-stained vacuoles in the tea bud were easily detected at the subcellular level, and the staining was not observed in the plastids (Figures 6A,B). The anti-galloylated catechin antibody was successively used to detect the subcellular localization of the galloylated catechins via immunohistochemistry. Interestingly, sepia-stained galloylated catechins in the tea bud were easily detected in vacuoles, whereas the chloroplasts were not stained (Figure 6C). This finding indicated that the galloylated catechins accumulated mainly in the vacuoles.

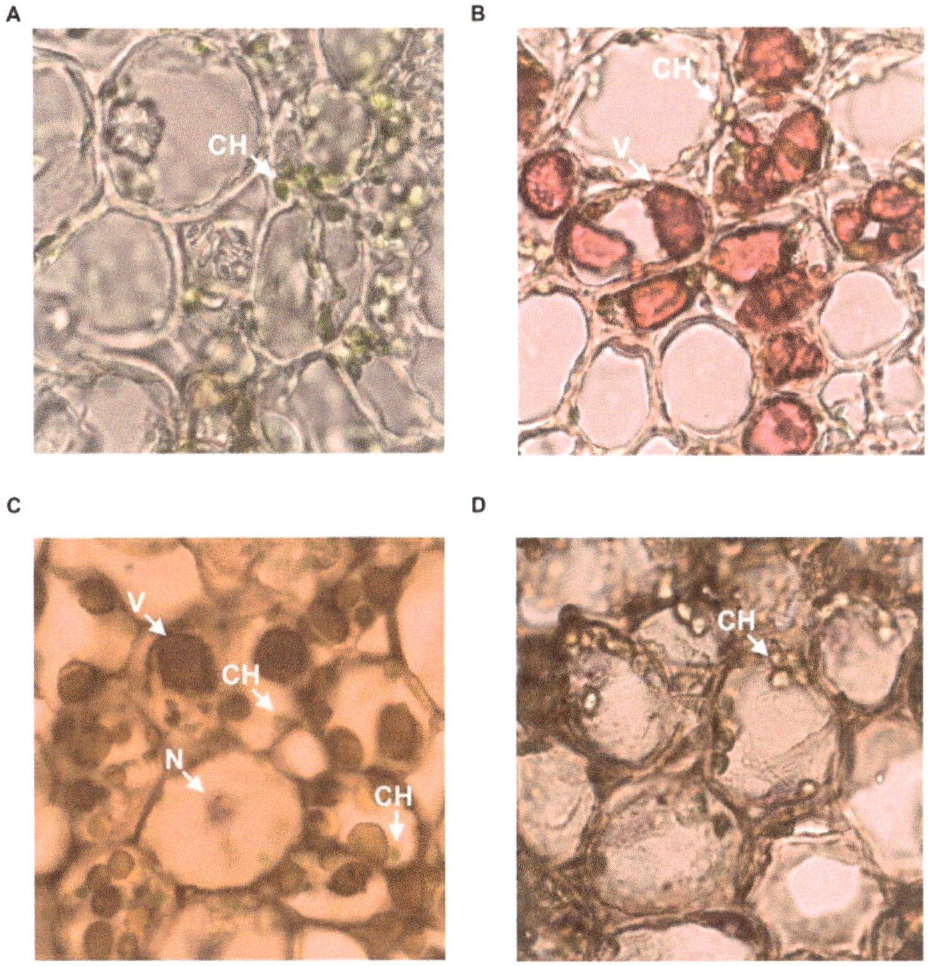

Figure 6: Subcellular localization of galloylated catechins in the tea bud. (A,B**)** Transverse bud sections before and after 0.5% neutral red staining, with red indicating the vacuoles. **(C,D)** Transverse bud sections after anti-galloylated catechin antibody and normal IgG antibody staining, respectively. Sepia represents galloylated catechin-accumulation areas. CH, chloroplast; V, vacuole; N, nucleus. Slice thickness, 20 µm. Oil microscopy.

To validate the immunohistochemistry data, a normal IgG antibody was selected as a control. Any general or plastid staining was not identified (Figure 6D). Similarly, no staining was identified in plastids. Taken together, these findings suggested that vacuoles are the main sites for galloylated catechins at the subcellular level. Finally, these data supported immunohistochemistry as a novel, specific, and sensitive method for the assessment of the subcellular localization of galloylated catechins in tea plant samples.

DISCUSSION

Immunohistochemistry is widely used in biomedical research to localize specific epitopes of molecules in cells and tissues (Hewitt et al., 2014). In addition, immunohistochemistry is advantageous for the localization of small molecules because the technique is substantially more specific than other standard histochemical methods using stains, such as vanillin-hydrochloric acid, which are not unique for a distinct small molecule, but rather an entire class of compounds, and false positives or side reactions may occur. Furthermore, immunohistochemistry has been used to determine effectively the localization of caffeine in young tea leaves (van Breda et al., 2013). Monoclonal antibodies are a superior choice for immunohistochemistry because they detect only one epitope in a particular antigen. Small changes in the compound of interest structure as a result of fixation protocols typically do not affect the binding affinity. In the present study, OTP, which contains EGCG as the major group, was first used for production of the anti-galloylated catechin mAb. The specificities of the mAbs were checked by direct ELISA and BLI assays, and, the binding affinities of the mAbs with EGCG and ECG were determined using ForteBio Octet Red 96 System. Most importantly, the anti-galloylated catechin mAb was used for the subcellular localization of galloylated catechins in the tea plant. Our experimental results indicated that the specific binding of the mAb to galloylated catechins with high affinities could be used to investigate efficiently the subcellular localization of these compounds via immunohistochemistry. Considering catechin structures, what's more, our findings suggest that the R1 galloyl group is necessary for anti-galloylated catechin antibody binding because both EGCG and ECG are the only catechins that contain this functional group (Figure 1). Therefore, immunohistochemistry is a useful method for assessing the subcellular localization of galloylated catechins in the tea plant. Using immunohistochemistry for galloylated catechins and neutral red staining for vacuoles, we demonstrated that the vacuoles were the primary sites for galloylated catechins at the subcellular level.

Although the galloylated catechins are the key secondary metabolites in the tea plant, the subcellular localization of galloylated catechins remains controversial. Using vanillin-HCl staining, Liu et al. (2009)demonstrated that catechins were primarily localized in the chloroplasts of mesophyll cells. However, catechins were simultaneously demonstrated to concentrate in callus vacuoles. In addition, Suzuki et al. (2003)demonstrated that catechins were primarily stored in the central vacuoles of the mesophyll cells as determined by Fe (II) staining. Till date, the subcellular localization of galloylated catechins remains unsolved, that is because none of the staining reagents could specifically detect galloylated catechins. Plant cells are distinguished from other eukaryotic cells by a rigid cellulose-based cell wall, chloroplasts, and a large central vacuole (Chi et al., 2015). The secondary metabolites may be considered chemical defense compounds against herbivores or microorganisms and are thus important for plant fitness. Several secondary metabolites are also toxic to the plant; thus, they need to be stored in a separate compartment (Wink, 1993). Polyphenol oxidase (PPO) is a ubiquitous copper metalloprotein in many plants, localized in chloroplasts, whereas flavonoid biosynthesis is speculated to occur in the cytoplasm (Roberts and Wood, 1950; Bokuchava et al., 1970; Buzun et al., 1970; Ono et al., 2006). We deduced that chloroplasts might not be the prime sites for galloylated catechin accumulation in the case of oxidization. As previously discussed, vacuoles were the primary sites for galloylated catechin accumulation at the subcellular level.

Recent studies have focused on the subcellular localization of galloylated catechins in the tea plant because these compounds possessed diverse biological activities and functions. Furthermore, multiple studies have identified promising preventative and therapeutic roles for galloylated catechins (Betts and Wareham, 2014; Chen et al., 2014; Cocci et al., 2014; Hodgson et al., 2014; Kim et al., 2014). Thus, the precise subcellular localization of galloylated catechins appears to be critical for unlocking valuable information regarding their biological roles. Our findings demonstrated that galloylated catechins accumulated in tea bud vacuoles, which indicates that vacuoles have a robust capacity to accumulate galloylated catechins. To assess the mode of transportation of synthesized galloylated catechins, sieve tube fluid of new shoots of tea plants was prepared via chelator-facilitated exudation (Dinant and Kehr, 2013), and the galloylated catechin content was determined by HPLC. Interestingly, galloylated catechins were detected in the sieve tube fluid (approximately 0.05% of the total amounts), which indicated that galloylated catechins may be transported through the sieve tube to vacuoles. The relative transportation mechanism need to be further studied.

CONCLUSION

This study reports production of a anti-galloylated catechin mAb which can recognize the galloylated catechins with high specificities and affinities. The high quality mAbs which exhibited excellent binding capability to galloylated catechins were further used to localize them in the tea plant. Our findings demonstrated that vacuoles were the primary sites of localization of galloylated catechins at the subcellular level.

Conflict of Interest Statement

The authors declare that the research was conducted in the absence of any commercial or financial relationships that could be construed as a potential conflict of interest.

The reviewer JPV and handling Editor declared their shared affiliation and the handling Editor states that the process nevertheless met the standards of a fair and objective review.

ACKNOWLEDGMENT

This research was financially supported by grants from the National Natural Science Foundation of China (No.31460392).

REFERENCES

1. Bayat, A. A., Yeganeh, O., Ghods, R., Zarnani, A. H., Ardekani, R. B., Mahmoudi, A. R., et al. (2013). Production and characterization of a murine monoclonal antibody against human ferritin. *Avicenna J. Med. Biotechnol.* 5, 212–219.
2. Betts, J. W., and Wareham, D. W. (2014). In vitro activity of curcumin in combination with epigallocatechin gallate (EGCG) versus multidrug-resistant *Acinetobacter baumannii. BMC Microbiol.* 14:172. doi: 10.1186/1471-2180-14-172
3. Bhattacharya, A., Sharma, M., Gulati, A., Joshi, R., Chanda, S. K., and Ahuja, P. S. (2015). Histochemical evaluation of catechins in PEG stressed transgenic tea plants using catechin-specific-diazotized sulfanilamide reagent. *Biotechnol. Histochem.* 90, 45–54. doi: 10.3109/10520295.2014.942369
4. Bigelow, R. L., and Cardelli, J. A. (2006). The green tea catechins, (-)-Epigallocatechin-3-gallate (EGCG) and (-)-Epicatechin-3-gallate (ECG), inhibit HGF/Met signaling in immortalized and tumorigenic breast epithelial cells. *Oncogene* 25, 1922–1930. doi: 10.1038/sj.onc.1209227

5. Bokuchava, M. A., Shalamberidze, T., and Soboleva, G. A. (1970). Localization of polyphenol oxidase in the tea leaf. *Dokl. Akad. Nauk SSSR.* 192, 1374–1375.

6. Braicu, C., Pilecki, V., Balacescu, O., Irimie, A., and Neagoe, I. B. (2011). The relationships between biological activities and structure of flavan-3-ols. *Int. J. Mol. Sci.* 12, 9342–9353. doi: 10.3390/ijms12129342

7. Buzun, G. A., Dzhemukhadze, K. M., and Mileshko, L. F. (1970). Some properties of tea polyphenol oxidase. *Biokhimiia* 35, 1002–1006.

8. Chen, W. C., Hsieh, S. R., Chiu, C. H., Hsu, B. D., and Liou, Y. M. (2014). Molecular identification for epigallocatechin-3-gallate-mediated antioxidant intervention on the H_2O_2-induced oxidative stress in H9c2 rat cardiomyoblasts. *J. Biomed. Sci.* 21:56. doi: 10.1186/1423-0127-21-56

9. Chi, W., Feng, P., Ma, J., and Zhang, L. (2015). Metabolites and chloroplast retrograde signaling. *Curr. Opin. Plant Biol.* 25, 32–38. doi: 10.1016/j.pbi.2015.04.006

10. Cocci, P., Mosconi, G., and Palermo, F. A. (2014). Partial cloning, tissue distribution and effects of epigallocatechin gallate on hepatic 3-hydroxy-3-methylglutaryl-CoA reductase mRNA transcripts in goldfish (*Carassius auratus*). *Gene* 545, 220–225. doi: 10.1016/j.gene.2014.05.030

11. Dinant, S., and Kehr, J. (2013). Sampling and analysis of phloem sap. *Methods Mol. Biol.* 953, 185–194. doi: 10.1007/978-1-62703-152-3_12

12. El-Shahawi, M. S., Hamza, A., Bahaffi, S. O., Al-Sibaai, A. A., and Abduljabbar, T. N. (2012). Analysis of some selected catechins and caffeine in green tea by high performance liquid chromatography. *Food Chem.* 134, 2268–2275. doi: 10.1016/j.foodchem.2012.03.039

13. Feucht, W., Treutter, D., and Christ, E. (1992). Localization and quantitative determination of catechins and proanthocyanidins in the phloem of elm and cherry. *Tree Physiol.* 10, 169–177. doi: 10.1093/treephys/10.2.169

14. Hewitt, S. M., Baskin, D. G., Frevert, C. W., Stahl, W. L., and Rosa-Molinar, E. (2014). Controls for immunohistochemistry: the histochemical society's standards of practice for validation of immunohistochemical assays. *J. Histochem. Cytochem.* 62,693–697. doi:10.1369/0022155414545224

15. Hodgson, A. B., Randell, R. K., Mahabir-Jagessar, T. K., Lotito, S., Mulder, T., Mela, D. J., et al. (2014). Acute effects of green tea extract intake on exogenous and endogenous metabolites in human plasma. *J. Agric. Food Chem.* 62, 1198–1208. doi: 10.1021/jf404872y

16. Huang, Y. W., Xu, H. H., Wang, S. M., Zhao, Y., Huang, Y. M., Li, R. B., et al. (2014). Absorption of caffeine in fermented Pu-er tea is inhibited in mice. *Food Funct.* 5, 1520–1528. doi: 10.1039/c4fo00051j

17. Jin, H., Gong, W., Zhang, C., and Wang, S. (2013). Epigallocatechin gallate inhibits the proliferation of colorectal cancer cells by regulating Notch signaling. *Onco Targets Ther.* 6, 145–153. doi: 10.2147/OTT.S40914

18. Kim, E., and Mahlberg, P. (1997). Immunochemical localization of tetrahydrocannabinol (THC) in cryofixed glandular trichomes of *Cannabis*(Cannabaceae). *Am. J. Bot.* 84, 336. doi: 10.2307/2446007

19. Kim, H. S., Montana, V., Jang, H. J., Parpura, V., and Kim, J. A. (2013a). Epigallocatechin gallate (EGCG) stimulates autophagy in vascular endothelial cells: a potential role for reducing lipid accumulation. *J. Biol. Chem.* 288, 22693–22705. doi: 10.1074/jbc.M113.477505

20. Kim, H. S., Quon, M. J., and Kim, J. A. (2014). New insights into the mechanisms of polyphenols beyond antioxidant properties; lessons from the green tea polyphenol, epigallocatechin 3-gallate. *Redox Biol.* 2, 187–195. doi: 10.1016/j.redox.2013.12.022

21. Kim, J. J., Tan, Y., Xiao, L., Sun, Y. L., and Qu, X. (2013b). Green tea polyphenol epigallocatechin-3-gallate enhance glycogen synthesis and inhibit lipogenesis in hepatocytes. *Biomed Res. Int.* 2013, 920128. doi: 10.1155/2013/920128

22. Liu, Y., Gao, L., Liu, L., Yang, Q., Lu, Z., Nie, Z., et al. (2012). Purification and characterization of a novel galloyltransferase involved in catechin galloylation in the tea plant (*Camellia sinensis*). *J. Biol. Chem.* 287, 44406–44417. doi: 10.1074/jbc.M112.403071

23. Liu, Y., Gao, L., Xia, T., and Zhao, L. (2009). Investigation of the site-specific accumulation of catechins in the tea plant (*Camellia sinensis* (L.) *O.* Kuntze) via vanillin-HCl staining. *J. Agric. Food Chem.* 57, 10371–10376. doi: 10.1021/jf902614n

24. Lu, Z., Liu, Y., Zhao, L., Jiang, X., Li, M., Wang, Y., et al. (2014). Effect of low-intensity white light mediated de-etiolation on the biosynthesis of polyphenols in tea seedlings. *Plant Physiol. Biochem.* 80, 328–336. doi: 10.1016/j.plaphy.2014.04.016

25. Moravcova, A., Cervinkova, Z., Kucera, O., Mezera, V., and Lotkova, H. (2014). Antioxidative effect of epigallocatechin gallate against D-galactosamine-induced injury in primary culture of rat hepatocytes. *Acta Med. (Hradec Kralove).* 57, 3–8. doi: 10.14712/18059694.2014.1

26. Ning, J. M., Zhang, Z. Z., Gu, X. G., Wan, X. C., and Sun, W. T. (2009). Study on HPLC fingerprint of Pu-erh crude tea in Yunnan. *Food Ferment. Ind.* 35, 36–40.

27. Ono, E., Hatayama, M., Isono, Y., Sato, T., Watanabe, R., Yonekura-Sakakibara, K., et al. (2006). Localization of a flavonoid biosynthetic polyphenol oxidase in vacuoles. *Plant J.* 45, 133–143. doi: 10.1111/j.1365-313X.2005.02625.x

28. Otles, S., and Yalcin, B. (2012). Phenolic compounds analysis of root, stalk, and leaves of nettle. *Sci. World J.* 2012:564367. doi: 10.1100/2012/564367

29. Roberts, E. A., and Wood, D. J. (1950). Oxidation of catechol by tea-oxidase. *Nature* 165:32. doi: 10.1038/165032b0

30. Roman, M. C. (2013). Determination of catechins and caffeine in camillia sinensis raw materials, extracts, and dietary supplements by HPLC-uv: single-laboratory

validation. *J. AOAC Int.* 96, 933–941. doi: 10.5740/jaoacint.10-488

31. Schramm, L. (2013). Going green: the role of the green tea component EGCG in chemoprevention. *J. Carcinog Mutagen.* 4:1000142. doi: 10.4172/2157-2518.1000142

32. Sonoda, J. I., Ikeda, R., Baba, Y., Narumi, K., Kawachi, A., Tomishige, E., et al. (2014). Green tea catechin, epigallocatechin-3-gallate, attenuates the cell viability of human non-small-cell lung cancer A549 cells via reducing Bcl-xL expression. *Exp. Ther. Med.* 8, 59–63. doi: 10.3892/etm.2014.1719

33. Suzuki, T., Yamazaki, N., Sada, Y., Oguni, I., and Moriyasu, Y. (2003). Tissue distribution and intracellular localization of catechins in tea leaves. *Biosci. Biotechnol. Biochem.* 67, 2683–2686. doi: 10.1271/bbb.67.2683

34. Tsutsumi, H., Kinoshita, Y., Sato, T., and Ishizu, T. (2011). Configurational studies of complexes of various tea catechins and caffeine in crystal state. *Chem. Pharm. Bull. (Tokyo).* 59, 1008–1015. doi: 10.1248/cpb.59.1008

35. van Breda, S. V., van der Merwe, C. F., Robbertse, H., and Apostolides, Z. (2013). Immunohistochemical localization of caffeine in young *Camellia sinensis* (L.) O. Kuntze (tea) leaves. *Planta.* 237, 849–858. doi: 10.1007/s00425-012-1804-x

36. Wang, Z., Raifu, M., Howard, M., Smith, L., Hansen, D., Goldsby, R., et al. (2000). Universal PCR amplification of mouse immunoglobulin gene variable regions: the design of degenerate primers and an assessment of the effect of DNA polymerase 3' to 5' exonuclease activity. *J. Immunol. Methods* 233, 167–177. doi: 10.1016/S0022-1759(99)00184-2

37. Wink, M. (1993). The plant vacuole: a multifunctional compartment. *J. Exp. Bot.* 44, 231–246.

38. Yang, C. S., Lambert, J. D., Ju, J., Lu, G., and Sang, S. (2007). Tea and cancer prevention: molecular mechanisms and human relevance. *Toxicol. Appl. Pharmacol.* 224, 265–273. doi: 10.1016/j.taap.2006.11.024

CHAPTER 14 TYROSINE HYDROXYLASE IMMUNOHISTOCHEMISTRY

Ryoma Morigaki and Satoshi Goto

Keywords: Putamen, matrix compartment, striosomes, tyrosine hydroxylase, human brain, immunohistochemistry

INTRODUCTION

The human neostriatum comprising the caudate nucleus (CN) and putamen is the primary input region of the basal ganglia, a group of subcortical nuclei that control a wide range of sensorimotor, cognitive and emotional functions (for review see, Graybiel, 2008; Amemori et al., 2011). It has so far been known that the basal ganglia are organized into several structurally and functionally distinct neural circuits that link the cortex, basal ganglia, and thalamus, with each circuit focused on a different frontal cortex territory (Alexander et al., 1986, 1990). Among these basal ganglia-thalamocortical circuits, the putamen participates in the "motor" circuits and is thereby important to basal ganglia motor control and movement disorders (Albin et al., 1989; DeLong, 1990). Parkinson's disease (PD) results from a striatal dopamine deficiency due to the neurodegenerative loss of dopamine-producing cells in the substantia nigra pars compacta (SNc; Hirsch et al., 1988). Kish et al. (1988)showed that the depletion of dopamine in patients with PD was most remarkable in the putamen, particularly in its caudal portions. Goto et al. (1989a, 1996) also documented that in parkinsonian patients, a pathological lesion was found specifically in the nigrostriatal loop that forms a link with the putamen.

The mammalian neostriatum is composed of two functional subdivisions known as the striosome (patch) and matrix compartments, which are developmentally, anatomically, and biochemically distinct (Graybiel and Ragsdale, 1978; Bolam et al., 1988; Graybiel, 1990; Gerfen, 1992). The striosome and matrix compartments make up about 15% and 85% of the volume of the striatum, respectively, in mammalian brains (Johnston et al., 1990). Although single dopaminergic afferent axons can terminate in both the compartments (Matsuda et al., 2009), the striosomes and matrix tend to receive dopaminergic afferents from distinct groups of SNc neurons. The striosomal cells are preferentially innervated by a group of dopamine-producing cells in the ventral tier of the SNc (Gerfen et al., 1987; Jimenez-Castellanos and Graybiel, 1987; Langer and Graybiel, 1989; Prensa and Parent, 2001), while the matrix cells preferentially receive the afferents arising from dopaminergic cells in the dorsal tier of the SNc, the ventral tegmental area and the retrorubral area (Gerfen et al., 1987; Jimenez-Castellanos and Graybiel, 1987; Prensa and Parent, 2001).

Accumulating evidence suggests that striosome-matrix dopaminergic systems exert a critical role in basal ganglia-thalamocortical circuits (Graybiel, 2008; Amemori et al., 2011). Interestingly, imbalanced dopamine activity between the striosome and matrix compartments has been suggested to underlie the genesis of pathological lesions and clinical symptoms that occur in multiple movement disorders (Graybiel, 2008; Goto et al., 2010; Crittenden and Graybiel, 2011), such as the L-DOPA-induced dyskinesia associated with PD (Graybiel et al., 2000). However, despite previous immunohistochemical studies using frozen sections (Ferrante and Kowall, 1987; Graybiel et al., 1987; Holt et al., 1997; Ciliax et al., 1999; Prensa et al., 1999, 2000), it remains undetermined whether or how striatal dopaminergic innervations might be organized into a discrete striosome-matrix axis in the human putamen.

To address this issue, we employed a highly-sensitive immunohistochemistry (IHC) method (Goto et al., 2015)

Citation: Morigaki R and Goto S (2016) Tyrosine Hydroxylase Immunohistochemistry. Front. Neuroanat. 10:34. doi: 10.3389/fnana.2016.00034.

to identify tyrosine hydroxylase (TH; EC 1.14.16.2) in formalin-fixed paraffin-embedded (FFPE) striatal tissues from autopsied human brains. TH serves as a reliable marker for visualizing dopaminergic axons and terminals in the striatum (Moss and Bolam, 2008). Here, we show that as in the CN, discrete compartmentalization of TH immunoreactivity occurs in the putamen, with a higher density of TH labeling in the matrix compartment relative to the striosomes. Our results provide anatomical evidence to support the hypothesis that compartment-specific dysfunction of the striosome-matrix dopaminergic systems might contribute to the genesis of human movement disorders.

MATERIALS AND METHODS

Western Blot Analysis on Mouse Brains

All procedural protocols that involve mouse experiments were approved by the Ethical Review Committee of the Tokushima University. We used male C57BL/6 mice (Nihon SLC Co., Shizuoka, Japan; $n = 3$) aged 8–10 weeks. Western blot analysis was performed with a rabbit polyclonal antibody against TH (Sato et al., 2008), according to the method that we previously ported (Morigaki and Goto, 2015). Blots were developed by chemiluminescent autoradiography (ECL plus kit; GE Healthcare, Buckingham, UK).

IHC for TH in Mouse Brains

After receiving an intraperitoneal injection of a lethal dose of pentobarbital (Sigma-Aldrich, St. Louis, MO, USA), mice ($n = 5$) were transcardially perfused with cold PBS, and followed by cold 4% paraformaldehyde in 0.1 M phosphate buffer (pH 7.2). Frozen sections with 16-μm thickness were processed for the IHC with the tyramide signal amplification (TSA) technique in a free-floating manner, as in our previous reports (Okita et al., 2012; Morigaki and Goto, 2015). Briefly, rabbit polyclonal antibody against TH (1:100,000) was used as a primary antibody. To detect the bound antibody, we used the Histofine Simple Stain Kit (Nichirei, Tokyo, Japan) and the TSA Plus Cyanine 3 System (Perkin Elmer, Shelton, CT, USA).

Human Brain Tissue Preparation for IHC

All procedural protocols that involve autopsied human brains were approved by the Ethical Review Committee of the Tokushima University. FFPE striatal sections with 4-μm-thickness were prepared from the autopsied brain tissues of neurologically-normal patients ($n = 5$; mean age ± SEM, 59 ± 8 years), as we previously described (Morigaki and Goto, 2015). After deparaffinization and rehydration, all sections were treated with 1% H_2O_2 in water for 5 min. For the antigen retrieval, they were then immersed in 0.01 M sodium citrate buffer (pH 6.0) and placed in a 700-W microwave for 15 min. Endogenous binding sites for avidin and biotin were blocked by using the Avidin/Biotin Blocking Kit (Vector, Burlingame, CA, USA). The sections were then immersed in 3% BSA-PBS for 60 min and they were processed for the IHC protocols described below.

IHC with 3,3′-Diaminobenzidine (DAB) in Human Brain Tissue

The sections were incubated for 18 h in 3% BSA-PBS containing a rabbit polyclonal antibody against TH (1:200,000; Sato et al., 2008) or [Met]-enkephalin (MEnk; 1:500,000; Millipore, St. Louis, MO, USA; Goto et al., 2015). They were then processed for a hybrid IHC protocol that implements aspects of both the polymer-staining and avidin-biotin-complex (ABC) methods combining with the biotin-TSA system, as we previously reported (Goto et al., 2015). Briefly, the sections were incubated for 30 min in the polymer-staining solution (Histofine Simple Stain Kit; Nichirei). After several rinses in PBS, they were incubated for 30 min with biotinyl TSA solution prepared from a TSA Biotin System kit (Perkin Elmer) with 1× Plus Amplification Diluent (Perkin Elmer). After several rinses in PBS, they were incubated for 30 min with the ABC reagent prepared from a Vectastain Elite ABC kit (Vector). After several rinses in PBS, the sections were immersed for 10 min in 0.05 M Tris-HCl (pH 7.4) containing 0.05% diaminobenzidine (DAB; Merck, Darmstadt, Germany) and 0.01% H_2O_2. After dehydration, the sections stained with DAB were cover-slipped with Malinol (Muto Pure Chemicals, Tokyo, Japan).

IHC with Fluorescents in Human Brain Tissue

The sections were first incubated for 18 h in 3% BSA-PBS containing rabbit polyclonal antibody against TH (1:100,000; Sato et al., 2008). After several rinses in PBS, the bound antibodies were visualized by using the Histofine Simple Stain Kit (Nichirei) and the TSA Plus Cyanine3 System (Perkin Elmer). The sections were then treated for 30 min in 0.1 M glycine-HCl (pH 2.2) to remove the first primary antibodies. After several rinses in PBS, they were incubated for 18 h in 3% BSA-PBS containing rabbit polyclonal antibody against MEnk (1:200,000; Millipore) or dopamine and cAMP-regulated phosphoprotein of 32 kDa (DARPP-32; 1:20,000; Cell Signaling, Denver, MA, USA). The bound antibodies were visualized by using the Histofine Simple Stain Kit (Nichirei) and the TSA Plus Fluorescein System (Perkin Elmer; Morigaki and Goto, 2015).

Digital Imaging and Morphometric Analysis

To capture macroscopic images, we used an Epson ES-2200 color image scanner (SEIKO EPSON Co., Nagano, Japan). Microscopic images were captured using an Olympus BX51 microscope (Olympus, Tokyo, Japan) equipped with a digital camera DP40 (Olympus). By means of Adobe Photoshop CS4, all captured images were digitally processed with minimal adjustments to contrast, brightness, and color balance.

Morphometric analysis was performed using an image-analyzer (MetaMorph, Molecular Device, Tokyo, Japan). We measured the optical density of TH-immunoreactive products in the striosome and matrix subfields represented by gray levels on non-colored digital images at low magnification, as previously reported (Sato et al., 2008; Morigaki and Goto, 2015). For each human striatum ($n = 5$), we measured five striatal subfields of the CN, rostral putamen, and caudal putamen.

We also measured the striosomal areas delineated by faint TH staining or dense MEnk staining in the CN ($n = 5$), rostral putamen ($n = 5$), and caudal putamen ($n = 5$) from each autopsied brain ($n = 5$). The mean values were used to quantify the percentage of the striatal area occupied by the striosome compartment.

To determine the cell density, we counted the numbers of neurons positive for TH or DARPP-32 in a 1 mm × 1 mm field in the human neostriatum, as described in our previous report (Goto et al., 2013). We examined five fields selected randomly in each of the CN and putamen from each patient ($n = 5$).

Statistical Analysis

All quantitative data are presented as the mean ± SEM. Two-group comparisons were made using the Student's t-test (two-tailed, paired). Significant differences were considered as $P < 0.05$.

RESULTS

Immunochemical Detection of TH in Mouse Brains

To determine the monospecificity of the anti-TH antibody used here, we first performed a western-blot analysis of the mouse brains. Immunoblots (IBs) of mouse striatal extracts showed a single protein band with an approximate molecular mass that corresponds to the predicted size of native TH protein (Figure 1A). The staining specificity was also assessed on frozen striatal sections from adult mouse brains with or without anti-TH antibody (Figures 1B–D). In the presence of the antibody, specific TH staining was detected in the striatum (Figure 1B), where numerous TH-positive puncta were densely found (Figure 1C). In agreement with our previous report (Sato et al., 2008), the distribution of TH labeling was diffuse and homogeneous throughout the striatum in adult mice. By contrast, TH immunoreactivity was not seen in striatal sections processed for the IHC protocol in the absence of the antibody (Figure 1D). In addition, strong TH labeling was also seen in the midbrain (Figure 1E), where SNc neurons exhibited intense TH immunoreactivity in their cell bodies and neurites (Figure 1F).

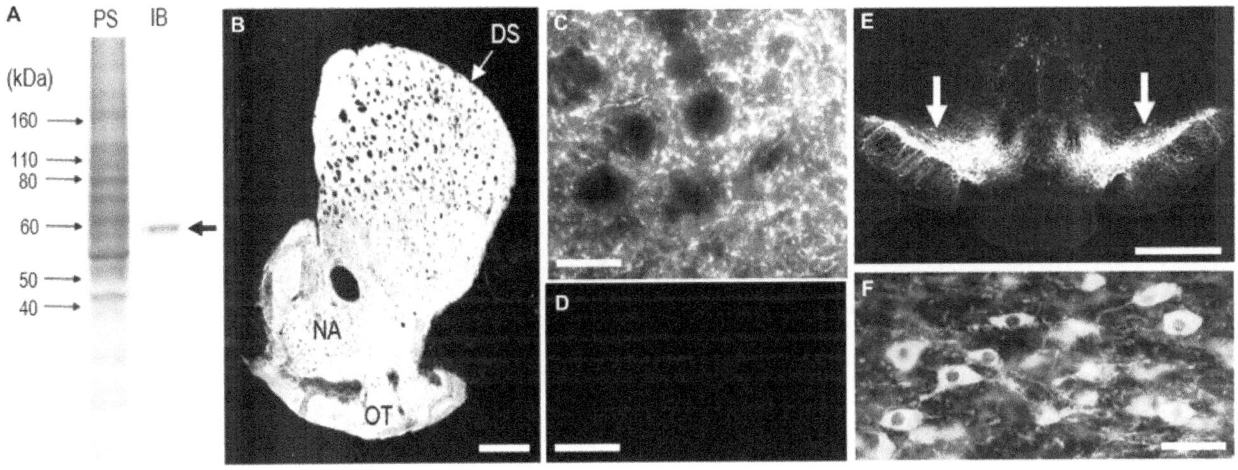

Figure 1: Identification of tyrosine hydroxylase (TH) in the mouse striatum. **(A)** Western blot assay. Crude homogenates of protein (10 μg) from the mouse striatum were separated on a 10% gel by SDS-PAGE and then immunoblotted using anti-TH antibody. An immunostained protein band (arrow) was selectively detected, with an approximate molecular mass corresponding to the predicted size of native TH protein. PS, protein staining; IB, immunoblot. **(B)** Photomicrograph of a striatal section stained for TH. TH immunoreactivity appears to be homogeneously distributed throughout the dorsal striatum (DS). **(C)** Photomicrograph of the striatal area stained for TH. Numerous tiny TH-positive dots were found in the striatum. **(D)** Photomicrograph of the DS processed using the immunostaining protocol without anti-TH antibody. **(E)** Photomicrograph of the midbrain stained for TH. Arrows indicate the substantia nigra pars compacta (SNc). **(F)**Photomicrograph of nigral dopaminergic cells positive for TH. Abbreviations: DS, dorsal striatum; NA, nucleus accumbens; OT, olfactory tubercle. Scale bars: **(B)** 500 μm, **(C,D)** 20 μm, **(E)** 1 mm, **(F)** 50 μm.

Putaminal Mosaic Pattern Visualized by TH-Immunostaining with DAB in Human Brains

A highly-sensitive IHC technique (Goto et al., 2015) allowed us to detect TH immunoreactivity in FFPE human autopsy tissue. Specific TH labeling was identified in the neostriatum composed of the CN and putamen. No TH labeling was detected in striatal sections processed for the IHC protocol without the anti-TH antibody. Bright-field (Figure 2A) and dark-field (Figure 2B) images are shown of a striatal section stained with DAB for TH. These macroscopic images reveal that in both the CN and putamen, TH labeling is distributed in a non-homogeneous pattern of low- and high-imunoreactive zones. Notably, patches of low TH immunoreactivity were evident in the putamen, as in the CN.

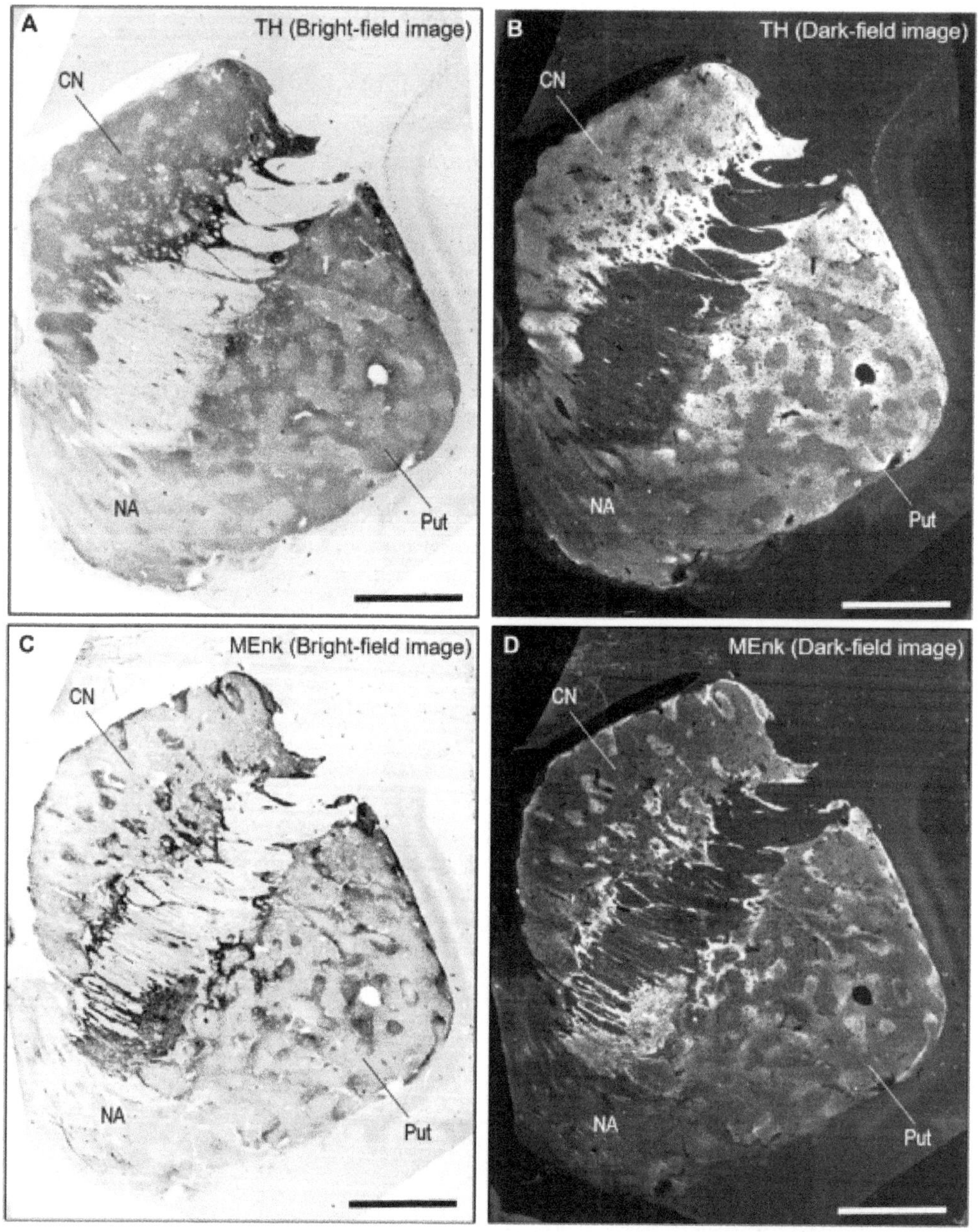

Figure 2: Non-homogeneous distribution of TH in the human neostriatum. **(A,B)** Bright-field **(A)**and dark-field **(B)** images taken from a frontal section of the striatum stained with diaminobenzidine (DAB) for TH. **(C,D)** Bright-field **(C)** and dark-field **(D)** images taken from a frontal section of the striatum stained with DAB for [Met]-enkephalin (MEnk), a marker for striosomes (patches). Note that they are contiguous to those shown in **(A,B)**. Abbreviations: CN, caudate nucleus; Put, putamen; NA, nucleus accumbens. Scale bars: 5 mm.

On FFPE striatal tissue obtained from autopsied human brains, MEnk is one of the most reliable IHC markers for visualizing striatal compartments with higher density of MEnk labeling in the striosomes than in the matrix (Goto et al., 2013, 2015). Bright-field and dark-field images of a striatal section stained with DAB for MEnk are shown in Figures 2C,D, respectively. Contiguous sections stained for TH (Figures 2A,B) and MEnk (Figures 2C,D) show a correspondence between zones of low TH labeling and those of heightened MEnk labeling in both the CN and putamen.

On dark-field microscopic images with low magnification, compartmental patterning of TH labeling was found in the rostral putamen (Figures 3A–D). A mosaic pattern of low- and high-immunoreactive zones that varied in their shapes and sizes was seen in both the dorsal (Figures 3A,B) and ventral (Figures 3C,D) portions of the rostral putamen. This was also evident in the graded color-converted images of dark-field (Figure 3E) and bright-field (Figure 3F) images of the putaminal area shown in Figure 3A.

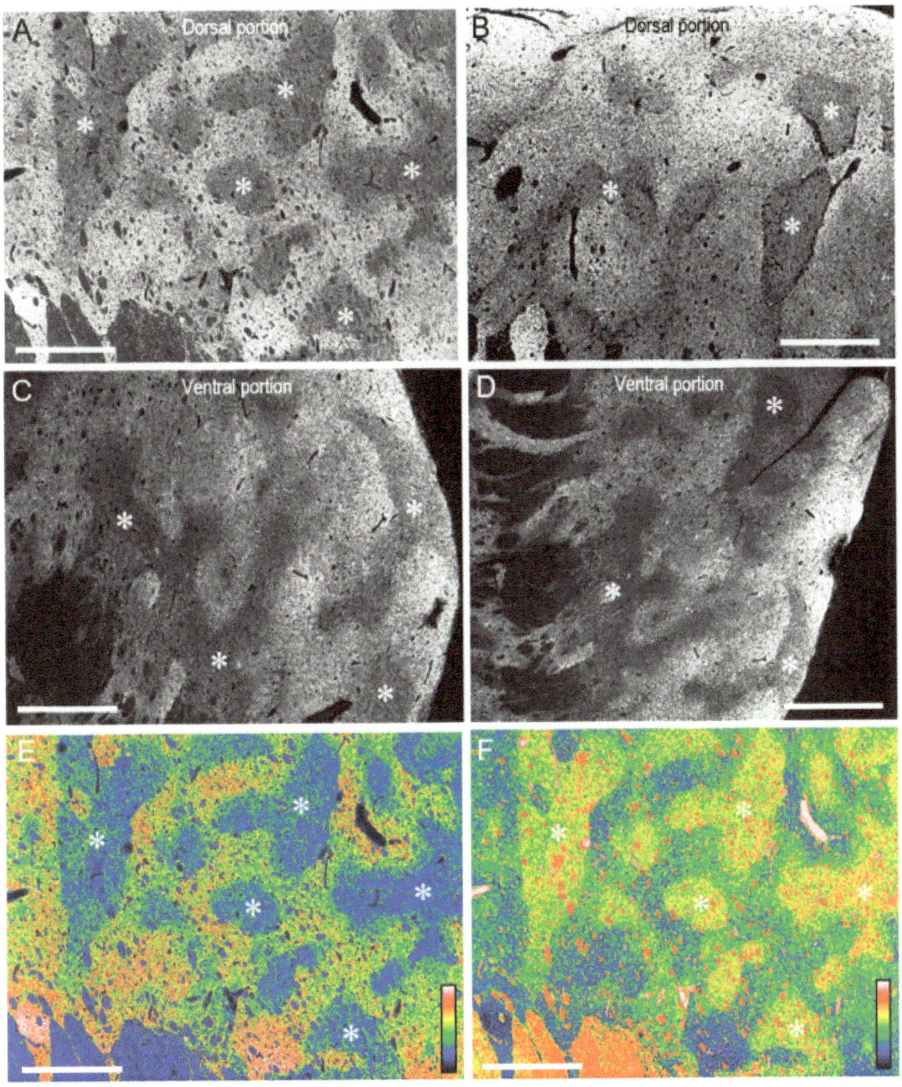

Figure 3: Mosaic pattern of TH-immunostaining in the rostral putamen of the human brains. **(A–D)** Photomicrographs of the dark-field images taken from the dorsal **(A,B)** and ventral portions **(C,D)** of the rostral putamen stained with DAB for TH. Asterisks indicate examples of striatal subfields with sparse TH labeling. **(E,F)** Graded color-converted representations of dark-field **(E)** and bright-field **(F)** images of the striatal area stained with DAB for TH, which is shown in **(A)**. A standard pseudocolor scale from blue (lowest level) through green, yellow, red, and white (highest level) was used. Asterisks indicate examples of corresponding zones poor in TH-labeling. Scale bars: 2 mm.

Dark-field macroscopic images of contiguous sections of the lenticular nucleus stained with DAB for TH and MEnk are shown in Figures 4A,B, respectively. They represent the complementary distribution of TH and MEnk in the caudal portion of the putamen. Microscopic images with low magnification (Figures 4C,D) also show a striking correspondence between the TH-poor zones and the MEnk-rich striosomes. A photomicrograph of the border between the striosome and matrix areas (Figure 4E) shows less dense TH immunoreactivity in the striosome compared to the matrix. Higher-magnification images also demonstrate that the matrix area contains a greater density of TH-positive fibers and puncta (Figure 4F), compared with the striosomal area (Figure 4G). To confirm this visual impression, the optical density was measured on areas of the striosome and matrix in the CN, rostral putamen, and caudal putamen (Figure 5). The results showed that in all the striatal areas examined, the density of TH-labeling in the matrix was significantly higher than that in the striosomes.

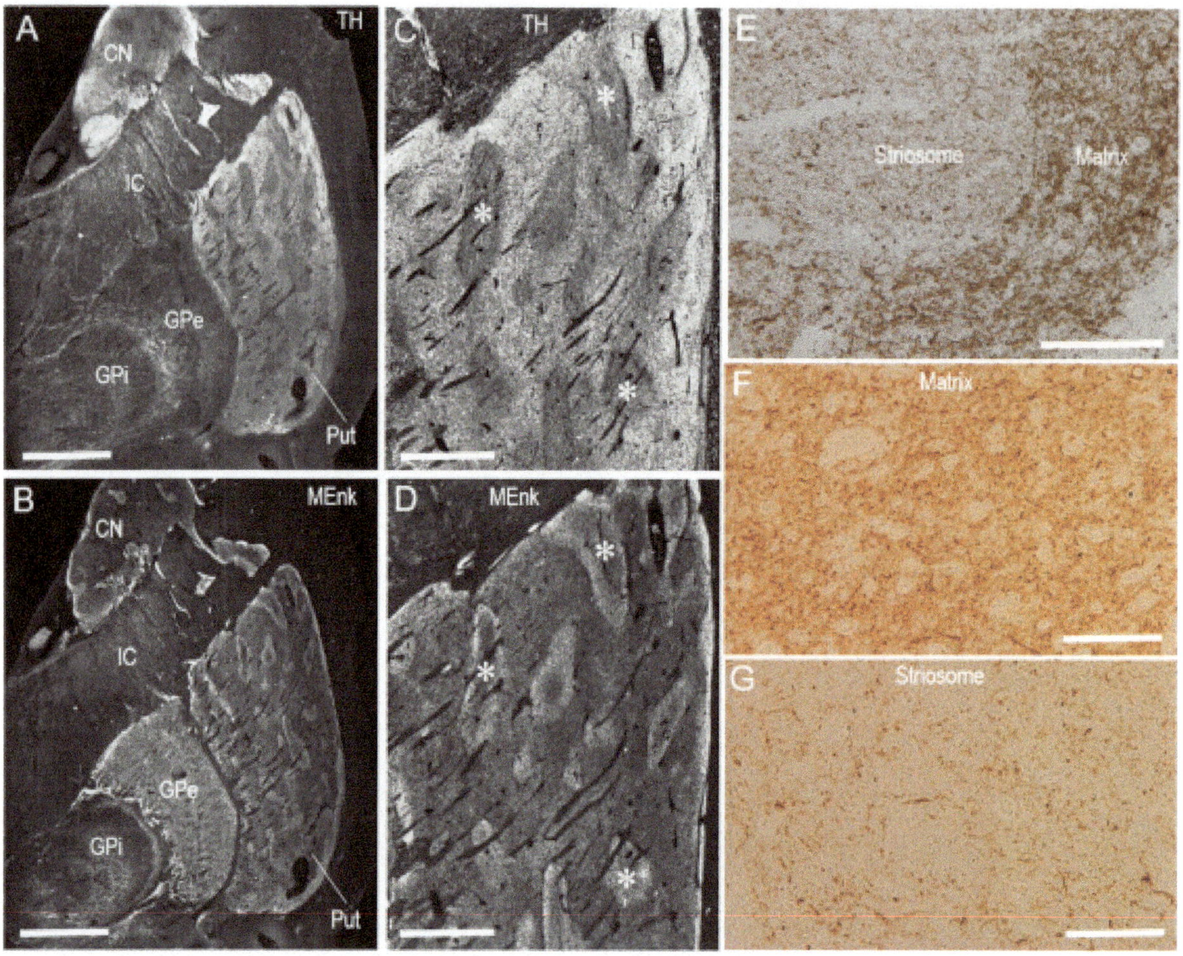

Figure 4: Compartmental distribution of TH immunoreactivity in the caudal putamen of the human brains. **(A–D)** Serial-section analysis of dark-field images of the lenticular nucleus **(A,B)** and caudal putamen **(C,D)** stained with DAB for TH **(A,C)** and MEnk **(B,D)**. Asterisks indicate examples of corresponding striosomes. **(E)** Photomicrograph at the border between the striosome and matrix in a putaminal area stained with DAB for TH. **(F,G)** Photomicrographs of the matrix **(F)** and striosome **(G)** in the putamen stained with DAB for TH. Note that the matrix area revealed a greater density of TH-positive fibers and puncta, compared with the striosomal area. Abbreviations: CN, caudate nucleus; Put, putamen; GPe, globus pallidus externa; GPi; globus pallidus interna; IC, internal capsule. Scale bars: **(A,B)** 5 mm, **(C,D)** 2 mm, **(E)** 500 μm, **(F,G)** 100 μm.

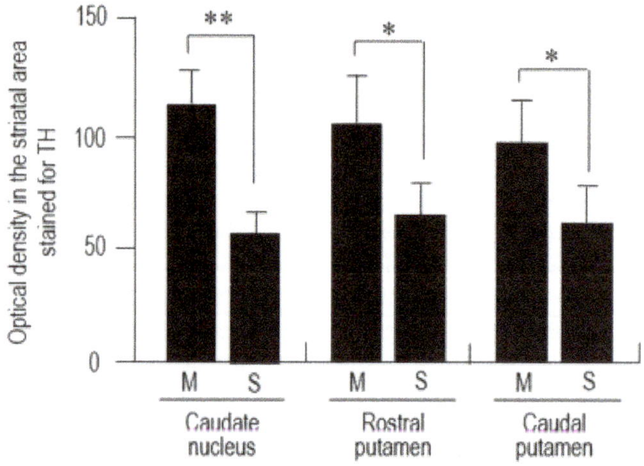

Figure 5: Densitometric analysis of the human striatum stained for TH. Measurements of the optical density of TH-immunoreactive DAB products were performed in the striosome (S) and matrix (M) compartments of the CN, rostral putamen and caudal putamen. Data represent means ± SEM (bars), $n = 25$. **indicates $P = 0.01$, M vs. S; *indicates $P = 0.05$, M vs. S.

Putaminal Mosaic Visualized by TH-Immunofluorescence in Human Brains

Specific immunoreactivity for TH in the human neostriatum was also identified by our IHC protocols using fluorescence. In a photomontage of the striatum stained with Cyanine 3 for TH (Figure 6A), mosaic patterns were clearly seen in both the CN and putamen, as shown in Figure 2. Microscopic images with low magnification also revealed the compartmentalized distribution of TH labeling in the CN (Figure 6B) and putamen (Figure 6C). At higher-magnification, abundant TH-immunoreactive fibers and puncta were seen in the matrix (Figure 6D), but less so in the striosomes (Figure 6E).

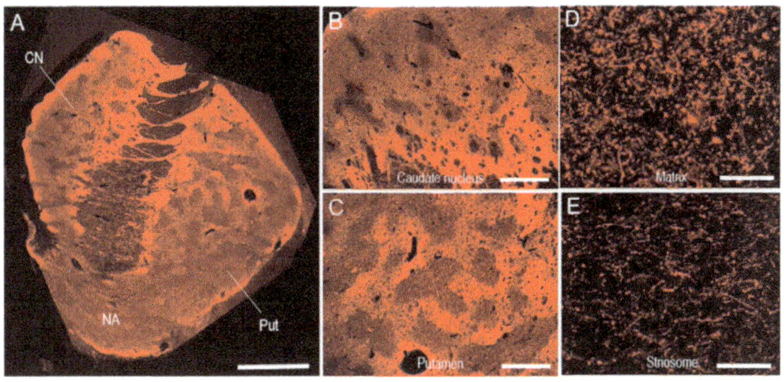

Figure 6: Neostriatal mosaic visualized by TH-immunostaining with Cyanine 3 in human brains. (A) A photomontage of a striatal section stained for TH. **(B,C)** Photomicrographs of the CN **(B)**and putamen **(C)** in the striatum stained for TH. **(D,E)** Photomicrographs of areas stained for TH in the matrix **(D)** and striosome **(E)** of the putamen. Abbreviations: CN, caudate nucleus; Put, putamen; NA, nucleus accumbens. Scale bars: **(A)** 5 mm, **(B,C)** 2 mm, **(D,E)** 50 μm.

Double immunofluorescence staining also revealed that TH immunoreactivity was sparse in the MEnk-enriched striosomes in the CN (Figures 7A,B) and putamen (Figures 7C,D). At higher-magnification, the margins of the TH-poor zones closely corresponded with the outer margins of the MEnk-rich zones (Figures 7E–G). Within the striosomes, there exist specialized zones rimming the striosomes, which are referred to as "annular" or "striocapsular" zones (Graybiel et al., 1981; Gerfen et al., 1985; Jakab et al., 1996; Holt et al., 1997; Brimblecombe and Cragg, 2015). These express higher levels of MEnk than the core (center) zones, as depicted in Figure 7H. Based on the findings shown here, it is likely that TH immunoreactivity is diffusely distributed within the striosomes, with no apparent difference in the TH-staining intensity between the annular and core zones (Figure 7H).

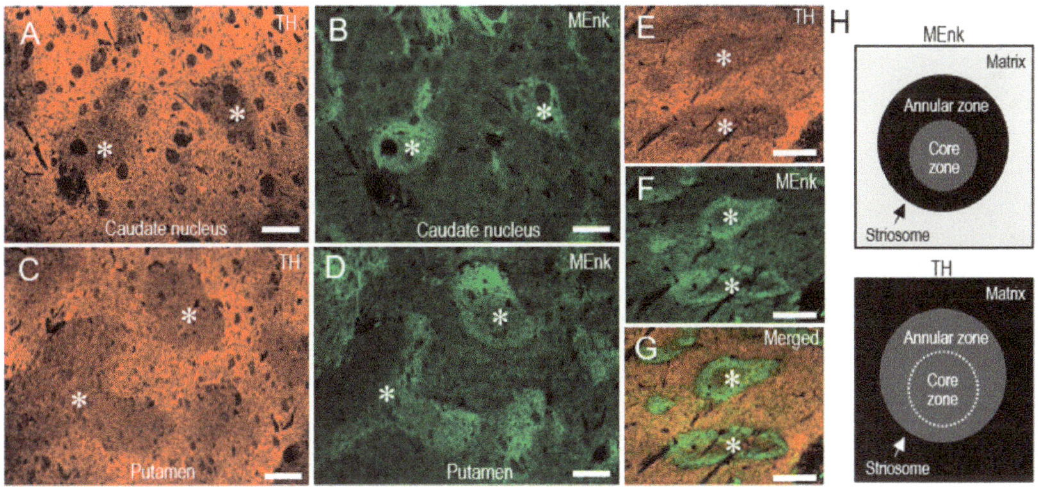

Figure 7: Pattern of localization of TH in the striosome-matrix domains of the human neostriatum. (A–D) Photomicrographs of the CN **(A,B)** and putamen **(C,D)** double-stained for TH **(A,C)** and MEnk **(B,D)**. Corresponding striosomes are indicated by asterisks. **(E–G)** Photomicrographs of an area of the putamen double-stained for TH **(E)** and MEnk **(F)**, with a merged image **(G)**. Corresponding striosomes are indicated by asterisks. Note that the margins of the TH-poor zones correspond to the outer margins of the striosomes enriched in MEnk. **(H)** Depicted are the patterns of localization of MEnk (*upper*) or TH (*lower*) in the striosome-matrix system. The striosome consists of annular and core zones. Higher densities of TH or MEnk-immunoreactive products are indicated by higher gray-scale levels. Scale bars: **(A–D)** 500 μm, **(E–G)** 250 μm.

Representative gray-scale images of the striatal areas stained for TH (Figures 8A–C) and MEnk (Figures 8D–F) are shown for the CN (Figures 8A,D), rostral putamen (Figures 8B,E), and caudal putamen (Figures 8C,F). These images (also see, Figures 2, 6) reveal an apparent difference in the striosome-to-matrix ratio among striatal areas. To confirm this visual impression, we carried out a morphometric analysis of the striatal sections. In the striatum stained for TH (Figure 8G), the percentage of the striatum occupied by the striosome compartment in the CN (18.2% ± 3.2%) was significantly different ($P < 0.05$) from that in both the rostral putamen (29.8% ± 6.7%) and caudal putamen (28.1% ± 5.2%). In the striatum stained for MEnk (Figure 8H), the percentage of the striatum occupied by the striosome compartment in the CN (14.0% ± 2.1%) was significantly different ($P < 0.05$) from that in both the rostral putamen (29.2% ± 6.4%) and caudal putamen (28.1% ± 5.1%). Thus, the striosome-to-matrix ratio of the putamen was 1.5~2.0 times that of the CN.

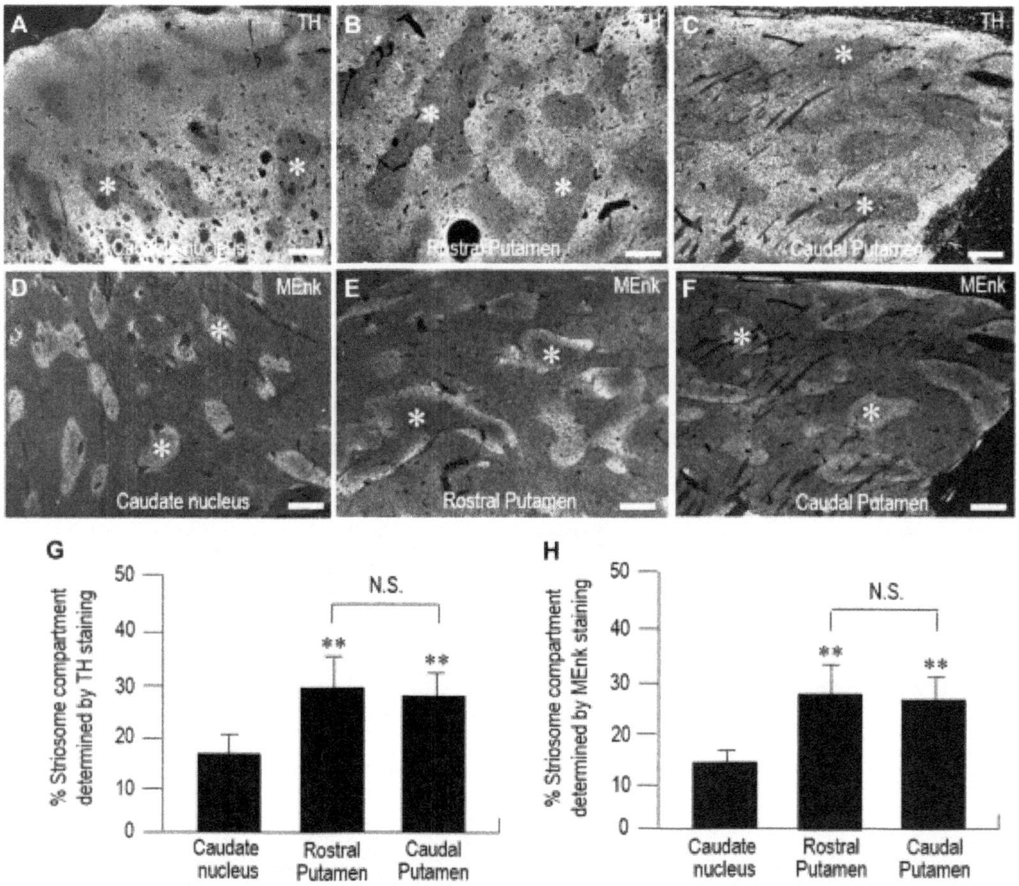

Figure 8: Morphometric analysis of the percentage of the striatum occupied by the striosome compartment in the human neostriatum. (A–F) Gray-scale-converted microscopic images of striatal areas stained with fluorescence for TH **(A–C)** and MEnk **(D–F)** in the CN **(A,D)**, rostral putamen **(B,E)**, and caudal putamen **(C,F)**. Asterisks indicate examples of striosomes. Scale bars: 1 mm. **(G)**Measurements of the percentage of the striatum occupied by the striosome compartment identified by TH-immunostaining in the CN, rostral putamen, and caudal putamen. Data represent means ± SEM (bars), $n = 25$. **indicates $P < 0.01$ vs. CN; N.S. (not significant) indicates $P > 0.05$, Rostral Putamen vs. Caudal Putamen. **(H)** Measurements of the percentage of the striatum occupied by the striosome compartment identified by MEnk-immunostaining in the CN, rostral putamen, and caudal putamen. Data represent means ± SEM (bars), $n = 25$. **indicates $P < 0.01$ vs. CN; N.S. (not significant) indicates $P > 0.05$, Rostral Putamen vs. Caudal Putamen.

Sparse Distribution of TH-Expressing Interneurons in the Human Neostriatum

It is known that the mammalian striatum contains a distinguished subgroup of GABAergic interneurons that express TH (for review see, Silberberg and Bolam, 2015). In this study, we also identified the TH-positive cells in both the CN and putamen (Figure 9). However, cell density analysis (Figures 9E,F) revealed that the TH cells were only sparsely distributed in the CN (1.8 ± 1.1 cells/mm^2) and putamen (1.6 ± 1.0 cells/mm^2), while striatal cells positive for DARPP-32, a marker for medium spiny neurons (Okita et al., 2012), were abundantly found in the CN (201 ± 22 cells/mm^2) and putamen (192 ± 31 cells/mm^2).

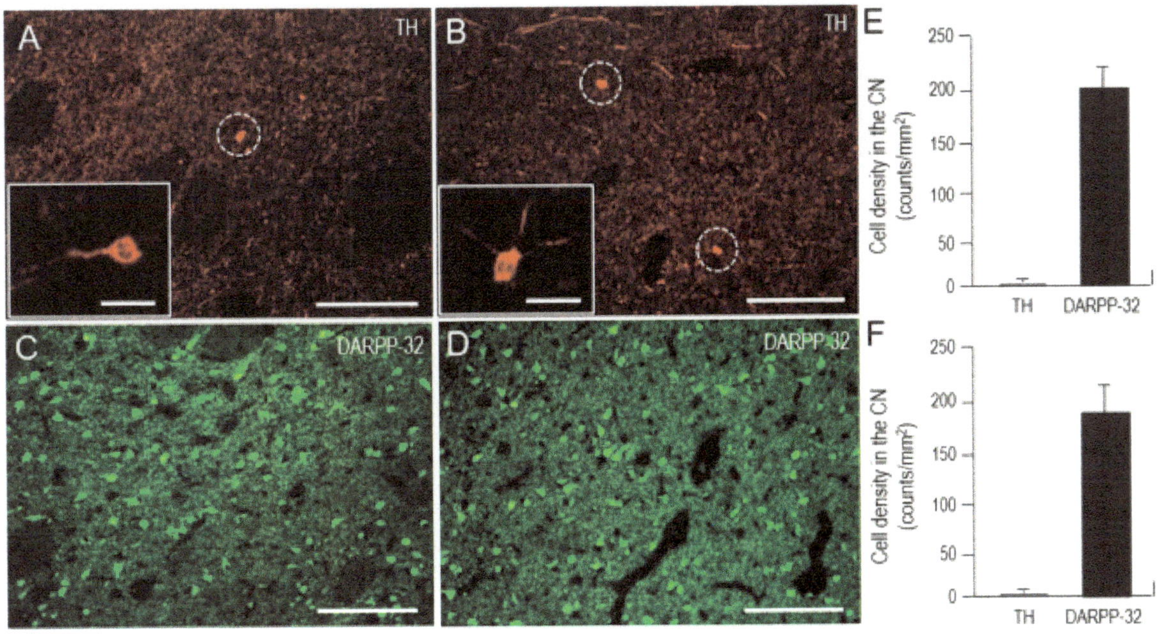

Figure 9: Scarcity of TH-positive interneurons in the human neostriatum. (A–D)Photomicrographs of the CN **(A,C)** and putamen **(B,D)** stained for TH **(A,B)** and DARPP-32 **(C,D)**. The TH-positive cells are indicated by dashed open circles **(A,B)**. Higher-magnification images of the TH-positive cells are also shown in the *insets* in **(A,B)**. Scale bars: **(A–D)** 200 μm, (*insets* in **A** and **B**) 20 μm. **(E,F)** Cell density measurements of striatal cells positive for TH or dopamine and cAMP-regulated phosphoprotein of 32 kDa (DARPP-32) in the CN **(E)** and putamen **(F)**. Values are means ± SEM (bars), $n = 25$.

DISCUSSION

In this study, we showed an immunohistochemical evidence that TH is compartmentally distributed in both the CN and putamen in FFPE human autopsy brains. By means of the serial section analysis and the double fluorescent labeling technique, the present study indicates that TH is enriched in the matrix compartment relative to the striosomes at the striatal levels from the rostral to the caudal throughout. We suggest that in the entire neostriatum, TH immunoreactivity forms the distinct striosome-matrix configurations in the same manner. This notion may contradict the previous report indicating that in the human striatum, striosomes are largely devoid of TH at rostral striatal levels while the inverse is found caudally (Prensa et al., 1999).

TH is highly concentrated in the neostriatum, where nearly all of it is expressed in axons of the dopaminergic nigrostriatal afferents. However, it has so far been known that in the mammalian striatum, there exists a subset of GABAergic interneurons that express TH (Silberberg and Bolam, 2015), although their roles in striatal dopamine systems have not yet been determined (Xenias et al., 2015). This means that striatal TH labeling is composed of not only the TH-positive afferents arising from the SNc but also the TH-immunoreactive products of such interneurons. Indeed, we here identified the TH-positive cells in the human neostriatum (Figure 9). In agreement with the previous report (Bernácer et al., 2012), our results, however, documented that the TH cells were only scarcely distributed in both the CN and putamen. The sparse density of the TH-positive cells casts doubts about their contribution to the mosaic organization of TH labeling in the human neostriatum.

Among striatal neurons, striosomal cells are unique because they send their GABAergic inhibitory projections directly or indirectly to the SNc, which contains dopaminergic neurons that project back to both the striosome and matrix compartments (Gerfen, 1984; Jiménez-Castellanos and Graybiel, 1989; Tokuno et al., 2002; Fujiyama et al., 2011; Watabe-Uchida et al., 2012). Accordingly, the striosome compartment could exert global control over striatal dopamine signals by inhibiting the activity of nigral dopaminergic cells (Crittenden and Graybiel, 2011). Considering possible mechanisms that underlie the inhomogeneous organization of TH immunoreactivity in the striatum of mature human brains, Graybiel et al. (1987) suggested an involvement of presynaptic differences between the striosome and matrix compartments in enzymatic regulation of dopamine content. We here showed that in the neostriatal sections stained for TH, the striosome-to-matrix ratio of the putamen is significantly higher ($P < 0.05$) than that of the CN (Figure 8). Taken together, we suggest that there might be a difference between the CN and putamen in the compartment-specific homeostatic regulation of striatal dopaminergic activities.

Given the evidence the patch (striosome) and matrix compartments comprised about 15% and 85% of the striatal volume, respectively, in the different species that included rat, rhesus monkey, and human, Johnston et al. (1990) suggested that a relatively constant ratio of 15% patch to 85% matrix area is maintained across mammalian species including humans. However, they also noted a slight, but significant increase (1.7 times) in the percentage of the striatum occupied by the striosome compartment from rat, through rhesus monkey, to human striatum (Johnston et al., 1990). Moreover, they also described that averaged across species, the rostral striatal sections were slightly richer in patch compartment (17%) than the caudal sections (9.8%) (Johnston et al., 1990). Our present study showed that in the human neostriatal sections stained for MEnk, the percentage of the striatum occupied by the striosome compartment in the CN (14.0%) was significantly different ($P < 0.05$) from that in both the rostral putamen (29.2%) and caudal putamen (28.1%). This indicates that the striosome-to-matrix ratio of the putamen was about 2.0 times that of the CN in the human neostriatum. In view of these observations, we posit that a species and regional difference of the small degree in the striosome-to-matrix ratio could be found in the striatum of mammals.

The putamen plays a critical role in the basal ganglia-thalamocortical circuit that regulates our voluntary movements and motor learning. Further anatomical and physiological research on the putamen is, therefore, important for elucidating the pathogenesis and symptomatology of human movement disorders. The putamen also serves as the most suitable site for the intrastriatal application of dopamine-producing transplants in PD patients (Lindvall, 2015), as previously suggested (Kish et al., 1988). There is a growing body of evidence that striosome-matrix dopaminergic systems might be involved in the disease-specific striatal pathology and symptoms of multiple human movement disorders (Crittenden and Graybiel, 2011). Indeed, human postmortem analyses have shown compartment-specific pathology in the striatum of patients with movement disorders, such as Huntington's disease (OMIM143100; Ferrante et al., 1987; Goto et al., 1989b; Goto and Hirano, 1990a; Morton et al., 1993; Hedreen and Folstein, 1995; Tippett et al., 2007), multiple system atrophy (OMIM146500) of the parkinsonian type (Goto and Hirano, 1990b; Sato et al., 2007), and X-linked dystonia-parkinsonism (OMIM314250; Goto et al., 2005, 2013). In this study, we performed an IHC study on FFPE tissues from autopsied human brains, and disclosed that striatal dopaminergic innervations labeled for TH are organized into discrete striosome-matrix configurations in the putamen. Our present findings provide anatomical evidence supporting the intriguing concept that compartment-specific dysfunction of dopamine-related neural circuits might underlie the genesis of human movement disorders.

Conflict of Interest Statement

The authors declare that the research was conducted in the absence of any commercial or financial relationships that could be construed as a potential conflict of interest.

ACKNOWLEDGMENTS

This work was supported in part by grants from the Ministry of Education, Culture, Sports, Science, and Technology of Japan (grants-in-aid for Scientific Research no. 24390223, 26461272, and 26430054).

REFERENCES

1. Albin, R. L., Young, A. B., and Penney, J. B. (1989). The functional anatomy of basal ganglia disorders. *Trends Neurosci.* 12, 366–375. doi: 10.1016/0166-2236(89)90074-X
2. Alexander, G. E., Crutcher, M. D., and DeLong, M. R. (1990). Basal ganglia-thalamocortical circuits: parallel substrates for motor, oculomotor, "prefrontal" and "limbic" functions. *Prog. Brain Res.* 85, 119–146. doi: 10.1016/s0079-6123(08)62678-3
3. Alexander, G. E., DeLong, M. R., and Strick, P. L. (1986). Parallel organization of functionally segregated circuits linking basal ganglia and cortex. *Annu. Rev. Neurosci.* 9, 357–381. doi: 10.1146/annurev.neuro.9.1.357
4. Amemori, K., Gibb, L. G., and Graybiel, A. M. (2011). Shifting responsibility: the importance of striatal modularity to reinforcement learning in uncertain environments. *Front. Hum. Neurosci.* 5:47. doi: 10.3389/fnhum.2011.00047
5. Bernácer, J., Prensa, L., and Giménez-Amaya, J. M. (2012). Distribution of GABAergic interneurons and dopaminergic cells in the functional territories of the human striatum. *PLoS One* 7:e30504. doi: 10.1371/journal.pone.0030504
6. Bolam, J. P., Izzo, P. N., and Graybiel, A. M. (1988). Cellular substrate of the histochemically defined striosome/matrix system of the caudate nucleus: a combined Golgi and immunocytochemical study in cat and ferret. *Neuroscience* 24, 853–875. doi: 10.1016/0306-4522(88)90073-5
7. Brimblecombe, K. R., and Cragg, S. J. (2015). Substance P weights striatal dopamine transmission differently within the striosome-matrix axis. *J. Neurosci.* 35, 9017–9023. doi: 10.1523/JNEUROSCI.0870-15.2015
8. Ciliax, B. J., Drash, G. W., Staley, J. K., Haber, S., Mobley, C. J., Miller, G. W., et al. (1999). Immunocytochemical localization of the dopamine transporter in human brain. *J. Comp. Neurol.* 409, 38–56. doi: 10.1002/(sici)1096-9861(19990621)409:1<38::aid-cne4>3.0.co;2-1
9. Crittenden, J. R., and Graybiel, A. M. (2011). Basal ganglia disorders associated with imbalances in the striatal striosome and matrix compartments. *Front. Neuroanat.* 5:59. doi: 10.3389/fnana.2011.00059
10. DeLong, M. R. (1990). Primate models of movement disorders of basal ganglia origin. *Trends Neurosci.* 13, 281–285. doi: 10.1016/0166-2236(90)90110-v
11. Ferrante, R. J., and Kowall, N. W. (1987). Tyrosine hydroxylase-like immunoreactivity is distributed in the matrix compartment of normal human and Huntington's disease striatum. *Brain Res.* 416, 141–146. doi: 10.1016/0006-8993(87)91506-x
12. Ferrante, R. J., Kowall, N. W., Beal, M. F., Martin, J. B., Bird, E. D., and Richardson, E. P., Jr. (1987). Morphologic and histochemical characteristics of a spared subset of striatal neurons in Huntington's disease. *J. Neuropathol. Exp. Neurol.* 46, 12–27. doi: 10.1097/00005072-198701000-00002
13. Fujiyama, F., Sohn, J., Nakano, T., Furuta, T., Nakamura, K. C., Matsuda, W., et al. (2011). Exclusive and common targets of neostriatofugal projections of rat striosome neurons: a single neuron-tracing study using a viral vector. *Eur. J. Neurosci.* 33, 668–677. doi: 10.1111/j.1460-9568.2010.07564.x
14. Gerfen, C. R. (1984). The neostriatal mosaic: compartmentalization of corticostriatal input and striatonigral output systems. *Nature* 311, 461–464. doi: 10.1038/312172a0
15. Gerfen, C. R. (1992). The neostriatal mosaic: multiple levels of compartmental organization in the basal

ganglia. *Annu. Rev. Neurosci.* 15, 285–320. doi: 10.1146/annurev.neuro.15.1.285

16. Gerfen, C. R., Baimbridge, K. G., and Miller, J. J. (1985). The neostriatal mosaic: compartmental distribution of calcium-binding protein and parvalbumin in the basal ganglia of the rat and monkey. *Proc. Natl. Acad. Sci. U S A* 82, 8780–8784. doi: 10.1073/pnas.82.24.8780
17. Gerfen, C. R., Herkenham, M., and Thibault, J. (1987). The neostriatal mosaic: II. Patch- and matrix-directed mesostriatal dopaminergic and non-dopaminergic systems. *J. Neurosci.* 7, 3915–3934.
18. Goto, S., and Hirano, A. (1990a). Synaptophysin expression in the striatum in Huntington's disease. *Acta Neuropathol.* 80, 88–91. doi: 10.1007/bf00294227
19. Goto, S., and Hirano, A. (1990b). Inhomogeneity of the putaminal lesion in striatonigral degeneration. *Acta Neuropathol.* 80, 204–207. doi: 10.1007/bf00308925
20. Goto, S., Hirano, A., and Matsumoto, S. (1989a). Subdivisional involvement of nigrostriatal loop in idiopathic Parkinson's disease and striatonigral degeneration. *Ann. Neurol.* 26, 766–770. doi: 10.1002/ana.410260613
21. Goto, S., Hirano, A., and Rojas-Corona, R. R. (1989b). An immunohistochemical investigation of the human neostriatum in Huntington's disease. *Ann. Neurol.* 25, 298–304. doi: 10.1002/ana.410250315
22. Goto, S., Kawarai, T., Morigaki, R., Okita, S., Koizumi, H., Nagahiro, S., et al. (2013). Defects in the striatal neuropeptide Y system in X-linked dystonia-parkinsonism. *Brain* 136, 1555–1567. doi: 10.1093/brain/awt084
23. Goto, S., Lee, L. V., Munoz, E. L., Tooyama, I., Tamiya, G., Makino, S., et al. (2005). Functional anatomy of the basal ganglia in X-linked recessive dystonia-parkinsonism. *Ann. Neurol.* 58, 7–17. doi: 10.1002/ana.20513
24. Goto, S., Matsumoto, S., Ushio, Y., and Hirano, A. (1996). Subregional loss of putaminal efferents to the basal ganglia output nuclei may cause parkinsonism in striatonigral degeneration. *Neurology* 47, 1032–1036. doi: 10.1212/wnl.47.4.1032
25. Goto, S., Morigaki, R., Okita, S., Nagahiro, S., and Kaji, R. (2015). Development of a highly sensitive immunohistochemical method to detect neurochemical molecules in formalin-fixed and paraffin-embedded tissues from autopsied human brains. *Front. Neuroanat.* 9:22. doi: 10.3389/fnana.2015.00022
26. Goto, S., Nagahiro, S., and Kaji, R. (2010). "Striosome-matrix pathology of dystonias: a new hypothesis for dystonia genesis," in *Dystonia: Causes, Symptoms and Treatment*, eds J. Kurstot and M. Forsstrom (New York, NY: Nova Science Publishers), 1–22.
27. Graybiel, A. M. (1990). Neurotransmitters and neuromodulators in the basal ganglia. *Trends Neurosci.* 13, 244–254. doi: 10.1016/0166-2236(90)90104-i
28. Graybiel, A. M. (2008). Habits, rituals and the evaluative brain. *Annu. Rev. Neurosci.* 31, 359–387. doi: 10.1146/annurev.neuro.29.051605.112851
29. Graybiel, A. M., Canales, J. J., and Capper-Loup, C. (2000). Levodopa-induced dyskinesias and dopamine-dependent stereotypies: a new hypothesis. *Trends Neurosci.* 23, S71–S77. doi: 10.1016/s1471-1931(00)00027-6
30. Graybiel, A. M., Hirsch, E. C., and Agid, Y. A. (1987). Differences in tyrosine hydroxylase-like immunoreactivity characterize the mesostriatal innervation of striosomes and extrastriosomal matrix at maturity. *Proc. Natl. Acad. Sci. U S A* 84, 303–307. doi: 10.1073/pnas.84.1.303
31. Graybiel, A. M., and Ragsdale, C. W., Jr. (1978). Histochemically distinct compartments in the striatum of human, monkeys and cat demonstrated by acetylcholinesterase staining. *Proc. Natl. Acad. Sci. U S A* 75, 5723–5726. doi: 10.1073/pnas.75.11.5723
32. Graybiel, A. M., Ragsdale, C. W., Jr., Yoneoka, E. S., and Elde, R. P. (1981). An immunohistochemical study of enkephalins and other neuropeptides in the striatum of the cat with evidence that the opiate peptides are arranged to form mosaic patterns in register with the striosomal compartments visible by acetylcholinesterase staining. *Neuroscience* 6, 377–397. doi: 10.1016/0306-4522(81)90131-7
33. Hedreen, J. C., and Folstein, S. E. (1995). Early loss of neostriatal striosome neurons in Huntington's disease. *J. Neuropathol. Exp. Neurol.* 54, 105–120. doi: 10.1097/00005072-199501000-00013
34. Hirsch, E., Graybiel, A. M., and Agid, Y. A. (1988). Melanized dopaminergic neurons are differentially susceptible to degeneration in Parkinson's disease. *Nature* 334, 345–348. doi: 10.1038/334345a0
35. Holt, D. J., Graybiel, A. M., and Saper, C. B. (1997). Neurochemical architecture of the human striatum. *J. Comp. Neurol.* 384, 1–25. doi: 10.1002/(sici)1096-9861(19970721)384:1<1::aid-cne1>3.0.co;2-5
36. Jakab, R. L., Hazrati, L. N., and Goldman-Rakic, P. (1996). Distribution and neurochemical character of substance P receptor (SPR)-immunoreactive striatal neurons of the macaque monkey: accumulation of SP fibers and SPR neurons and dendrites in "striocapsules" encircling striosomes. *J. Comp. Neurol.* 369, 137–149. doi: 10.1002/(sici)1096-9861(19960520)369:1<137::aid-cne10>3.0.co;2-o
37. Jimenez-Castellanos, J., and Graybiel, A. M. (1987). Subdivisions of the dopamine-containing A8–A9-A10 complex identified by their differential mesostriatal innervation of striosomes and extrastriosomal matrix. *Neuroscience* 23, 223–242. doi: 10.1016/0306-4522(87)90285-5
38. Jiménez-Castellanos, J., and Graybiel, A. M. (1989). Compartmental origins of striatal efferent projections in the cat. *Neuroscience* 32, 297–321. doi: 10.1016/0306-4522(89)90080-8
39. Johnston, J. G., Gerfen, C. R., Haber, S. N., and van der Kooy, D. (1990). Mechanisms of striatal pattern formation: conservation of mammalian compartmentalization. *Brain Res. Dev. Brain Res.* 57, 93–102. doi: 10.1016/0165-3806(90)90189-6

40. Kish, S. J., Shannak, K., and Hornykiewicz, O. (1988). Uneven pattern of dopamine loss in the striatum of patients with idiopathic Parkinson's disease. Pathophysiologic and clinical implications. *N. Engl. J. Med.* 318, 876–880. doi: 10.1056/nejm198804073181402

41. Langer, L. F., and Graybiel, A. M. (1989). Distinct nigrostriatal projection systems innervate striosomes and matrix in the primate striatum. *Brain Res.* 498, 344–350. doi: 10.1016/0006-8993(89)91114-1

42. Lindvall, O. (2015). Treatment of Parkinson's disease using cell transplantation. *Philos. Trans. R. Soc. Lond. B Biol. Sci.* 370:20140370. doi: 10.1098/rstb.2014.0370

43. Matsuda, W., Furuta, T., Nakamura, K. C., Hioki, H., Fujiyama, F., Arai, R., et al. (2009). Single nigrostriatal dopaminergic neurons form widely spread and highly dense axonal arborizations in the neostriatum. *J. Neurosci.* 29, 444–453. doi: 10.1523/JNEUROSCI.4029-08.2009

44. Morigaki, R., and Goto, S. (2015). Postsynaptic density protein 95 in the striosome and matrix compartments of the human neostriatum. *Front. Neuroanat.* 9:154. doi: 10.3389/fnana.2015.00154

45. Morton, A. J., Nicholson, L. F., and Faull, R. L. (1993). Compartmental loss of NADPH diaphorase in the neuropil of the human striatum in Huntington's disease. *Neuroscience* 53, 159–168. doi: 10.1016/0306-4522(93)90294-p

46. Moss, J., and Bolam, J. P. (2008). A dopaminergic axon lattice in the striatum and its relationship with cortical and thalamic terminals. *J. Neurosci.* 28, 11221–11230. doi: 10.1523/JNEUROSCI.2780-08.2008

47. Okita, S., Morigaki, R., Koizumi, H., Kaji, R., Nagahiro, S., and Goto, S. (2012). Cell type-specific localization of optineurin in the striatal neurons of mice: implications for neuronal vulnerability in Huntington's disease. *Neuroscience* 202, 363–370. doi: 10.1016/j.neuroscience.2011.11.059

48. Prensa, L., Cossette, M., and Parent, A. (2000). Dopaminergic innervation of human basal ganglia. *J. Chem. Neuroanat.* 20, 207–213. doi: 10.1016/s0891-0618(00)00099-5

49. Prensa, L., Giménez-Amaya, J. M., and Parent, A. (1999). Chemical heterogeneity of the striosomal compartment in the human striatum. *J. Comp. Neurol.* 413, 603–618. doi: 10.1002/(SICI)1096-9861(19991101)413:4<603::AID-CNE9>3.0.CO;2-K

50. Prensa, L., and Parent, A. (2001). The nigrostriatal pathway in the rat: a single-axon study of the relationship between dorsal and ventral tier nigral neurons and the striosome/matrix striatal compartments. *J. Neurosci.* 21, 7247–7260.

51. Sato, K., Kaji, R., Matsumoto, S., Nagahiro, S., and Goto, S. (2007). Compartmental loss of striatal medium spiny neurons in multiple system atrophy of parkinsonian type. *Mov. Disord.* 22, 2365–2370. doi: 10.1002/mds.21732

52. Sato, K., Sumi-Ichinose, C., Kaji, R., Ikemoto, K., Nomura, T., Nagatsu, I., et al. (2008). Differential involvement of striosome and matrix dopamine systems in a transgenic model of dopa-responsive dystonia. *Proc. Natl. Acad. Sci. U S A* 105, 12551–12556. doi: 10.1073/pnas.0806065105

53. Silberberg, G., and Bolam, J. P. (2015). Local and afferent synaptic pathways in the striatal microcircuitry. *Curr. Opin. Neurobiol.* 33, 182–187. doi: 10.1016/j.conb.2015.05.002

54. Tippett, L. J., Waldvogel, H. J., Thomas, S. J., Hogg, V. M., van Roon-Mom, W., Synek, B. J., et al. (2007). Striosomes and mood dysfunction in Huntington's disease. *Brain* 130, 206–221. doi: 10.1093/brain/awl243

55. Tokuno, H., Chiken, S., Kametani, K., and Moriizumi, T. (2002). Efferent projections from the striatal patch compartment: anterograde degeneration after selective ablation of neurons expressing mu-opioid receptor in rat. *Neurosci. Lett.* 332, 5–8. doi: 10.1016/s0304-3940(02)00837-6

56. Watabe-Uchida, M., Zhu, L., Ogawa, S. K., Vamanrao, A., and Uchida, N. (2012). Whole-brain mapping of direct inputs to midbrain dopamine neurons. *Neuron* 74, 858–873. doi: 10.1016/j.neuron.2012.03.017

57. Xenias, H. S., Ibáñez-Sandoval, O., Koós, T., and Tepper, J. M. (2015). Are striatal tyrosine hydroxylase interneurons dopaminergic? *J. Neurosci.*35, 6584–6599. doi: 10.1523/JNEUROSCI.0195-15.2015

CHAPTER 15 IMMUNOHISTOCHEMISTRY FOR MYC

Christopher W. Toon, Angela Chou, Adele Clarkson, Keshani DeSilva, Michelle Houang, Joseph C. Y. Chan, Loretta L. Sioson, Lucy Jankova, Anthony J. Gill

INTRODUCTION

Dysregulation of MYC (HGNC:7553) is an early consequence of activating mutations in APC(HGNC:583), a key driver mutation in the adenoma-carcinoma pathway in colorectal cancer (CRC). Mediated by beta-catenin via the canonical Wnt pathway, aberrant over-expression of MYC and CYCLIN D1 results in uncontrolled cellular proliferation, conferring a growth advantage to cancer cells [1], [2]. The role of MYC over-expression in driving CRC tumorigenesis has been confirmed by gene expression profiling studies [3], and more recently by CRC genome-wide analysis as part of the Cancer Genome Atlas Network initiative [4].

Interestingly MYC over-expression as determined by Northern blot analysis was reported as a biomarker of good outcome in colorectal cancer as far back as 1996. [5] Currently its use as a prognostic biomarker is difficult to justify because of the limited availability and expense involved of molecular testing. Therefore testing for MYC over-expression in CRC is not currently available, feasible or warranted in the routine clinical setting.

Recently a novel highly sensitive and specific rabbit monoclonal antibody directed against the myc protein (clone Y69) has become available. This antibody has been validated in the routine clinical setting in formalin fixed paraffin embedded tissue, where myc immunohistochemsitry in combination with bcl2 immunohistochemistry, has been used to identify the poor prognostic subgroup of non-Hodgkin lymphoma known as 'double hit lymphoma'. [6], [7] In fact MYC and BCL2 expression as determined by immunohistochemsitry in formalin fixed paraffin embedded tissue has rapidly become part of the routine diagnostic assessment of patients with high grade B-cell lymphoma. [8].

We sought to revisit the use of MYC expression as biomarker in CRC by correlating outcome with MYC expression as determined by this widely available rabbit monoclonal antibody.

MATERIALS AND METHODS

Our CRC cohort has been previously described. [9] Briefly, retrospective CRC cases were recruited by searching the pathology database of the Department of Anatomical Pathology, Royal North Shore Hospital, Sydney for patients who had definitive operations for CRC between 2004 and 2009. During this period this center performed centralized pathological testing for two quaternary referral hospitals with dedicated colorectal surgery units and 4 community hospitals. Therefore this patient cohort represents a true snapshot of CRC cases encountered in the Australian community as a whole.

Exclusion criteria were tumors of extra-colonic and appendiceal location, tumors treated exclusively endoluminally and histological types other than adenocarcinoma defined by the WHO 2010 system. [10].

Tumors were independently reviewed by three pathologists (CT, KDS and AG) to confirm the diagnosis and to restage the tumors according to 7th edition 2009 AJCC/TNM. [11] For resections involving synchronous tumors, the tumor with the highest pathologic stage was selected and annotated. Tissue microarrays (TMA) containing duplicate 1 mm cores were then constructed from available tumor tissue blocks.

Citation: Toon CW, Chou A, Clarkson A, DeSilva K, Houang M, Chan JCY, et al. (2014) Immunohistochemistry for Myc. PLoS ONE 9(2): e87456. doi:10.1371/journal.pone.0087456.

Immunohistochemistry was performed on the TMA using a commercially available rabbit anti-myc antibody (clone Y69, cat:ab32072, Abcam, Burlingame CA USA) using the Leica BondIII autostainer (Leica microsystems, Mount Waverley, Victoria, Australia) according to the manufacturer's protocol. The slides were dewaxed in Bond Dewax solution (AR9222, Leica Microsystems) and hydrated in Bond Wash solution (AR9590, Leica Microsystems). Heat induced epitope retrieval was performed for 60 minutes in the manufacturer's alkaline retrieval solution ER2 (VBS part no: AR9640, Leica Microsystems). Slides were then incubated with the primary antibody at a dilution of 1 in 100 for 30 minutes at room temperature. Antibody detection was performed using the biotin free Bond Polymer Defined Detection System (DS9713 Leica Microsystems) according to the manufacturer's protocol. Slides were then counterstained with hematoxylin.

MYC over-expression was assessed by myc IHC, scored using a two-tiered visual system by a practicing surgical pathologist (CT) blinded to all clinical, pathological and outcome information. Nuclear staining of any intensity in greater than 10% of neoplastic cells was scored as positive (over-expressed). All other patterns of staining were scored as negative. An external control (a MYC amplified lymphoma) was run with each batch of slides.

DNA mismatch repair (MMR) and BRAF IHC status were determined by immunohistochemistry as previously described [9], [12].

In order to examine the accuracy of TMA IHC interpretation, Myc IHC was performed on whole sections of CRCs on a subcohort of 98 consecutive CRCs from 2004, interpreted by same assessor on TMA (CT) blinded to all clinical, pathological and TMA data.

Correlation between MYC over-expression and CRC patient clinicopathological variables were examined in 2×2 contingengy tables for categorical variables or using the Mann-Whitney test for age (Table 1). Variables which showed a significance of $p<0.10$ were included in a binary logistic regression model to further examine the relationship between MYC over-expression and DNA mismatch repair (MMR)/ BRAF status IHC phenotype (Table 2).

Table 1: Clinical and pathological characteristics of 1421 consecutive CRC patients (2004–2009)

Variable	myc IHC positive	myc IHC negative	p-value*
Gender, n (valid %)			0.717
Female	514 (52.4)	226 (51.2)	
Male	466 (47.6)	215 (48.8)	
Age at diagnosis, median (range)	73 (17–100)	75 (33–98)	0.071
Anatomic location, n (valid %)			0.771
Rectum	247 (25.5)	113 (25.7)	
Caecum	218 (22.5)	94 (21.4)	
Ascending colon	142 (14.6)	76 (17.3)	
Transverse colon	119 (12.3)	48 (10.9)	
Descending colon	33 (3.4)	18 (4.1)	
Sigmoid colon	211 (21.8)	91 (20.7)	
Histologic grade, n (valid %)			0.755
Low	553 (79.0)	269 (80.1)	
High	147 (21.0)	67 (19.9)	
Lymphovascular space invasion, n (valid %)			0.663
Absent	362 (36.9)	173 (39.2)	
Present	303 (30.9)	155 (35.1)	
Peritumoral lymphocyte reaction, n (valid %)			0.316
Absent	34 (4.8)	11 (3.3)	
Present	669 (95.2)	326 (96.7)	
Overall Stage AJCC/TNM 7th ed, n (valid %)			0.003
I	181 (18.5)	53 (12.0)	
IIA	298 (30.4)	116 (26.3)	
IIB	52 (5.3)	33 (7.5)	
IIC	11 (1.1)	4 (0.9)	
IIIA	49 (5.0)	15 (3.4)	
IIIB	237 (24.2)	136 (30.8)	
IIIC	116 (11.8)	58 (13.2)	
IVA	20 (2.0)	12 (2.7)	
IVB	16 (1.6)	14 (3.2)	
MMR IHC status, n (valid %)			0.008
Proficient	770 (78.6)	374 (84.8)	
Deficient	210 (21.4)	67 (15.2)	
BRAFV600E IHC status, n (valid %)			0.035
Wild type	776 (79.2)	371 (84.1)	
Mutant	204 (20.8)	70 (15.9)	
IHC phenotypes, n (valid %)			0.001
MMRp/BRAFwt	714 (72.9)	339 (76.9)	
MMRd/BRAFwt	61 (6.2)	32 (7.3)	
MMRd/BRAFV600E	149 (15.2)	35 (7.9)	
MMRp/BRAFV600E	56 (5.7)	35 (7.9)	

*Reports on the significance of differences between myc positive and negative groups for each variable, using either Pearson chi-square test (with continuity correction for 2×2 tables) for categorical variables or Mann-Whitney U test for age.

Table 2: Multivariable binary logistic regression showing adjusted effect of MMR/BRAF IHC phenotype on myc over-expression in 1421 CRCs

Variable	Multivariable analysis
	OR (95%CI), p
Age at diagnosis	0.99 (0.98–1.00), 0.02
Overall Stage AJCC/TNM 7th edition	
I	1.00
IIA	0.72 (0.49–1.05), 0.09
IIB	0.48 (.28–.82), <0.01
IIC	0.70 (0.21–2.34), 0.57
IIIA	0.93 (0.48–1.80), 0.83
IIIB	0.51 (0.45–0.74), <0.01
IIIC	0.60 (0.38–0.94), 0.02
IVA	0.49 (0.22–1.07), 0.08
IVB	0.34 (0.15–0.75), <0.01
MMR/BRAF IHC phenotype	
MMRp/BRAFwt	1.00
MMRd/BRAFwt	0.88 (0.58–1.38), 0.57
MMRd/BRAFV600E	2.17 (1.45–3.24), <0.01
MMRp/BRAFV600E	0.85 (0.54–1.34), 0.48

Follow-up was obtained by the examination of hospital medical records, those from surgeons' private rooms and archival public death notices and obituaries in the state of New South Wales, Australia. Overall survival was defined as the duration alive from time of definitive surgery. Patients were followed up until death or their last date of follow-up not more than 7 years after definitive surgery.

Kaplan Meier analysis was used to report 5-year overall survivals for CRCs with and without MYC over-expression, with the difference assessed by Log Rank Test. Multivariable cox regression was used to explore the association between adjusted effect of MYC over-expression on overall survival, in a full model which included age at diagnosis, gender, anatomic site of tumor, tumor stage, combined mismatch repair deficiency and BRAF IHC status, tumor size, histologic grade, presence or absence of lymphovascular space invasion and peritumoral lymphocyte response status.

A $p<0.05$ was taken as significant, except in the initial modeling using binary logistic regression (mentioned above). Statistical analyses were performed using IBM SPSS Statistics v21 on OSX.

RESULTS

A total of 1421 CRCs were assessed on TMA. The clinical and pathological features are summarized in Table 1. Briefly, there was approximately equal gender distribution, with a median age of diagnosis at 74 years (range 17–100 years). The 5-year overall survival for the cohort was 66.3%, with a mean of 52.9% (95%CI=5.14–5.44).

Myc IHC showed consistent nuclear immuno-localisation, and there was a visible distinction between cases which were negative (scored as negative for over-expression), and those which showed weak to strong staining in 10% or more neoplastic cells (scored as positive for over-expression). Examples of myc IHC staining characteristics are presented in Figure 1. The prevalence of MYC over-expression in CRC was 69%.

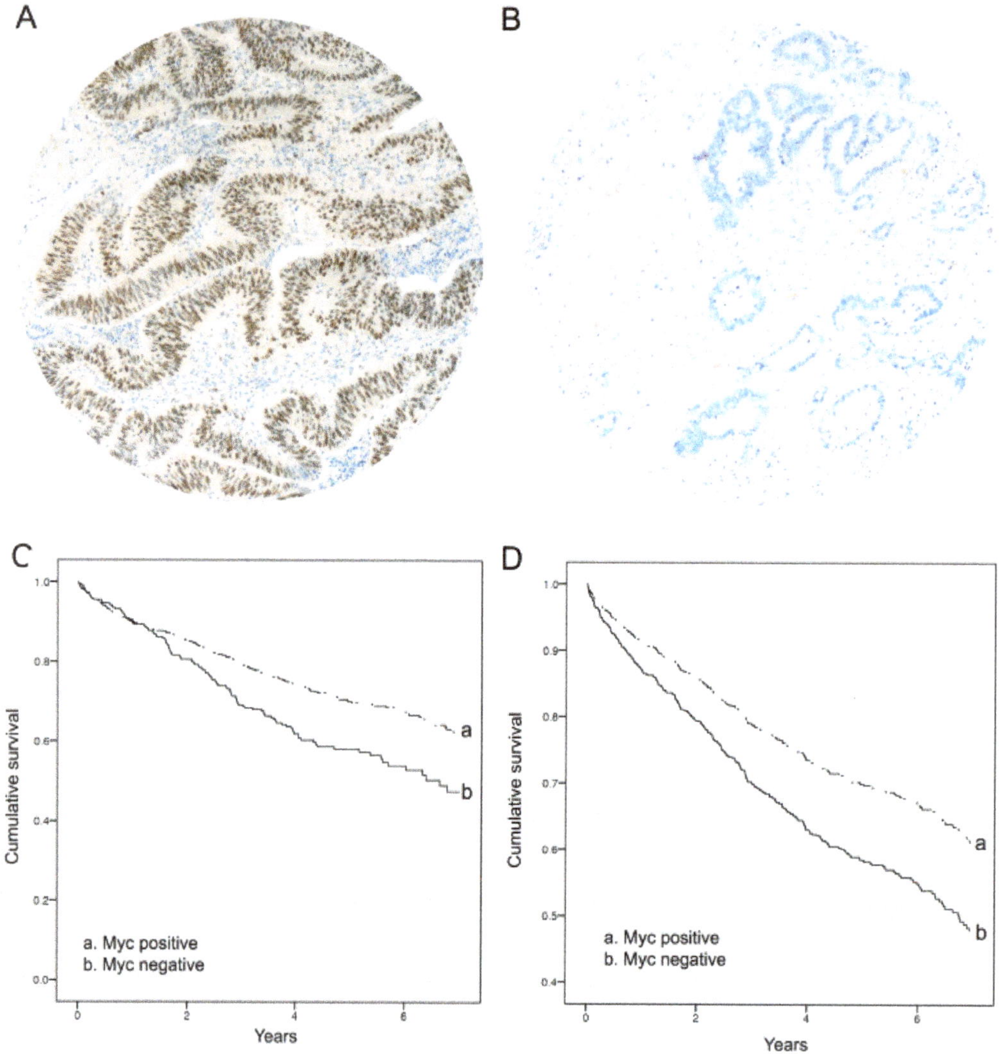

Figure 1: Panel A: Myc positive IHC staining; Panel B: Myc negative IHC staining; Panel C: Kaplan Meier analysis (Log Rank test p=0.01); Panel D: Univariable Cox regression.

The clinical and pathological features of myc IHC negative (n=441, 31.0%) and myc IHC positive (MYC over-expressed, n=980, 69.0%) CRCs are summarized in Table 1. MYC over-expression was significantly associated with tumor stage and MMR/BRAF IHC phenotype, but not gender, anatomic location, histologic grade, presence or absence of lymphovascular space invasion, nor peritumoral lymphocyte reaction status. The relationship between MYC over-expression and age at diagnosis tended to significance (p=0.07).

Table 2 shows the adjusted effect of of MMR/BRAF IHC phenotype on myc IHC status. MYC over-expression was strongly associated with the MMRd/BRAFV600E IHC phenotype [odds ratio=2.17 (95%CI=1.45–3.24), p<0.01].

The 5 year survival for CRCs with MYC over-expression was 93.2% (overall 50th centile survival 3.06 years, interquartile range 0.56–5.22), compared with myc negative CRC of 57.3% (overall 50th centile survival 2.32 years, interquartile range 0.31–4.26).

The effect of myc status on CRC overall survival is displayed in Figure 1. CRCs with MYC over-expression showed significantly better survival compared to myc negative cases (Log Rank test p<0.01), with a crude effect (univariable model) hazard ratio of 0.67 [(95%CI=0.54–0.83), p<0.01]. This crude effect on overall survival remained significant even when stratified by MMR/BRAF IHC phenotype [hazard ratio=0.68 (96%CI=0.54–0.84), p<0.01].

In the full multivariable model, the adjusted effect of MYC over-expression on overall survival became insignificant [hazard ratio=0.91 (95%CI=0.69–1.20), p=0.52] due to the dominant effect of age at diagnosis, tumor stage and lymphovascular space invasion status and the MMR deficient/ BRAFV600E mutant IHC phenotype on survival (Table 3). Table 4 displays the full model including interaction between myc IHC and MMR/BRAF status.

Table 3: Multivariable Cox regression proportional hazards analysis of 1421 CRCs

Variable	Multivariable analysis
	HR (95%CI), p
Gender	
Female	1.00
Male	1.25 (0.94–1.65), 0.12
Age at diagnosis	1.04 (1.03–1.05), <0.01
Anatomic location	
Left colon	1.00
Right colon	1.10 (0.83–1.45), 0.52
Histologic grade	
Low	1.00
High	1.28 (0.90–1.83), 0.18
Lymphovascular space invasion	
Absent	1.00
Present	1.60 (1.14–2.30), <0.01
Peritumoral lymphocyte reaction	
Absent	1.00
Present	1.93 (0.75–4.97), 0.18
Overall Stage AJCC/TNM 7th edition	
I	1.00
IIA	2.22 (1.20–4.11), 0.01
IIB	2.67 (1.21–5.90), 0.02
IIC	11.91 (4.68–30/29), <0.01
IIIA	0.96 (0.27–3.39), 0.95
IIIB	2.70 (1.46–4.99), <0.01
IIIC	5.78 (3.06–10.89), <0.01
IVA	11.0 (4.61–26.27), <0.01
IVB	15.34 (6.47–36.37), <0.01
MMR/BRAF IHC phenotype	
MMRp/BRAFwt	1.00
MMRd/BRAFwt	0.58 (0.29–1.16), 0.13
MMRd/BRAFV600E	0.60 (0.37–0.97), 0.04
MMRp/BRAFV600E	1.07 (0.67–1.70), 0.78
Myc IHC status	
Negative	1.00
Positive	0.91 (0.69–1.20), 0.49

Table 4: Multivariable Cox regression proportional hazards analysis of 1421 CRCs including myc IHC status and MMR/BRAF IHC phenotype interaction terms

Variable	Multivariable analysis
	HR (95%CI), p
Gender	
Female	1.00
Male	1.24 (0.93–1.64), 0.14
Age at diagnosis	1.04 (1.03–1.05), <0.01
Anatomic location	
Left colon	1.00
Right colon	1.11 (0.84–1.48), 0.47
Histologic grade	
Low	1.00
High	1.29 (0.90–1.85), 0.17
Lymphovascular space invasion	
Absent	1.00
Present	1.60 (1.14–2.23), <0.01
Peritumoral lymphocyte reaction	
Absent	1.00
Present	1.98 (0.77–5.13), 0.16
Overall Stage AJCC/TNM 7th edition	
I	1.00
IIA	2.22 (1.20–4.11), 0.01
IIB	2.68 (1.21–5.93), 0.02
IIC	12.14 (4.77–30.88), <0.01
IIIA	0.97 (0.27–3.41), 0.96
IIIB	2.70 (1.46–4.99), <0.01
IIIC	5.83 (3.09–11.00), <0.01
IVA	10.84 (4.53–25.94), <0.01
IVB	15.67 (6.59–37.22), <0.01
MMR/BRAF IHC phenotype	
MMRp/BRAFwt	1.00
MMRd/BRAFwt	0.29 (0.07–1.21), 0.09
MMRd/BRAFV600E	0.77 (0.36–1.67), 0.77
MMRp/BRAFV600E	0.91 (0.47–1.75), 0.77
Myc IHC status	
Negative	1.00
Positive	0.87 (0.64–1.20), 0.39
Interaction terms	
Myc *MMRp/BRAFwt	1.00
Myc *MMRd/BRAFwt	2.77 (0.55–13.88), 0.22
Myc *MMRd/BRAFV600E	0.70 (0.28–1.74), 0.44
Myc *MMRp/BRAFV600E	1.38 (0.58–3.32), 0.47

MMRd – DNA mismatch repair deficient; MMRp – DNA mismatch repair proficient; BRAFwt – BRAF wild type; BRAFV600E – BRAFV600E mutant.

There was substantial agreement between TMA and whole section myc IHC scores (kappa=0.742, $p<0.01$). All positive TMA cases were positive on whole sections. There were 11 discordant cases (negative on TMA, positive on whole section), all due to patchy staining. Univariable Cox regression was also performed on whole sections, confirming the improved overall survival of CRCs showing MYC over-expression (Figure 2).

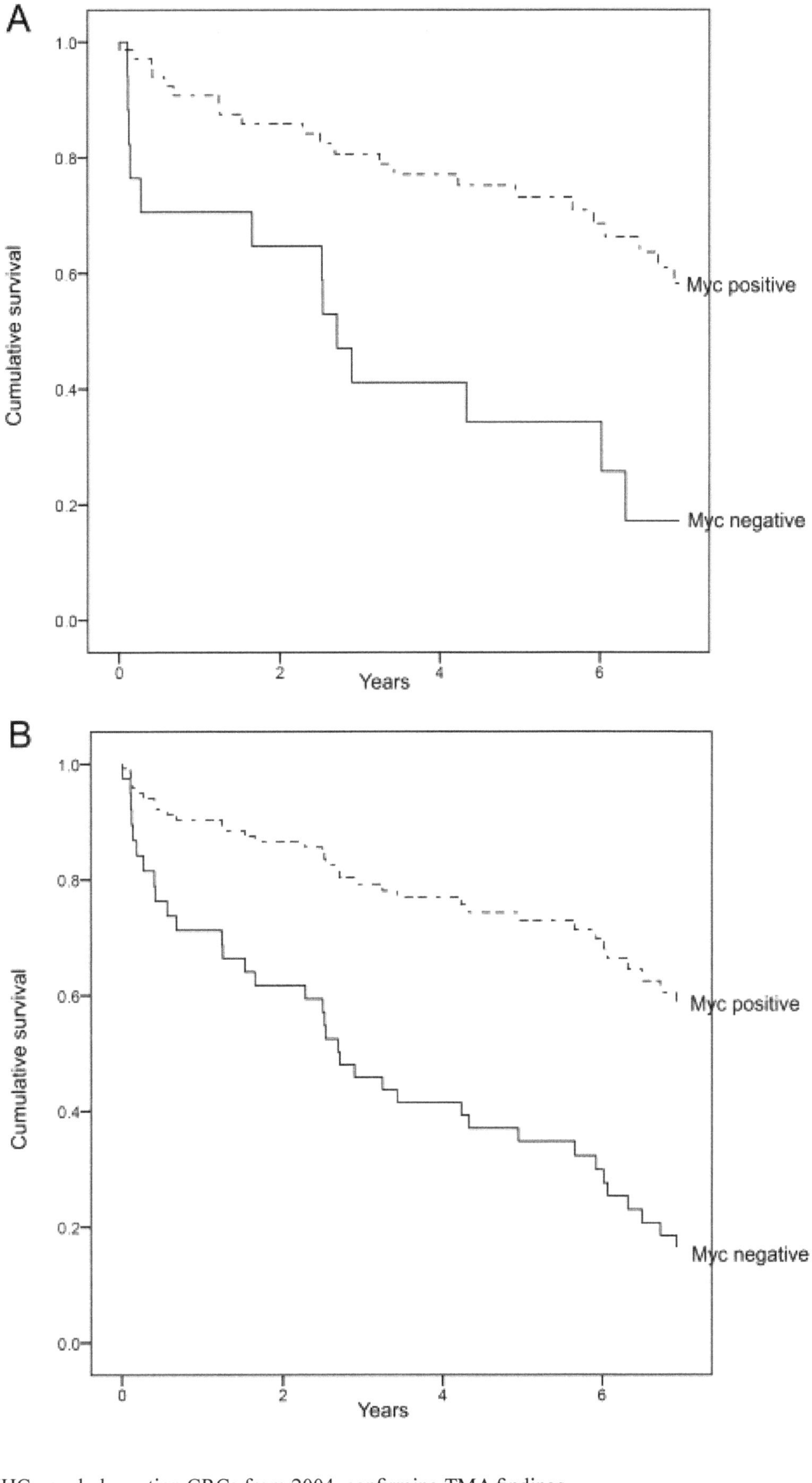

Figure 2: Myc IHC on whole section CRCs from 2004, confirming TMA findings.

Panel A: Kaplan Meier curves showing superior overall survival of CRCs with MYC over-expression compared to myc negative CRCs (Log Rank test $p<0.01$); Panel B: Univariable Cox regression analysis showing MYC over-expression significantly correlated with improved overall survival [hazard ratio=0.30 (95%CI=0.15–0.60), $p<0.01$].

DISCUSSION

Previous studies on MYC expression in CRC have been inconsistent and conflicting presumably due to the use of small cohorts (n ranging from 38 to 310) and the use of a variety of detection methods including IHC, fluorescent in-situ hybridization (FISH), RNA-based analysis and DNA copy number. [5], [13]–[17]. Older studies using IHC have been limited by the use of antibodies which demonstrated aberrant (cytoplasmic) immuno-localisation presumably due to poor specificity. [18].

The development and validation of a highly specific rabbit monoclonal antibody for myc has made a major impact in lymphoma diagnosis where the combination of MYC and BCL2 overexpression as determined by immunohistochemistry alone has been used to define a poor prognosis group of B-cell non Hodgkin lymphoma known as double hit lymphomas. [6], [7] Interestingly, in these lymphoma studies where myc IHC and FISH assessment have resulted in conflicting results, MYC expression as determined by IHC has been a better predictor of outcome than the previous gold standard FISH. Presumably this is because MYC over-expression can be due to a variety of cellular processes rather than just simple amplification.

In this context, our study, which is based on a very large and unselected cohort on 1421 CRC cohorts using this next generation of specific rabbit monoclonal antibody, demonstrates the high prevalence of MYC over-expression in CRCs, and more importantly, the potential role of myc as a powerful prognostic biomarker in CRCs. The fact that MYC over-expression is significantly associated with better overall survival in univariable analysis is perhaps surprising given current understanding of the tumorigenic potential of MYC dysregulation [1]–[4]. Only one previous study has shown this effect in CRC [5]. While there is insufficient data to postulate as to the underlying mechanism, the correlation between tumorigenic potential (oncogenesis) and survival, at least for MYC, is like to be more complex than initially thought.

In this study we have chosen to examine MYC over-expression in the context of CRCs grouped according to their MMR and BRAF status, rather than MMR and BRAF status individually. It is now well established that MMR and BRAF interact in complex ways in relation to their effect on survival. For example, in MMR proficient CRCs, the presence of BRAFV600E mutation confers a worse survival, whereas in MMR deficient CRCs, BRAFV600E is a marker of the methylator phenotype, a group of CRCs which show excellent prognosis [12], [19].

Interestingly, although MYC over-expression was strongly associated with the MMRd/BRAFV66E phenotype, their lack of interaction in the full multivariable model shows that MYC's effect on survival cannot be explained entirely just by its association with MMR/BRAF status. This suggests that the predictive effect of MYC over-expression on survival is mediated in part, by mechanisms independent of MMR/BRAF status.

One of the major drawbacks of our study is the over-simplification by which MYC over-expression is determined. The semi-quantitative nature of IHC is such that changes in IHC intensity need to be significant (in the logarithmic scale, otherwise known as the Weber-Fechner law) in order that the human eye be able to appreciate a change. This method of IHC scoring does however lend itself to more straightforward correlative analysis such as binary logistic regression, and is the predominant methodology by which most IHC is scored in the diagnostic clinical setting. Significantly, despite this drawback we were able to demonstrate significant overall survival differences on univariable analysis of myc IHC status.

Another significant drawback is the lack of disease specific outcomes and cancer specific mortality in our study cohort. Future studies employing these endpoints will provide important information which may significantly inform on clinical practice.

In summary, our study shows that myc status, as determined by IHC using a simple semi-quantitative scoring methodology readily deployed in the clinical setting can be used as a predictor of prognosis in CRC. The refinement of this predictive utility awaits further elucidation in cohorts with disease specific outcomes.

REFERENCES

1. He T-C, Sparks AB, Rago C, Hermeking H, Zawel L, et al. (1998) Identification of c-MYC as a Target of the APC Pathway. Science 281: 1509–1512. doi: 10.1126/science.281.5382.1509
2. Powell SM, Zilz N, Beazer-Barclay Y, Bryan TM, Hamilton SR, et al. (1992) APC mutations occur early during colorectal tumorigenesis. Nature 359: 235–237. doi: 10.1038/359235a0
3. Chan SK, Griffith OL, Tai IT, Jones SJM (2008) Meta-analysis of colorectal cancer gene expression profiling studies identifies consistently reported candidate biomarkers. Cancer Epidemiology Biomarkers & Prevention 17: 543–552. doi: 10.1158/1055-9965.epi-07-2615
4. Muzny DM, Bainbridge MN, Chang K, Dinh HH, Drummond JA, et al. (2012) Comprehensive molecular characterization of human colon and rectal cancer. Nature 487: 330–337.
5. Smith DR, Goh HS (1996) Overexpression of the c-myc proto-oncogene in colorectal carcinoma is associated with a reduced mortality that is abrogated by point mutation of the p53 tumor suppressor gene. Clin Cancer Res 2: 1049 1053.
6. Green TM, Young KH, Visco C, Xu-Monette ZY, Orazi A, et al. (2012) Immunohistochemical Double-Hit Score Is a Strong Predictor of Outcome in Patients With Diffuse Large B-Cell Lymphoma Treated With Rituximab Plus Cyclophosphamide, Doxorubicin, Vincristine, and Prednisone. Journal of Clinical Oncology 30: 3460–3467. doi: 10.1200/jco.2011.41.4342

7. Johnson NA, Slack GW, Savage KJ, Connors JM, Ben-Neriah S, et al. (2012) Concurrent Expression of MYC and BCL2 in Diffuse Large B-Cell Lymphoma Treated With Rituximab Plus Cyclophosphamide, Doxorubicin, Vincristine, and Prednisone. Journal of Clinical Oncology 30: 3452–3459. doi: 10.1200/jco.2011.41.0985

8. Hu S, Xu-Monette ZY, Tzankov A, Green T, Wu L, et al.. (2013) MYC/BCL2 protein coexpression contributes to the inferior survival of activated B-cell subtype of diffuse large B-cell lymphoma and demonstrates high-risk gene expression signatures: a report from The International DLBCL Rituximab-CHOP Consortium Program. Blood 121: 4021–4031; quiz 4250.

9. Toon CW, Walsh MD, Chou A, Capper D, Clarkson A, et al. (2013) BRAFV600E immunohistochemistry facilitates universal screening of colorectal cancers for Lynch syndrome. Am J Surg Pathol 37: 1592–1602. doi: 10.1097/pas.0b013e31828f233d

10. FT Bosman FC, RH Hruban, ND Theise (2010) WHO classification of Tumors of the DIgestive System 4th ed Lyon, France: IARC press; 2010.

11. Edge SB, Byrd DR, Compton CC (2009) AJCC Cancer Staging Manual, Springer, New York, NY, USA, 7th edition, 2009.

12. Toon CW, Chou A, Desilva K, Chan J, Patterson J, et al.. (2013) BRAFV600E immunohistochemistry in conjunction with mismatch repair status predicts survival in patients with colorectal cancer. Mod Pathol.

13. Erisman MD, Litwin S, Keidan RD, Comis RL, Astrin SM (1988) Noncorrelation of the Expression of the C-Myc-Oncogene in Colorectal-Carcinoma with Recurrence of Disease or Patient Survival. Cancer Research 48: 1350–1355.

14. Al-Kuraya K, Novotny H, Bavi P, Siraj AK, Uddin S, et al. (2007) HER2, TOP2A, CCND1, EGFR and C-MYC oncogene amplification in colorectal cancer. J Clin Pathol 60: 768–772. doi: 10.1136/jcp.2006.038281

15. Miller F, Heimann TM, Quish A, Pyo DJ, Szporn A, et al. (1992) ras and c-myc protein expression in colorectal carcinoma. Study of cancer-prone patients. Dis Colon Rectum 35: 430–435. doi: 10.1007/bf02049398

16. Nagai MA, Habr-Gama A, Oshima CT, Brentani MM (1992) Association of genetic alterations of c-myc, c-fos, and c-Ha-ras proto-oncogenes in colorectal tumors. Frequency and clinical significance. Dis Colon Rectum 35: 444–451. doi: 10.1007/bf02049400

17. Bhatavdekar JM, Patel DD, Ghosh N, Chikhlikar PR, Trivedi TI, et al. (1997) Coexpression of Bcl-2, c-Myc, and p53 oncoproteins as prognostic discriminants in patients with colorectal carcinoma. Dis Colon Rectum 40: 785–790. doi: 10.1007/bf02055433

18. Williams ARW, Piris J, Wyllie AH (1990) Immunohistochemical Demonstration of Altered Intracellular-Localization of the C-Myc Oncogene Product in Human Colorectal Neoplasms. Journal of Pathology 160: 287–293. doi: 10.1002/path.1711600404

19. Lochhead P, Kuchiba A, Imamura Y, Liao X, Yamauchi M, et al. (2013) Microsatellite instability and BRAF mutation testing in colorectal cancer prognostication. J Natl Cancer Inst 105: 1151–1156. doi: 10.1093/jnci/djt173

CHAPTER 16

GAUGING NOTCH1 ACTIVATION IN CANCER USING IMMUNOHISTOCHEMISTRY

Michael J. Kluk, Todd Ashworth, Hongfang Wang[1] , Birgit Knoechel, Emily F. Mason, Elizabeth A. Morgan, David Dorfman[1] , Geraldine Pinkus, Oliver Weigert, Jason L. Hornick, Lucian R. Chirieac, Michelle Hirsch, David J. Oh, Andrew P. South, Irene M. Leigh, Celine Pourreyron, Andrew J. Cassidy, Daniel J. DeAngelo, David M. Weinstock, Ian E. Krop, Deborah Dillon, Jane E. Brock, Alexander J. F. Lazar, Myron Peto, Raymond J. Cho, Alexander Stoeck, Brian B. Haines, Sriram Sathayanrayanan, Scott Rodig, Jon C. Aster[1]

INTRODUCTION

Notch receptors participate in a conserved signaling pathway that regulates many cellular phenotypes, including cell fate, cell proliferation, and cell survival (for review, see [1]). Mammals possess four Notch genes (*NOTCH1-4*), each with distinct patterns of expression and different knockout phenotypes in mice. Canonical signaling through all four receptors relies on a series of ligand-dependent proteolytic cleavages, the last of which is carried out by a multisubunit protease called gamma-secretase, which cleaves Notch receptors within the inner half the receptor's transmembrane domain. This liberates the Notch intracellular domain, NICD, which translocates to the nucleus and forms a short-lived transcriptional activation complex.

Outcomes produced by Notch signaling in normal cells vary dramatically with cellular context, presumably because epigenetic patterning of genomes leads to varied effects of NICD on transcriptional outputs. Genotypic data from humans and experimental results from mice indicate that *NOTCH1* also has varied roles in cancer, acting as either an oncogene or a tumor suppressor gene depending on cellular context. Gain-of-function mutations of *NOTCH1* are common in T lymphoblastic leukemia/lymphoma (T-LL) [2,3], and have also been described in subsets of chronic lymphocytic leukemia (CLL) [4–6], mantle cell lymphoma (MCL) [7], diffuse large B cell lymphoma [8], peripheral T cell lymphoma (PTCL) [9], breast cancer [10], and non-small cell lung cancer (NSCLC) [11]. These activating mutations include diverse point substitutions, deletions, and translocations that produce ligand-independent NOTCH1 proteolysis and activation, as well as mutations that remove a C-terminal PEST degron domain and thereby stabilize NICD1. In addition, data emerging from deep sequencing of cancer genomes has identified frequent mutation of genes encoding Notch pathway components in high-grade ovarian serous carcinomas [12], although the functional consequences of these mutations on Notch signaling is uncertain. There is also evidence that NOTCH1 has important functional roles in endothelium and other stromal components that may contribute to the malignant behavior of cancers [13,14]. Conversely, loss-of-function mutations distributed over a large part of the *NOTCH1* locus are common in squamous cell carcinomas of the skin [15] and head and neck [16,17] and also occur in a smaller subset of squamous cell carcinomas of the lung [15,18]. Similarly, loss of *notch1* function in vascular endothelium leads to angiosarcoma-like proliferations in mice [19,20].

There is interest in therapeutic targeting of NOTCH1 in cancers in which it has an oncogenic role with antagonists such as inhibitory antibodies and gamma-secretase inhibitors (GSI)

Citation: Kluk MJ, Ashworth T, Wang H, Knoechel B, Mason EF, Morgan EA, et al. (2013) Gauging NOTCH1 Activation in Cancer Using Immunohistochemistry. PLoS ONE 8(6): e67306. doi:10.1371/journal.pone.0067306.

[21]. Ideally, such trials would focus on treatment of patients whose tumors show evidence of ongoing NOTCH1 activation. Given the large size of the *NOTCH1* locus and the diversity of genetic aberrations that produce ligand-independent activation of NOTCH1 or stabilize NICD1, genetic screening for oncogenic *NOTCH1* alterations is challenging, particularly when working with archival FPE samples. Moreover, it is suspected that ligand-mediated NOTCH1 activation also contributes to tumor cell growth and survival, and such tumors would go undetected by genetic screening.

An ideal biomarker test would detect NICD1 within tumor cells directly, regardless of the underlying mechanism of NOTCH1 activation. To this end, we developed a robust, specific immunohistochemical (IHC) staining method that detects NICD1 in archival samples. The test relies on a commercial rabbit monoclonal antibody, previously used only in Western blot analyses, that is specific for a neoepitope in NICD1 created by gamma-secretase-mediated proteolysis of NOTCH1, the event that triggers NOTCH1 signaling. Following optimization and validation of the test using cancer xenografts bearing diverse *NOTCH1* aberrations and normal tissues, we screened a large series of human cancers of unknown *NOTCH1* mutational status for activated NOTCH1. Most T-LLs and CLLs showed evidence of ongoing NOTCH1 activation, as did many peripheral T cell lymphomas and a small subset triple-negative breast cancers. Activation of NOTCH1 was also detected in a majority of angiosarcomas, in line with the observation that NICD1 is readily detectable in normal endothelial cells within tumor stroma. By contrast, little or no NOTCH1 activation was observed in mantle cell lymphoma, diffuse large B cell lymphoma, non-small cell lung cancers, and ovarian carcinoma. These findings indicate that NOTCH1 activation among B cell tumors is both more sharply restricted to and more prevalent in CLL than would be predicted from prior genotypic data, raise questions about the proposed tumor suppressive role for NOTCH1 in vascular neoplasms, and suggest that IHC testing for NICD1 can be used to select patients for clinical trials of Notch pathway inhibitors, particularly those involving patients with tumors such as triple-negative breast cancer, in which NOTCH1 activation is confined to a small subset of tumors.

MATERIALS AND METHODS

Use of Human Tissues

Human tissues specimens were approved for use by Institutional Review Boards as follows. All tissues involved by lymphoid neoplasms (save one) were collected and used without informed consent under Brigham and Women's Hospital IRB protocol 2010-P002736. A non-small cell lung carcinoma microarray was constructed with tissues obtained from patients without consent under Brigham and Women's Hospital IRB protocol 2006-P001929. A serous ovarian cancer microarray was constructed with tissues obtained from patients without consent under Brigham and Women's Hospital IRB protocol 2006-P000321. An angiosarcoma microarray was constructed with tissues obtained from patients without informed consent under the University of Texas M. D. Anderson Cancer Center IRB protocol LAB04-0890. In each of these instances, the studies were granted waivers of consent on the following bases: 1) samples were gathered retrospectively from pathology archives and resulted from routine surgical procedures performed for diagnostic purposes; 2) patient identities were anonymized and completely delinked from unique identifiers; and 3) there was no risk to the participants (only anonymized tissues were used). One T-lymphoblastic lymphoma sample collected as part of a trial of the Merck GSI MK-0752 was used with the written informed consent of the affected patient under Dana Farber/Partners Cancer Center protocol 2004-P002170. A breast cancer microarray containing triple negative tumors (negative for estrogen receptor, progesterone receptor, and *HER2* amplification) was constructed with tissues obtained from patients who provided written informed consent under Dana Farber Cancer Institute IRB protocol 93-085.

Use of Mice in Xenograft Studies

REC-1 and KOPT-K1 cell subcutaneous xenograft studies were performed under Dana Farber Cancer Institute IACUC protocol 04-111. HCC1599, HCC1587, and MB-157 cell subcutaneous xenograft studies were performed under a protocol approved by the IACUC at Merck Oncology. Animal work was conducted according to NIH guidelines. All xenograft-bearing animals were monitored daily by veterinary staff for abnormal behaviors/conditions that might require attention to minimize suffering. Animals were sacrificed by CO_2 asphyxiation per recommendations of the American Veterinary Medical Association. All animals were maintained in CO_2 for a minimum of 5 minutes following cessation of respiratory motions.

Cell Lines

Cell lines were obtained from the American Tissue Culture Collection (REC-1, MAVER-1, HCC1599, HCC1587, and MB-157 cells) or the Leibniz-Institute DSMZ-German Collection of Microorganisms and Cell Lines (KOPT-K1).

Test Development and Validation Studies

These studies relied on: 1) cell lines with mutations in *NOTCH1* that produce either gain or loss of NOTCH1 function, that were grown as xenografts in mice; 2) normal human squamous mucosae and thymus, in which the anatomic distributions of cells with activated NOTCH1 are known; and 3) a primary human T-ALL of known *NOTCH1* genotype (described below). Xenografted cell lines and associated *NOTCH1* genotypes are given in Table 1. All xenografted tumors were fixed in a phosphate buffered solution containing 10% formalin or 4% paraformaldehyde (squamous cell carcinomas) and embedded in paraffin, and were retrieved from the tissue archives of individual laboratories in which xenograft studies were undertaken as part of other studies. Bones were decalcified following formalin fixation using RDO Rapid Decalcification Solution (Sigma, St. Louis, MO).

Table 1: Cancer xenografts and associated gain-of-function mutations in NOTCH1

Cell Line	Tumor Type	NOTCH1 Mutation	Effect on NOTCH1 Signaling	Reference
KOPT-K1	T-LL	L1600P/del(P)*	Gain	[3]
REC-1	MCL	del(ECN1)/del(P)*	Gain	this paper/ [7]
MAVER-1	MCL	None	N.A.	[7]
HCC1599	Breast Carci-noma	del(ECN1)	Gain	[10]
MB-157	Breast Carci-noma	del(ECN1)	Gain	Unpublished data
HCC1587	Breast Carci-noma	None	N.A.	[10]

* X/Y indicates paired mutations created by aberrations in *cis* in the same *NOTCH1* alleledel(ECN1) indicates the present of a deletion that removes the coding sequence for the extracellular domain of NOTCH1del(P) indicates the presence of frameshift or stop codon mutations that remove the C-terminal NOTCH1 PEST degron domainT-LL, T lymphoblastic leukemia/ lymphoma; MCL, mantle cell lymphoma; N.A., not applicable

Archival Human Cancer Samples

All FPE samples were used following approval of institutional review boards (see ethic statements). A primary T-ALL sample known to bear activating mutations in *NOTCH1* was collected as part of a clinical trial of the gamma-secretase inhibitor MK-0754 in patients with relapsed/refractory T-ALL [22]. Archival "discarded" T-LL, CLL, MCL, angiosarcoma, and normal tissue samples were selected from the paraffin-embedded tissues archives of Brigham and Women's Hospital based solely on the availability of tissue fixed in 10% formalin or in B+, a buffered fixative containing 3.7% formaldehyde and zinc chloride that is widely used for tissues involved by lymphoid neoplasms. FPE non-small cell lung cancer [23], diffuse large B cell lymphoma [24], angiosarcoma [25], and ovarian cancer [26] specimens were studied by staining previously described tissue microarrays. A new tissue microarray containing a set of 78 triple negative breast cancers was assembled as follows. Archival formalin-fixed, paraffin-embedded breast cancers were collected and best blocks and best areas for coring were identified and selected by a breast pathologist (DD). Results of immunohistochemical studies for estrogen (ER) and progesterone receptor (PR) and HER2 and FISH assay results for HER2 were extracted from pathology reports. Seventy-eight triple negative (ER/PR/HER2 negative) invasive breast cancers were identified with adequate tumor tissue for tissue microarray (TMA) construction, which was carried out in the Dana Farber/Harvard Cancer Center Tissue Microarray Core Facility. Three 0.6 mm cores were taken from marked areas and placed into a recipient block using a manual arrayer (Beecher Instruments).

Immunohistochemistry

Standard 4-micron paraffin embedded tissue sections were stained using the Ventana Benchmark XT platform (Ventana Medical Systems, Inc., Tucson, AZ.) with extended heat-induced epitope retrieval (CC1 Buffer). Slides were incubated for 1hr at room temperature with anti-NICD1 rabbit monoclonal antibody (clone D3B8, catalog #4147, Cell Signaling Technology, Beverly, MA; final concentration, 8.5microgram/mL). Signals were then amplified (Ventana Amplification Kit, #760-080) and visualized (Ventana Ultraview Universal DAB detection kit, #760-500) per the manufacturer's instructions. All staining runs included two positive control samples (REC-1 cell xenograft and tonsillar mucosa). Scoring was performed by two pathologists (MJK, JCA). Staining results were also reviewed with pathologists with subspecialty expertise in hematopathology (MJK, JCA, GP, DD, EAM, EFM), lung pathology (LC), gynecologic pathology (MH), breast pathology (DD), and soft tissue pathology (JH, AL), all of whom also contributed to case selection.

NOTCH1 Sequencing

DNA was prepared from fresh-frozen samples using the QiaAmp DNA Mini kit (Qiagen, Valencia, CA). Sanger sequencing of *NOTCH1* mutational hotspots in a case of T-lymphoblastic lymphoma was performed as described [3]; sequencing traces with analyzed with Mutation Surveyor Software (Softgenetics, State College, PA). Deep sequencing of *NOTCH1* mutational hotspots was performed as follows. Primers were designed and validated by Fluidigm (Fluidigm Corporation, San Francisco, CA) for exons 25-28 and 34 of *NOTCH1* per recommended guidelines for Roche Titanium sequencing (Roche, Mannheim, Germany). A total of 2304 amplicons representing 48 unique samples amplified with 48 target specific primer pairs were generated in each sequencing run. Each primer included sample-specific Fluidigm 454 bar code primer and adapter sequences. Reactions contained 50ng genomic DNA, forward and reverse tagged amplification primers (1microM), forward and reverse bar code primers (400nM), 1x Access Array Loading Reagent, 1x FastStart High Fidelity Reaction Buffer, 4.5mM $MgCl_2$, 5% DMSO, 0.05U FastStart High Fidelity Enzyme Blend and PCR-grade nucleotide mix (200microM, Roche). Thermal cycling was performed on the Fluidigm FC1 Cycler per manufacturer guidelines. The resultant libraries were harvested and collected on a microtiter plate, where they were quantified using the Qubit® dsDNA BR Assay Kit on a Qubit® 2.0 Fluorometer (Invitrogen, UK). Libraries were normalized and pooled before purification using Agencourt AMPure XP system (Beckman, UK) per the manufacturer's protocol. Library components were clonally amplified using the GS Junior emPCR Lib-A Kit (Roche) by inputting 1 molecule of library DNA per capture bead. Pyrosequencing was performed using the GS Junior system (Roche/454 Life Sciences).

To selectively detect the codon 2514 del(CT) mutation in *NOTCH1*, a pyrosequencing assay was developed. Briefly, *NOTCH1* exon 34 target sequence was amplified in a PCR containing 30ng of genomic DNA, a biotinylated forward primer (5›-CTCCTCGCCTGTGGACAA) and a reverse primer (5›-GGGACGAGCTGGACCACT) using the following cycling parameters: 94°C x 2 minutes, followed 94°C x 30 seconds, 62°C x 30 seconds, 72°C x 30 seconds for 45 cycles, followed by a final extension at 72°C for 10 minutes. The PCR amplification product was captured on streptavidin sepharose beads, denatured, transferred to a pyrosequencing plate, annealed to a reverse sequencing primer (5› CACTGGTCAGGGGACT 3›), and sequenced per a standard protocol (PyroMark Q96 MD, Qiagen, Germantown, MD). The decision to use a reverse sequencing primer was based on the fortuitous presence of a run of 3 G residues immediately 3' of the ΔG antisense codon 2514 mutation, which acts to increase the sensitivity of the assay roughly 3-fold. In line with this prediction, control studies using the cell line KOPT-K1, a T-LL cell line with a heterozygous del(CT) codon 2514 mutation [3], showed reliable detection of this sequence variant when diluted down to a level of 2.5% mutated alleles with DNA containing wild type *NOTCH1* alleles.

Molecular Characterization of an Intragenic NOTCH1 Deletion in REC-1 cells

5' rapid amplification of cDNA ends (RACE) was performed on RNA prepared from REC-1 cells and control DND-41 T-ALL cells as described [27]. Genomic DNA was isolated from REC-1 cells using the QIAamp genomic DNA isolation kit (Qiagen, Valencia, CA). Exon1 sense (5'-CCTGCTCTGCCTGGCGCTG) and exon 28 (5'-CCACGAAGAACAGAAGCACA) antisense primers were used to amplify the intragenic Notch1 deletion from 100ng of genomic DNA using the Expand Long Template PCR system (Roche, Branford, CT). The PCR amplification conditions were 94°C x 2 minutes, followed by 94°C x 15 seconds, 60°C x 30 seconds, and 68°C x 45 seconds for 30 cycles, followed by a 68°C extension for 7 minutes. The resulting PCR product was purified, cloned into the pCR2.1-TOPO plasmid (Invitrogen, Carlsbad, CA), and Sanger sequenced.

Western Blot Analysis

Whole cell detergent lysates of cell lines prepared as described [27] were stained for NICD1 (catalog # 4147), total NOTCH1 (catalog #4380), or actin (catalog #4970) using antibodies obtained from Cell Signaling Technologies (Beverly, MA).

Xenograft Studies

REC-1 cells and MAVER-1 cells were inoculated subcutaneously into 6-week old SCID/beige mice (Charles River Laboratory, Wilmington, MA) ($1x10^7$ cells per mouse) in 30% Matrigel basement membrane matrix (Becton Dickinson, Franklin Lakes, NJ). Tumor volume was determined by caliper measurements. When tumors reached a volume of 100-200 mm^3, mice were treated with the gamma-secretase inhibitor diaminobenzidine (DBZ) at 10microM/kg by intraperitoneal injection or with vehicle (DMSO) for 3 days. Tissues were harvested 2hr after the last drug dose. KOPT-K1 cells transduced with a lentivirus that expresses firefly luciferase were injected by tail vein into NOD/SCID/gamma-chain (NSG) mice bred at the Lurie Family Imaging Center (Dana Farber Cancer Institute). Mice were monitored for development of leukemia by bioluminescence and then treated with DBZ or DMSO as above. HCC1587 and HCC1599 human breast cancer cell line xenografts were developed in CB17 mice as described [10], while MB157 cell line xenografts were developed in Swiss nu/nu (nude) mice, all at Merck Oncology. Animal studies were carried out in strict accordance with the recommendations in the Guide for the Care and Use of Laboratory Animals of the National Institutes of Health.

RESULTS

Development of an Immunohistochemical Stain for Activated NOTCH1

Although canonical Notch signaling relies on nuclear translocation of its intracellular domain (NICD), detection of nuclear NICD *in situ* in human tissues has been difficult. Polyclonal antibodies that detect the neoepitope created at the amino-terminus of NICD1 by cleavage of NOTCH1 at conserved site within its transmembrane domain have been widely used to identify NICD1 in cell lysates, but have not yielded reliable IHC tests. Recent development of a rabbit monoclonal antibody against the NICD1 neoepitope encouraged us to revisit the possibility of using IHC to detect NICD1 in FPE tissues. To limit run-to-run staining variation and to enable possible clinical translation, we evaluated staining on two widely used automated immunostaining platforms, the Ventana Discovery XT and the Leica Bond. Both performed similarly, but we noted that staining interpreted as specific (as per below) appeared stronger on the Ventana platform (data not shown), which was used for all of the studies reported herein.

To develop a reliable staining method for NICD1, we made use of control FPE tissues from mice xenografted with human tumor cell lines bearing oncogenic *NOTCH1* mutations that result in ligand-independent generation of NICD1 (Table 1). Tumors studied with gain-of-function *NOTCH1* mutations included a T-LL cell line, KOPT-K1, which has an activating point substitution in the NOTCH1 negative regulatory region aligned in *cis* with a codon 2514 del(CT) mutation that results in deletion of the C-terminal NOTCH1 PEST degron domain [3]; the MCL cell line REC-1, which bears a *NOTCH1* allele with a previously uncharacterized activating deletion removing most of the coding sequence for the NOTCH1 ectodomain aligned in *cis* with a nonsense mutation in codon 2428 (described below) that also results in deletion of the C-terminal PEST degron domain; and two breast cancer cell lines, HCC1599 and MB-157, which bear *NOTCH1* alleles with deletions that remove most of the NOTCH1 ectodomain coding sequences ([10]; and data not shown). Formalin FPE sections of all four xenografts bearing activating *NOTCH1* mutations showed strong diffuse nuclear reactivity when stained with the NICD1-specific antibody (Figure 1A–D). Notably, NICD1 staining in KOPT-K1 and REC-1 xenografts was markedly reduced by treatment of animals with the GSI DBZ (Figure 1E, F), which blocks the generation of NICD1 ([3]). In addition, no NICD1 staining was seen in sections of the MCL cell line MAVER-1 (Figure 1G), which has wild type *NOTCH1* alleles and is devoid of NICD1 [7], or in the breast cancer cell line HCC1587 (Figure 1H), which has wild type *NOTCH1* alleles and instead has an activating deletion involving *NOTCH2* [10].

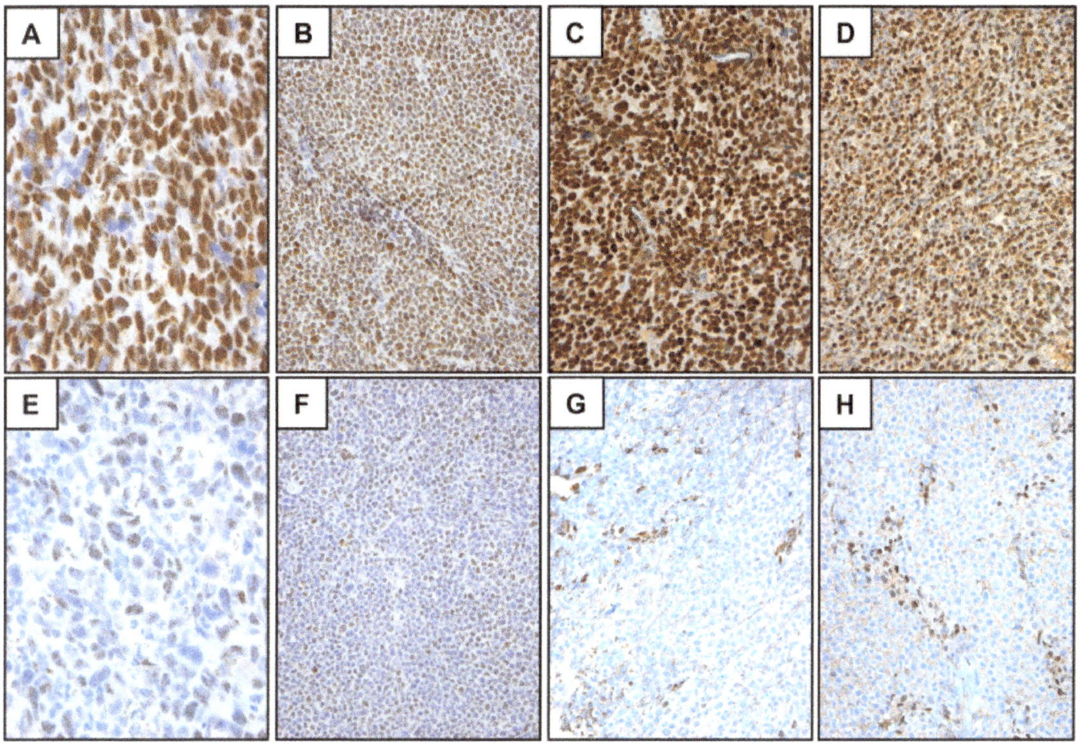

Figure 1: Validation of IHC staining of NICD1 using formalin FPE tumor xenografts.

Sections were stained for NICD1 using an IHC method that produces a brown nuclear stain and counterstained with hematoxylin. A) KOPT-K1 T-ALL cells. B) REC-1 mantle cell lymphoma cells. C) HCC1599 breast carcinoma cells. D) MB-157 breast carcinoma cells. E, F) KOPT-K1 and REC-1 cell staining, respectively, in tissues harvested from animals treated with the GSI DBZ. G) MAVER-1 mantle cell lymphoma cells. H) HCC1587 breast cancer cells. Genotypes of these cell lines are given in Table 1.

To further evaluate the sensitivity of the method and the stability of the NICD1 neoepitope in archival tissues, we performed IHC for NICD1 on sections prepared from a T-LL specimen obtained in the year 2004 from a patient enrolled in a trial of the Merck GSI MK-0754 [22]. Sanger sequencing of DNA isolated from this specimen revealed a heterozygous point mutation that results in a L1574P substitution, as well as two additional subclonal point mutations aligned in *cis* with the L1574P substitution that create L1600P and F1592S substitutions (Figure 2A). All of these mutations fall in exon 26 of *NOTCH1* and correspond to previously characterized gain-of-function mutations in the NOTCH1 negative regulatory region [28], a portion of the NOTCH1 ectodomain that must be intact to keep the receptor in the off-state in the absence of ligand [29]. Tandem mutations aligned in *cis* in the NOTCH1 ectodomain have been reported previously [3] and are likely a manifestation of continued selection for increased NOTCH1 signaling during T-ALL progression. IHC staining of this T-ALL produced strong diffuse nuclear positivity, suggesting that the NICD1 epitope detected by the rabbit monoclonal antibody is stable for a period of years in routinely stored FPE samples (Figure 2B).

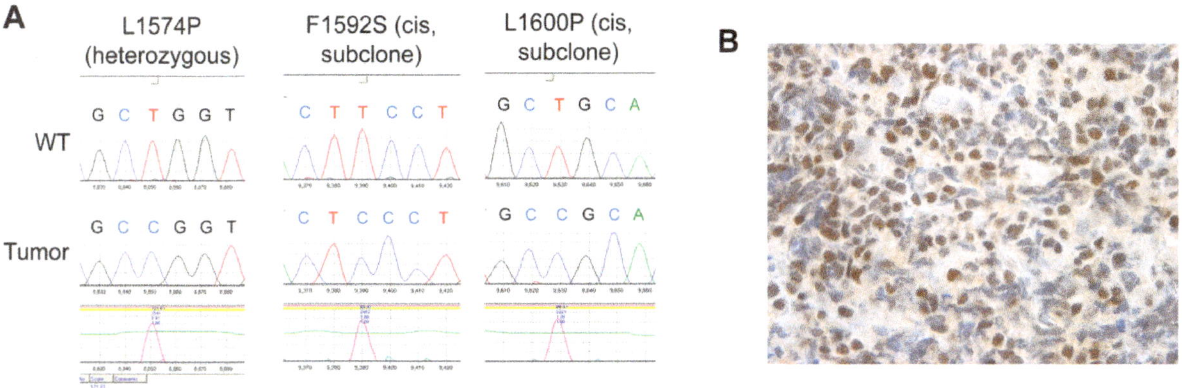

Figure 2: NICD1 staining in an archival human T-LL of known genotype.

A) Identification of activating mutations involving exon 26 of *NOTCH1*. Of 24 individual cloned PCR products, 13 gave wild type sequences, 9 showed a mutation producing a L to P substitution in residue 1574, 1 showed the L1574P mutation in *cis* with a mutation producing a F to S substitution in residue 1592, and 1 showed the L1574P mutation in *cis* with a variant producing a L to P substitution in residue 1600. B) IHC staining for NICD1 in the same tumor, a formalin-fixed paraffin-embedded biopsy of a mediastinal mass. There is crush artifact, but strong nuclear staining is seen in intact cells.

We also noted in sections of xenografted tumors that murine endothelial cells and scattered stromal cells showed nuclear reactivity with the NICD1 antibody (best seen in Figure 1G and H). These observations are in line with data indicating roles for notch1 in vascular endothelium [30] and peripheral T cells [31], and suggested that our IHC method can detect physiologic levels of NICD1. To evaluate this, we stained normal sections of human squamous mucosa, skin, and thymus (Figure 3). Prior work has shown that notch1 is transiently activated in suprabasilar cells in squamous epithelia [32], in which it promotes cell cycle exit and differentiation [33], an activity that may contribute to NOTCH1's tumor suppressive roles in squamous cell carcinomas of the skin and head and neck. As expected, NICD1 staining in squamous epithelia was confined to suprabasilar cells (Figure 3A, B). In thymocytes, notch1 activation rises to a maximum in CD4/CD8 double-negative cells undergoing beta-selection [34], which are located within the thymic cortex just deep to the thymic capsule [35]. In prior work, we noted that cells in this region of the thymus have the highest level of immunoreactivity with antibodies that recognize total notch1, without regard to its activation status [36]. As predicted from the reported pattern of NOTCH1 activation in thymocytes, NICD1 staining in human thymus was most prominent in cortical thymocytes lying immediately below the capsule (Figure 3C, D). These results demonstrate that our IHC method is sufficiently sensitive to detect physiologic levels of activated NOTCH1 in at least some normal tissues. To further explore NOTCH1 activation in normal lymphoid tissues, staining of tonsil was also carried out. We noted that germinal centers containing reactive B cells were devoid of immunoreactivity, whereas surrounding mantle zones showed weak staining for NICD1 (data not shown).

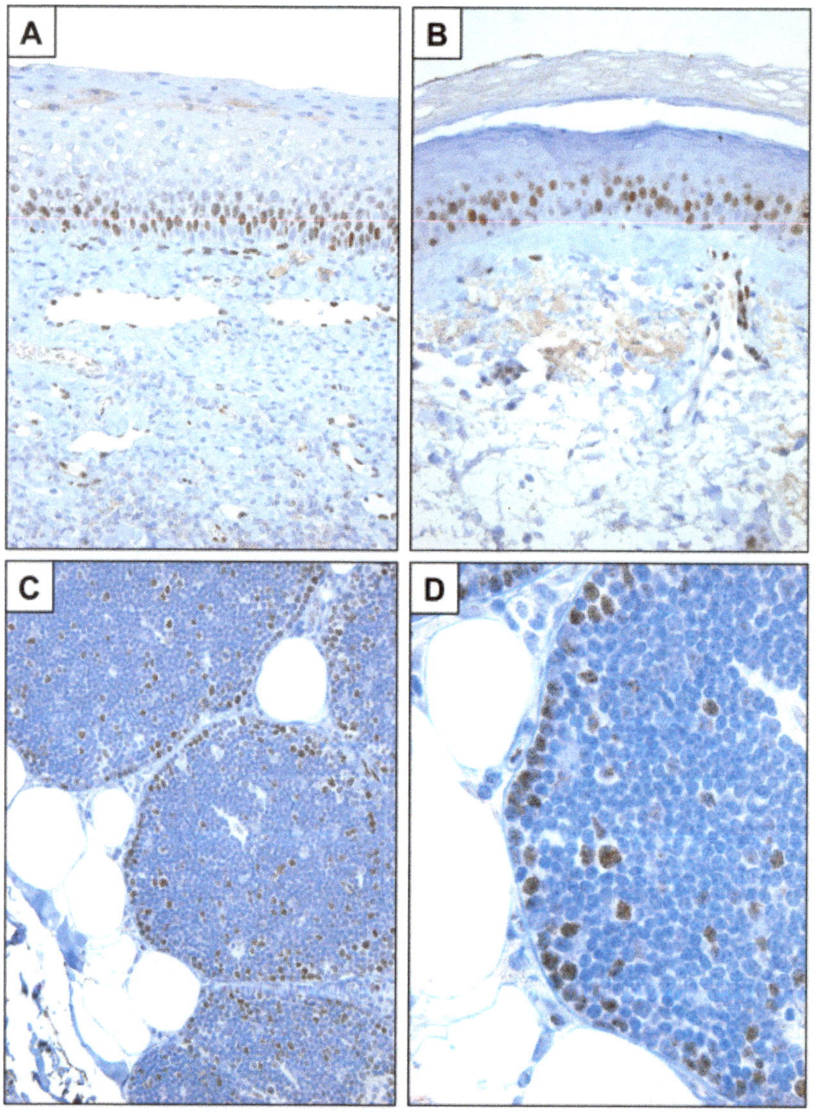

Figure 3: NICD1 staining in normal formalin FPE human tissues.

A) Oropharyngeal squamous mucosa. B) Skin. C, D) Thymus.

Detection of NOTCH1 Activation in Archival Cancer Specimens

Building on these validation studies, we next used IHC to screen a series of FPE human cancers for evidence of NOTCH1 activation, focusing on tumor types in which *NOTCH1* gain-of-function mutations have been described. We also studied angiosarcoma, based on the observation that normal endothelial cells frequently stained positively for NICD1 and prior studies suggesting that *notch1* has a tumor suppressive function in murine vascular endothelium [19,20]; hence, we were curious to see if NOTCH1 activation might be lost in human angiosarcomas. We used NICD1 staining of normal endothelial cells as an internal control to judge the preservation of immunoreactivity in the tissues studied. In exploratory studies, we noted that archival samples fixed in Zenker's solution, a mercuric fixative used at our institution to decalcify bone marrow biopsies, negated NICD1 immunoreactivity in endothelium. Loss of immunoreactivity was not caused by decalcification *per se*, since bone marrow involved by xenografted KOPT-K1 cells that was fixed in formalin and then rapidly decalcified with a strong acid retained immunoreactivity (Figure 1A). Because of this limitation, we confined our studies to tumors involving soft tissues for which FPE samples were available. Some lymph nodes involved by CLL samples were fixed in B+, a fixative that contains formaldehyde and zinc chloride. Samples fixed in B+ retained NICD1 staining in normal endothelial cells and thus were included in the analysis. Results are summarized in Table 2 and are described in the sections below.

Table 2: Summary of NICD1 staining in human FPE cancer specimens

Tumor (Number of Cases)	NICD1 Staining Results
T-LL (N=14)	57% positive (N=8; all diffusely positive)
CLL (N=52)	89% positive (N=46; 15% diffusely positive, 74% subset positive)
Peripheral T cell lymphoma (N=55)	38% positive (N=21; 1.8% diffusely positive, 36% subset positive)
Mantle cell lymphoma (N=53)	0% positive
Diffuse large B cell lymphoma (N=68)	0% positive
Triple negative breast carcinoma (N=78)	3.8% positive (N=3; all diffusely positive)
Non-small cell lung carcinoma (N=151)	0% positive
Ovarian carcinoma (N=147)	0% positive
Angiosarcoma (N=57)	77% positive (N=44; 47% diffusely positive, 30% subset positive)

Diffusely positive, ≥80% of cells positive; subset positive, ≤80% of cells positive

T lymphoblastic leukemia/lymphoma (T-LL)

NOTCH1 gain-of-function mutations occur in roughly 50% to 60% of human T-LL [3] and a high fraction of murine T-LL models. Consistent with the known incidence of *NOTCH1* gain-of-function mutations in human disease, 8 of 14 T-ALLs screened (57%) showed diffuse nuclear staining for NICD1 (Figure 4A). In tumors that were negative, little or no staining was observed. This black and white distinction—diffuse positivity or no staining—is consistent with the idea that T-LL falls into two major classes, one in which NOTCH1 is "on" by virtue of acquired gain-of-function mutations and a second that is unrelated to NOTCH1 activation and free of *NOTCH1* mutations.

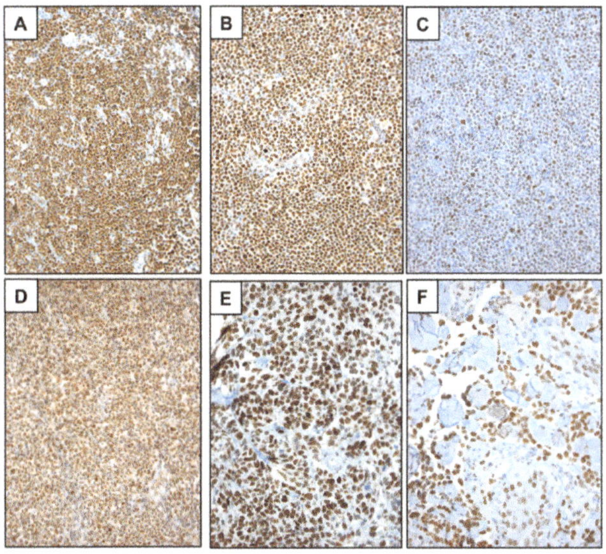

Figure 4: NICD1 immunoreactivity in archival FPE human cancers.

A) T-ALL. B) CLL, diffuse pattern. C) CLL, subset pattern. D) Adult T-cell leukemia/lymphoma. E) Triple-negative breast carcinoma. F) Angiosarcoma.

Mantle cell lymphoma (MCL)

A recent report identified *NOTCH1* exon 34 mutations in 11% of MCL and in the MCL cell line REC-1, while certain other MCL cell lines such as MAVER1 were free of NOTCH1 mutations [7]. The high levels of NICD1 in REC-1 cell line extracts [7] and the intense immunoreactivity of xenografted REC-1 cells stained for NICD1 suggested that this cell line might harbor additional mutations leading to ligand-independent activation of NOTCH1, since exon 34 mutations affecting the NOTCH1 PEST domain have no effect on NICD1 generation *per se*[3,28]. The most common mutations leading to ligand-independent activation of NOTCH1 in human T-LL are point mutations in the extracellular negative regulatory region, but sequencing of REC-1 failed to identify mutations in this region [7]. We previously noted that murine T-LLs often have activating deletions that remove the coding sequences for the notch1 extracellular negative regulatory region [27], and similar lesions in human NOTCH1 occur in a subset of human breast cancers and breast cancer cell lines such as HCC1599 and MB-157 [10].

We thus asked whether REC-1 cells might harbor a *NOTCH1* deletion leading to expression of an aberrant *NOTCH1* mRNA. Using 5'-rapid amplification of cDNA ends (5'-RACE), we identified an abnormal transcript consisting of an in-frame fusion of *NOTCH1* exon 1 and exon 28 sequences (Figure 5A, C). PCR amplification of genomic REC-1 DNA produced a product with the same sequence (Figure 5B, C), consistent with the presence of a *NOTCH1* deletion created by DNA breaks in exon 1 and exon 28 followed by non-homologous end joining. Virtual translation of the aberrant REC-1 transcript produces a membrane-tethered form of NOTCH1 closely resembling truncated forms of NOTCH1 that are potent leukemogens in mice [37] and that undergo ligand-independent cleavage by gamma-scretase to yield NICD1 [38]. In line with this prediction, treatment of REC-1 cells with GSI led to accumulation of a truncated NOTCH1 protein and disappearance of NICD1 (Figure 5D).

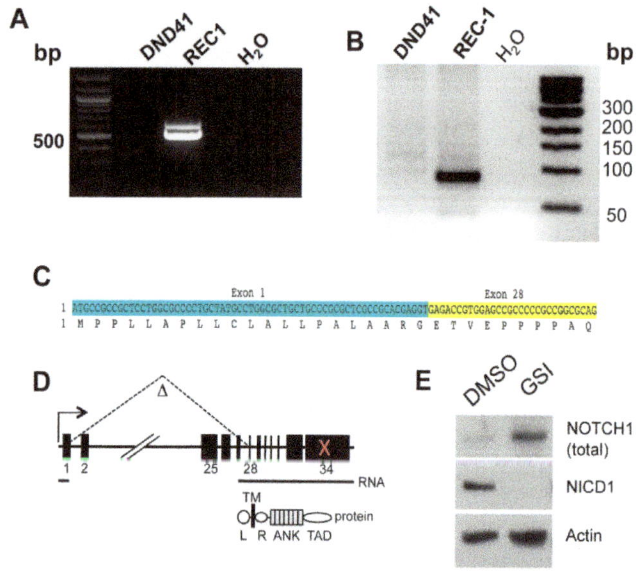

Figure 5: Identification of an activating deletion in *NOTCH1* **in REC-1 mantle cell lymphoma cells.**

A) 5'-RACE products synthesized from input RNA from REC-1 MCL cells and DND-41 T-ALL cells; the latter have intact *NOTCH1* alleles. B) Results of PCR of genomic REC-1 and DND-41 cell DNA with a *NOTCH1* exon 1/exon 28-specific primer pair. C) Sequence of the 5'-RACE product in A and the genomic PCR product in B. Both showed an in-frame fusion of exon 1 and exon 28 *NOTCH1* coding sequences. D) Cartoon depicting the intragenic *NOTCH1* deletion in REC-1 cells and its consequences at the level of NOTCH1 RNA and protein. The red X denotes the position of a frame-shift mutation in exon 34 of *NOTCH1*. L, leader peptide; TM, transmembrane domain; R, RAM domain; ANK, ankyrin repeat domain; TAD, transcriptional activation domain. E) Western blot showing the effect of treatment of REC-1 cells with the gamma-secretase inhibitor (GSI) compound E for 72 hours versus DMSO control. GSI depletes NICD1 (detected with the NICD1-specific V1744 antibody) and leads to the accumulation of a polypeptide of the size predicted by virtual translation of the aberrant *NOTCH1* mRNA. Total NOTCH1 was detected with a polyclonal antibody raised against the NOTCH1 TAD.

Based on the findings in REC-1 cells and the report of *NOTCH1* mutations in 11% of MCLs [7], we anticipated that NICD1 staining would be observed in a significant subset of MCLs. However, IHC staining in 53 cases of MCL was uniformly negative, suggesting that NOTCH1 activation and (by extension, *NOTCH1* mutations) were absent from our cohort of cases, which were diagnosed by experienced hematopathologists using standard World Health Organization criteria. In line with the IHC results, deep sequencing of DNAs prepared from all MCLs for which frozen tissue was available (N=45) failed to detect any mutations in *NOTCH1* exons encoding the extracellular negative regulatory region (exons 25-27), the gamma-secretase cleavage site (exon 28), or the C-terminal PEST degron domain (exon 34) (data not shown). Based on prior structure: function studies [28,39], these exons span all regions of *NOTCH1*that are predicted to potentially harbor gain-of-function point mutations and small insertions and deletions. Thus, although activating *NOTCH1* mutations clearly occur in MCL, they may be less common than originally thought.

Chronic lymphocytic leukemia (CLL)

In contrast to T-LL and MCL, staining for NICD1 in CLL was both more frequent and more variable. In total, 89% of CLLs (46 of 52 cases) stained positively for NICD1 in >10% of tumor cells; of these 33% (17 of 52) stained positively in >50% of tumor cells, and 15% (8 of 52) showed diffusely positive staining (defined as staining in >80% of cells). Examples of diffusely positive cases and subset-positive cases are shown in Figure 4B and 4C, respectively. From 10% to 18% of CLLs have been reported to have *NOTCH1* gain-of-function mutations in prior studies [4–6]; thus, the frequency of NOTCH1 activation as judged by NICD1 staining in our tumor cohort greatly exceeds what would be expected if activation were confined to CLLs with *NOTCH1* mutations.

To evaluate genotype/phenotype relationships directly, deep sequencing was performed on all CLL samples evaluated by NICD1 staining for which fresh-frozen tissue was available (N=46). Fold coverage of reads in most samples was >100, sufficient to allow detection of minor subclones.

We detected *NOTCH1* gain-of-function mutations in 8 of 46 cases (17%), all in exon 34. Seven corresponded to a del(CT) mutation in codon 2514 that is highly prevalent in CLL, and one corresponded to a nonsense mutation in codon 2444 (Figure 6A); mutations at both of these sites result in disruption of the C-terminal PEST degron domain. Six mutations were present in dominant clones (defined as >20% mutated reads), whereas two mutations were present in minor subclones (defined as <5% mutated reads). All seven codon 2514 del(CT) mutations were confirmed using a pyrosequencing assay capable of detecting approximately 2.5% mutated sequences diluted into wild type DNA; representative pyrosequencing results are shown in Figure 6B. The *NOTCH1* codon 2444 nonsense mutation was confirmed by repeat deep sequencing of DNA from two additional frozen pieces of tissue from this case. In the first piece of tissue analyzed, the codon 2444 mutation was present in 46% of reads, and in the two additional pieces the same mutation was present in 33% and 48% of the reads (data not shown), confirming that this mutation is also real.

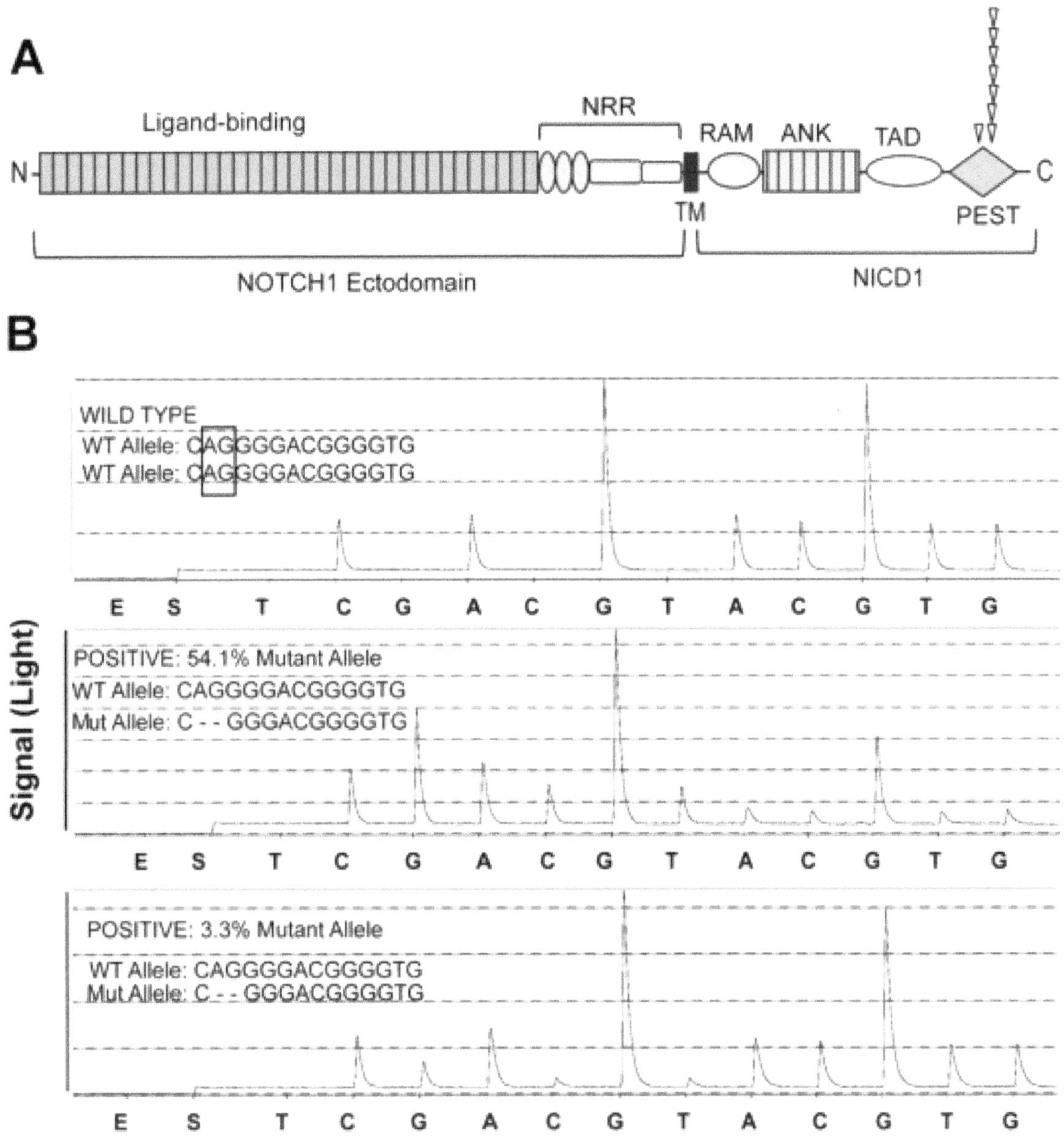

Figure 6: ***NOTCH1* mutations in CLL.**

A) Position of *NOTCH1* mutations, superimposed on a cartoon showing the NOTCH1 protein. NRR, negative regulatory region; RAM, RAM domain; ANK, ankyrin repeat domain; TAD, transcriptional activation domain; PEST, degron domain. B) Representative confirmatory pyrosequencing results in CLL cases positive by deep sequencing for the *NOTCH1* codon 2514 del(CT) mutation. Results for a case with wild type codon 2514 sequences is shown in the upper panel. The lower two panels are cases in which deep sequencing revealed high (54.1%) or low numbers of mutated reads (3.3%). Reverse-sequences of the wild type (WT) and mutant (MUT) del(CT) alleles are shown for reference. "E" corresponds to the addition of enzyme to the reaction chamber, while "S" corresponds to the addition of the substrate. In this sequencing by synthesis assay, nucleotides are added to the reaction chamber sequentially in the order shown.

Nucleotide incorporation releases pyrophosphate, which catalyses a reaction in which the number of photons produced is proportional to the number of nucleotides incorporated. The codon 2514 del(CT) mutation causes the appearance of a new signal corresponding to the incorporation of 3 G residues.

We then correlated NOTCH1 activation with *NOTCH1* genotype. The fraction of reads with *NOTCH1* mutations in a particular sample was strongly correlated with NICD1 staining (Figure 7A), in line with the expectation that PEST deletions should stabilize NICD1 and increase its levels. Cases with *NOTCH1* mutations had significantly more widespread staining for NICD1 than cases with wild type alleles (Figure 7B, $p<0.05$); however, there was substantial overlap between these two groups of tumors, and some tumors with wild type *NOTCH1* alleles were diffusely positive for NICD1 (>80% of cells positive). We also assessed the relationship between NOTCH1 activation and cytogenetic abnormalities, which are widely used markers of prognosis in CLL. Prior work showed enrichment for *NOTCH1* mutations in CLLs associated with trisomy 12 [40,41], suggesting that this group of tumors might have higher levels of NOTCH1 activation. Among CLLs for which cytogenetic results were available, however, we did not observe any significant difference in NICD1 staining between tumors with trisomy 12, del(13q), or del(17p) (Figure 7C). The most notable observation was low NICD1 positivity in tumors associated with del(11q) relative to other cytogenetics subtypes ($p<0.02$).

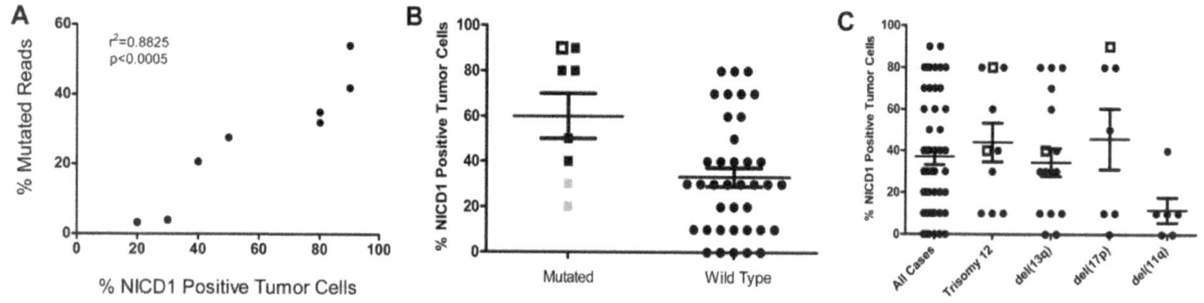

Figure 7: Relationship of NICD1 staining, *NOTCH1* **genotype, and karyotype in CLL.**

A) Correlation between the fraction of mutated *NOTCH1* exon 34 reads and NICD1 staining. B) NICD1 staining in CLLs with and without mutated *NOTCH1* alleles. Filled squares correspond to CLLs with the NOTCH1 codon 2514 del(CT) mutation; black squares are tumors with a "high" fraction (>20%) of mutated reads, while gray squares are tumors with a "low" fraction (<5%) of mutated reads. The open square corresponds to a CLL with a nonsense mutation in codon 2444. C) Relationship of NICD1 staining to CLL karyotype. Open squares correspond to tumors with *NOTCH1* mutations.

Frequent activation of NOTCH1 in CLLs with wild type *NOTCH1* alleles suggests that microenvironmental factors (e.g., Notch ligands) mediate NOTCH1 activation in this disease. Little is known about Notch ligand expression in lymph nodes, and reliable IHC staining methods for the full set of Notch ligands (Jagged1, Jagged2, Delta-like-1, Delta-like-3, and Delta-like-4) have yet to be developed, limiting our ability to directly assess the possible involvement of ligands. However, several "experiments of nature" in our tumor set point to a role for intranodal factors in NOTCH1 activation. In 13 of the CLL cases studied, tumor cells extended beyond the lymph node capsule into perinodal soft tissue. In 12 of these 13 cases, we noted that NICD1 staining was much weaker in tumor cells in perinodal soft tissue than it was within tumor cells in the immediately adjacent lymph node, including one case associated with a the *NOTCH1* codon 2514 del(CT) in 35% of sequencing reads (Figure 8A). In addition, the case with a NOTCH1 codon 2444 nonsense mutation in 42% of sequencing reads subsequently recurred as a tumor with wild type *NOTCH1* alleles (Figure 8B, C). The original mutated sample showed evidence of transformation to a more aggressive histologic grade as judged by the presence of frequent large cells, a feature associated with *NOTCH1* mutations in a prior report [5], whereas the later lymph node biopsy showed only a few scattered large cells. NICD1 staining was somewhat stronger in the earlier tumor with mutated *NOTCH1*, but both biopsies showed diffusely positive NICD1 staining. These observations are consistent with past work showing that exon 34 mutations producing C-terminal PEST domain deletions have no effect on receptor activation *per se* [3,28]; thus, they are only selected for in contexts in which there is already ongoing NOTCH1 activation, which may be caused by mutations in exons 25-28 (apparently absent in CLL) or by ligand-mediated NOTCH1 activation.

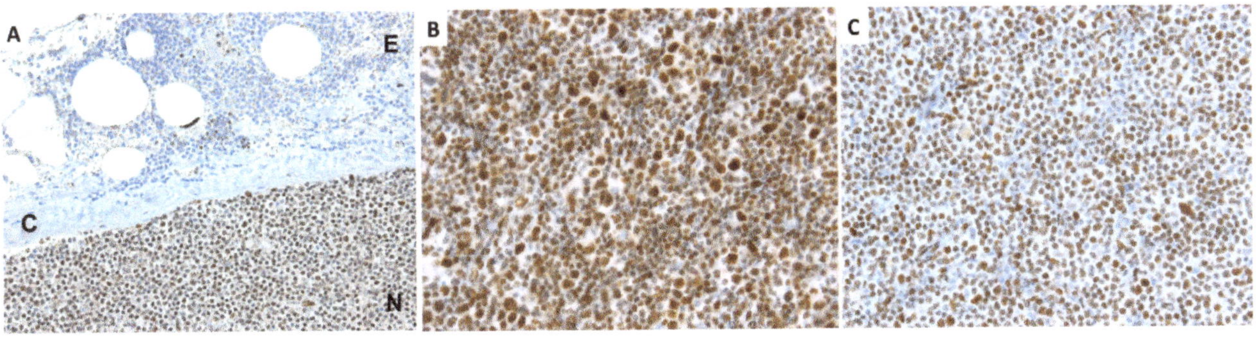

Figure 8: Salient observations from archival CLL biopsies stained for NICD1.

A) Loss of NICD1 positivity in extranodal tumor. This case was associated with a *NOTCH1* codon 2514 del(CT) mutation (35% of sequencing reads). E, extranodal fibrofatty tissue; C, lymph node capsule; N, lymph node. B, C) NICD1 staining in sequential biopsies involved by CLL with (B) and without (C) the *NOTCH1* codon 2444 nonsense mutation. The specimen in (B) was associated with 42% mutated sequencing reads; no mutated reads were detected in the subsequent biopsy shown in (C).

Diffuse large B cell lymphoma

Mutations in *NOTCH1* have been reported in a minor subset of diffuse large B cell lymphoma [8]. However, staining of a tissue microarray containing 68 well-characterized diffuse large B cell lymphomas revealed no NICD1 positive tumors (Table 2). Thus, NOTCH1 activation is uncommon in diffuse large B cell lymphoma.

Adult T-cell leukemia/lymphoma and other peripheral T cell lymphomas

Staining of a diverse collection of peripheral T cell lymphomas, subclassified by World Health Organization criteria, revealed NICD1 positivity in 21 of 55 cases (38%; Table 3), including diffuse nuclear positivity in 1 case of adult T cell leukemia/lymphoma (Figure 4D). Also noted was a variable pattern of NICD1 immunoreactivity in 12 of 14 cases (86%) of angioimmunoblastic lymphoma, a T cell lymphoma derived from follicular T helper cells (Figure 9). As with CLL, NICD1 staining was diminished in angioimmunoblastic lymphoma cells in extranodal soft tissues, suggesting that NICD1 production is also stimulated in this tumor-type by factors in the nodal microenvironment (Figure 9).

Table 3: NICD1 staining in peripheral T cell lymphomas.

Tumor Type (N=55 Total Cases)	NICD1 Staining Results
Angioimmunoblastic lymphoma (N=14)	86% positive (N=12; all subset positive)
Peripheral T cell lymphoma, NOS (N=12)	42% positive (N=5; all subset positive)
Cutaneous T cell lymphoma (N=12)	17% positive (N=2; all subset positive)
Anaplastic large cell lymphoma (ALCL, N=7)	14% positive (N=1; subset positive, ALK+ tumor)
	86% negative (N=6, 1 ALK+ tumor, 5 ALK- tumors)
Adult T cell leukemia/lymphoma (N=5)	20% positive (N=1; diffusely positive)
EBV+ T/NK extranodal lymphoma (N=4)	0% positive
Subcutaneous paniculitis-like T cell lymphoma (N=1)	0% positive

NOS, not otherwise specified; ALK, anaplastic lymphoma kinase; EBV, Epstein–Barr virus; NK, natural killer cell

Diffusely positive, ≥80% of cells positive; subset positive, ≤80% of cells positive

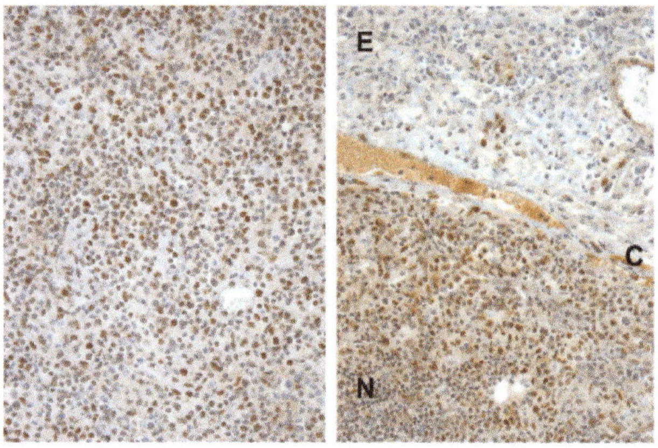

Figure 9: Representative NICD1 staining in angioimmunoblastic T cell lymphoma.

Left, intranodal tissue, showing variable staining of resident cells. Right, micrograph showing a sharp decrease in NICD1 staining in extranodal (E) tumor cells as compared to nodal (N) tumor cells, which are separated by the nodal capsule (C).

Triple-Negative Breast Cancer

Activating deletions in either *NOTCH1* or *NOTCH2* have been identified in a minority of breast cancers, most of which are triple-negative (ER/PR/HER2 negative) tumors [10]. Staining of a tissue microarray containing 78 triple negative breast cancers for NICD1 identified 3 tumors (3.8%) with strong diffuse nuclear staining (Figure 4E), a pattern similar to that in xenografted breast cancer cell lines with activating deletions of *NOTCH1* (Figure 1C and D).

Non-small cell lung cancer (NSCLC) *and Ovarian Carcinoma*

None of 151 NSCLCs or 147 ovarian serous carcinomas had detectable NICD1 staining (Table 2). All cases scored demonstrated staining for NICD1 in vascular endothelium, indicating that lack of staining in tumor cells was unlikely to have resulted from loss of tissue immunoreactivity. Thus, despite reports of NOTCH1 PEST domain mutations in lung cancer [11] and *NOTCH3* amplification and acquired mutations in genes encoding other NOTCH pathway signaling components in ovarian cancer [12,42], NOTCH1 activation does not appear to be common in either of these tumors.

Angiosarcoma

An initial screen of 3 well-differentiated angiosarcomas of the scalp revealed diffuse NICD1 positivity in all 3 tumors (Figure 4F), prompting us to study NOTCH1 activation in an arrayed collection of 54 additional angiosarcomas. Overall, these studies revealed diffuse or focal positive staining for NICD1 in 77% (44 of 57) of angiosarcomas (Table 2). In general, well-differentiated vasoformative tumors showed more diffuse and stronger staining than tumors with epithelioid morphologies or solid growth patterns, both of which are associated with more aggressive behavior.

DISCUSSION

The method described here for detecting NICD1 in FPE tissues should find wide utility in evaluating NOTCH1 activation in clinical samples and experimental models of human disease. It relies on a commercial rabbit monoclonal antibody and can be performed using standardized reagents on widely used automated staining platforms. The antibody detects a neoepitope at the amino terminus of NICD1 that is created by gamma-secretase cleavage of human NOTCH1 and murine notch1, and which appears to be stable in FPE samples stored routinely for a decade or more. We anticipate that this IHC stain should be useful in a number of contexts, including: i) studies using tissue archives to explore the role of NOTCH1 in various neoplastic and non-neoplastic disorders; ii) selection of patients for trials of gamma-secretase inhibitors (GSIs) [21], the lead Notch pathway antagonists being tested in cancer patients, particularly trials involving diseases such as triple-negative breast cancer in which NOTCH1 activation is confined to a small subset of tumors; and iii) judging the efficacy of NOTCH1 antagonists in experimental models and in patients. Staining for NICD1 may also prove useful in identifying tumors with *NOTCH1* loss-of-function mutations, which are present in a subset of squamous cell carcinomas.

The IHC test that we described has certain limitations. Decalcification of bone marrow with some agents (e.g., Zenker's solution) seems to negate immunoreactivity, based on staining of T-ALLs for which both soft tissue samples and involved bone marrow were available (data not shown). In addition, the assay is specific for NOTCH1, and therefore cannot be used to assess activation of other NOTCH receptors, which have been implicated in certain cancers. Specifically, activating *NOTCH2* mutations have been identified in marginal zone B-cell lymphoma [43–45] and diffuse large B-cell lymphoma [8], and biochemical analyses have detected activation of NOTCH2 as well as NOTCH1 in CLL [46,47]. Similarly, amplification of *NOTCH3* has been described in ovarian cancers [42,48]. It may be possible to overcome this limitation by developing IHC stains for activated NOTCH2-4, which is feasible in principle since the neoepitopes created by gamma-secretase cleavage of NOTCH1-4 are unique. Finally, a role for NOTCH1 in maintenance of cancer stem cells has been proposed in some tumors [49–52]; if such cells are rare, assessment of NICD1 in bulk tumor cell populations may underestimate the contribution of NOTCH1 to the malignant phenotype.

In addition to a small subset of breast cancers and (as expected) more than half of T-LLs, our screen of human cancers indicates that NOTCH1 activation is prevalent in CLL and also occurs in a subset of peripheral T cell lymphomas and a high fraction of angiosarcomas. An unexpected finding, based on prior results of genomic sequencing studies, was the much more widespread activation of NOTCH1 in CLL than in other two other B cell tumors, mantle cell lymphoma [7] and diffuse large B cell lymphoma [8]. NOTCH1 activation in CLL is not confined to tumors with *NOTCH1* mutations and appears to be augmented by factors expressed in the nodal microenvironment. These findings raise questions about how best to gauge and target NOTCH1 activation in CLL patients who are being considered for treatment with Notch pathway inhibitors. It would be desirable to be able to stratify patients based on analysis of circulating CLL cells, but our findings raise several questions about analyses conducted on peripheral blood. On the one hand, the loss of NICD1 immunoreactivity in CLL cells in soft tissues adjacent to lymph nodes suggests that the levels of NOTCH1 activation differ in CLL cells in different microenvironments within an individual patient. It will be of interest to compare levels of NOTCH1 activation in lymph nodes and peripheral blood cells obtained from patients at the same time point. On the other hand, it appears that *NOTCH1* mutational analysis may underestimate the involvement of NOTCH1 in CLL, based on the presence of readily detectable NOTCH1 activation in the nodal microenvironment in cases with wild type *NOTCH1*alleles. The latter observations suggest that NOTCH1 activation in CLL may be largely ligand-mediated; if true, this would have significant therapeutic implications, since ligand-specific blocking antibodies with antitumor activity have been developed [53,54]. Our observations point to the need for further work on nodal factors that trigger NOTCH1 activation in CLL cells and potentially in other tumors as well. By contrast, while our identification of a novel activating *NOTCH1* deletion in the mantle cell lymphoma cell line REC-1 and prior identification of *NOTCH1* mutations in primary cases of mantle cell lymphoma [7] clearly indicate an oncogenic role for NOTCH1, our failure to detect NOTCH1 activation or *NOTCH1* mutations in 53 well characterized mantle cell lymphomas suggests that involvement of NOTCH1 in this disease is rare.

NOTCH1 has an important role in regulating the differentiation and function of diverse peripheral T cell subsets [55], but its role in peripheral T cell lymphomas is largely unknown. Detection of NICD1 in a substantial subset of peripheral T cell lymphomas suggest that Notch antagonists merit study as potential treatments for these tumors, which have poor outcomes with current therapies.

NOTCH1 is a double-edged sword with respect to tumorigenesis, being capable of serving as a tumor suppressor as well as an oncoprotein. Indeed, inhibition of notch signaling in rodents with inhibitory antibodies directed against the Notch ligand DLL4 leads to tumors in several organs that may be of vascular origin [56], and conditional knockout of *notch1* in endothelial cells causes the appearance of vascular proliferations in the liver [19,20], suggesting that NOTCH1 is a tumor suppressor in endothelium. However, we observed ongoing NOTCH1 activation in a high fraction of human angiosarcomas, particularly in those that are well differentiated. Thus, while loss of NOTCH1 function may be associated with progression of angiosarcoma, it may not be essential for its genesis. These findings suggest that the role of NOTCH1 in transformed endothelium cells merits additional study.

In addition to cancer cells, we observed widespread activation of NOTCH1 in normal endothelial cells and variable activation in mononuclear cells that may represent T cells, macrophages or dendritic cells. Given that NOTCH1 signaling has been implicated in a number of non-neoplastic immunologic, inflammatory and vascular conditions [14,57], the method described here should find widespread use in studying NOTCH1 activation in a broad range of human disorders and corresponding experimental models.

ACKNOWLEDGMENTS

The authors wish to recognize technical support of Desiree Rutschow and the Genetics Core Service at Dundee University and the Dana Farber/Harvard Cancer Center Specialized Histopathology Core Laboratory.

REFERENCES

1. Kopan R, Ilagan MX (2009) The canonical Notch signaling pathway: unfolding the activation mechanism. Cell 137: 216-233. doi:10.1016/j.cell.2009.03.045. PubMed: 19379690.
2. Ellisen LW, Bird J, West DC, Soreng AL, Reynolds TC et al. (1991) TAN-1, the human homolog of the Drosophila notch gene, is broken by chromosomal translocations in T lymphoblastic neoplasms. Cell 66: 649-661. doi:10.1016/0092-8674(91)90111-B. PubMed: 1831692.
3. Weng AP, Ferrando AA, Lee W, Morris JP, Silverman LB et al. (2004) Activating mutations of NOTCH1 in human T cell acute lymphoblastic leukemia. Science 306: 269-271. doi:10.1126/science.1102160. PubMed: 15472075.
4. Di Ianni M, Baldoni S, Rosati E, Ciurnelli R, Cavalli L et al. (2009) A new genetic lesion in B-CLL: a NOTCH1 PEST domain mutation. Br J Haematol 146: 689-691. doi:10.1111/j.1365-2141.2009.07816.x. PubMed: 19604236.
5. Fabbri G, Rasi S, Rossi D, Trifonov V, Khiabanian H et al. (2011) Analysis of the chronic lymphocytic leukemia coding genome: role of NOTCH1 mutational activation. J Exp Med 208: 1389-1401. doi:10.1084/jem.20110921. PubMed: 21670202.
6. Puente XS, Pinyol M, Quesada V, Conde L, Ordóñez GR et al. (2011) Whole-genome sequencing identifies recurrent mutations in chronic lymphocytic leukaemia. Nature 475: 101-105. doi:10.1038/nature10113. PubMed: 21642962.
7. Kridel R, Meissner B, Rogic S, Boyle M, Telenius A et al. (2012) Whole transcriptome sequencing reveals recurrent NOTCH1 mutations in mantle cell lymphoma. Blood 119: 1963-1971. doi:10.1182/blood-2011-11-391474. PubMed: 22210878.
8. Lohr JG, Stojanov P, Lawrence MS, Auclair D, Chapuy B et al. (2012) Discovery and prioritization of somatic mutations in diffuse large B-cell lymphoma (DLBCL) by whole-exome sequencing. Proc Natl Acad Sci U S A 109: 3879-3884. doi:10.1073/pnas.1121343109. PubMed: 22343534.
9. Pancewicz J, Taylor JM, Datta A, Baydoun HH, Waldmann TA et al. (2010) Notch signaling contributes to proliferation and tumor formation of human T-cell leukemia virus type 1-associated adult T-cell leukemia. Proc Natl Acad Sci U S A 107: 16619-16624. doi:10.1073/pnas.1010722107. PubMed: 20823234.
10. Robinson DR, Kalyana-Sundaram S, Wu YM, Shankar S, Cao X et al. (2011) Functionally recurrent rearrangements of the MAST kinase and Notch gene families in breast cancer. Nat Med 17: 1646-1651. doi:10.1038/nm.2580. PubMed: 22101766.

11. Westhoff B, Colaluca IN, D'Ario G, Donzelli M, Tosoni D et al. (2009) Alterations of the Notch pathway in lung cancer. Proc Natl Acad Sci U S A 106: 22293-22298. doi:10.1073/pnas.0907781106. PubMed: 20007775.

12. The cancer genome atlas consortium (2011) Integrated genomic analyses of ovarian carcinoma. Nature 474: 609-615.

13. Ridgway J, Zhang G, Wu Y, Stawicki S, Liang WC et al. (2006) Inhibition of Dll4 signalling inhibits tumour growth by deregulating angiogenesis. Nature 444: 1083-1087. doi:10.1038/nature05313. PubMed: 17183323.

14. Radtke F, Fasnacht N, Macdonald HR (2010) Notch signaling in the immune system. Immunity 32: 14-27. doi:10.1016/j.immuni.2010.01.004. PubMed: 20152168.

15. Wang NJ, Sanborn Z, Arnett KL, Bayston LJ, Liao W et al. (2011) Loss-of-function mutations in Notch receptors in cutaneous and lung squamous cell carcinoma. Proc Natl Acad Sci U S A 108: 17761-17766. doi:10.1073/pnas.1114669108. PubMed: 22006338.

16. Stransky N, Egloff AM, Tward AD, Kostic AD, Cibulskis K et al. (2011) The mutational landscape of head and neck squamous cell carcinoma. Science 333: 1157-1160. doi:10.1126/science.1208130. PubMed: 21798893.

17. Agrawal N, Frederick MJ, Pickering CR, Bettegowda C, Chang K et al. (2011) Exome sequencing of head and neck squamous cell carcinoma reveals inactivating mutations in NOTCH1. Science 333: 1154-1157. doi:10.1126/science.1206923. PubMed: 21798897.

18. Hammerman PS, Hayes DN, Wilkerson MD, Schultz N, Bose R et al. (2012) Comprehensive genomic characterization of squamous cell lung cancers. Nature 489: 519-525. doi:10.1038/nature11404. PubMed: 22960745.

19. Liu Z, Turkoz A, Jackson EN, Corbo JC, Engelbach JA et al. (2011) Notch1 loss of heterozygosity causes vascular tumors and lethal hemorrhage in mice. J Clin Invest 121: 800-808. doi:10.1172/JCI43114. PubMed: 21266774.

20. Dill MT, Rothweiler S, Djonov V, Hlushchuk R, Tornillo L et al. (2012) Disruption of Notch1 induces vascular remodeling, intussusceptive angiogenesis, and angiosarcomas in livers of mice. Gastroenterology 142: 967-977 e962. doi:10.1053/j.gastro.2011.12.052. . PubMed : 22245843. doi: 10.1053/j.gastro.2011.12.052

21. Aster JC, Blacklow SC (2012) Targeting the notch pathway: twists and turns on the road to rational therapeutics. J Clin Oncol 30: 2418-2420. doi:10.1200/JCO.2012.42.0992. PubMed: 22585704.

22. DeAngelo DJ, Stone RM, Silverman LB, Aster JC (2006) A phase I clinical trial of the Notch inhibitor MK-0752 in patients with T-cell acute lympho-blastic leukemia/lymphoma (T-ALL) and other leukemias. J Clin Oncol 24: 6585.

23. Barletta JA, Perner S, Iafrate AJ, Yeap BY, Weir BA et al. (2009) Clinical significance of TTF-1 protein expression and TTF-1 gene amplification in lung adenocarcinoma. J Cell Mol Med 13: 1977-1986. doi:10.1111/j.1582-4934.2008.00594.x. PubMed: 19040416.

24. Bogusz AM, Baxter RH, Currie T, Sinha P, Sohani AR et al. (2012) Quantitative Immunofluorescence Reveals the Signature of Active B-cell Receptor Signaling in Diffuse Large B-cell Lymphoma. Clin Cancer Res 18: 6122-6135. doi:10.1158/1078-0432.CCR-12-0397. PubMed: 22966017.

25. Lahat G, Dhuka AR, Hallevi H, Xiao L, Zou C et al. (2010) Angiosarcoma: clinical and molecular insights. Ann Surg 251: 1098-1106. doi:10.1097/SLA.0b013e3181dbb75a. PubMed: 20485141.

26. Liu JF, Hirsch MS, Lee H, Matulonis UA (2009) Prognosis and hormone receptor status in older and younger patients with advanced-stage papillary serous ovarian carcinoma. Gynecol Oncol 115: 401-406. doi:10.1016/j.ygyno.2009.08.023. PubMed: 19796795.

27. Ashworth TD, Pear WS, Chiang MY, Blacklow SC, Mastio J et al. (2010) Deletion-based mechanisms of Notch1 activation in T-ALL: key roles for RAG recombinase and a conserved internal translational start site in Notch1. Blood 116: 5455-5464. doi:10.1182/blood-2010-05-286328. PubMed: 20852131.

28. Malecki MJ, Sanchez-Irizarry C, Mitchell JL, Histen G, Xu ML et al. (2006) Leukemia-associated mutations within the NOTCH1 heterodimerization domain fall into at least two distinct mechanistic classes. Mol Cell Biol 26: 4642-4651. doi:10.1128/MCB.01655-05. PubMed: 16738328.

29. Gordon WR, Roy M, Vardar-Ulu D, Garfinkel M, Mansour MR et al. (2009) Structure of the Notch1-negative regulatory region: implications for normal activation and pathogenic signaling in T-ALL. Blood 113: 4381-4390. doi:10.1182/blood-2008-08-174748. PubMed: 19075186.

30. Takeshita K, Satoh M, Ii M, Silver M, Limbourg FP et al. (2007) Critical role of endothelial Notch1 signaling in postnatal angiogenesis. Circ Res 100: 70-78. doi:10.1161/01.RES.0000254788.47304.6e. PubMed: 17158336.

31. Eagar TN, Tang Q, Wolfe M, He Y, Pear WS et al. (2004) Notch 1 signaling regulates peripheral T cell activation. Immunity 20: 407-415. doi:10.1016/S1074-7613(04)00081-0. PubMed: 15084270.

32. Lefort K, Dotto GP (2004) Notch signaling in the integrated control of keratinocyte growth/differentiation and tumor suppression. Semin Cancer Biol 14: 374-386. doi:10.1016/j.semcancer.2004.04.017. PubMed: 15288263.

33. Rangarajan A, Talora C, Okuyama R, Nicolas M, Mammucari C et al. (2001) Notch signaling is a direct determinant of keratinocyte growth arrest and entry into differentiation. EMBO J 20: 3427-3436. doi:10.1093/emboj/20.13.3427. PubMed: 11432830.

34. Yashiro-Ohtani Y, Ohtani T, Pear WS (2010) Notch regulation of early thymocyte development. Semin Immunol 22: 261-269. doi:10.1016/j.smim.2010.04.015. PubMed: 20630772.

35. Petrie HT, Zúñiga-Pflücker JC (2007) Zoned out: functional mapping of stromal signaling microenvironments in the thymus. Annu Rev Immunol 25: 649-679. doi:10.1146/annurev.immunol.23.021704.115715. PubMed:

17291187.

36. Hasserjian RP, Aster JC, Davi F, Weinberg DS, Sklar J (1996) Modulated expression of notch1 during thymocyte development. Blood 88: 970-976. PubMed: 8704256.

37. Pear WS, Aster JC, Scott ML, Hasserjian RP, Soffer B et al. (1996) Exclusive development of T cell neoplasms in mice transplanted with bone marrow expressing activated Notch alleles. J Exp Med 183: 2283-2291. doi:10.1084/jem.183.5.2283. PubMed: 8642337.

38. Weng AP, Millholland JM, Yashiro-Ohtani Y, Arcangeli ML, Lau A et al. (2006) c-Myc is an important direct target of Notch1 in T-cell acute lymphoblastic leukemia/ lymphoma. Genes Dev 20: 2096-2109. doi:10.1101/ gad.1450406. PubMed: 16847353.

39. Chiang MY, Xu ML, Histen G, Shestova O, Roy M et al. (2006) Identification of a conserved negative regulatory sequence that influences the leukemogenic activity of NOTCH1. Mol Cell Biol 26: 6261-6271. doi:10.1128/ MCB.02478-05. PubMed: 16880534.

40. Balatti V, Bottoni A, Palamarchuk A, Alder H, Rassenti LZ et al. (2012) NOTCH1 mutations in CLL associated with trisomy 12. Blood 119: 329-331. doi:10.1182/ blood-2011-10-386144. PubMed: 22086416.

41. Del Giudice I, Rossi D, Chiaretti S, Marinelli M, Tavolaro S et al. (2012) NOTCH1 mutations in +12 chronic lymphocytic leukemia (CLL) confer an unfavorable prognosis, induce a distinctive transcriptional profiling and refine the intermediate prognosis of +12 CLL. Haematologica 97: 437-441. doi:10.3324/ haematol.2011.060129.

42. Park JT, Li M, Nakayama K, Mao TL, Davidson B et al. (2006) Notch3 gene amplification in ovarian cancer. Cancer Res 66: 6312-6318. doi:10.1158/0008-5472. CAN-05-3610. PubMed: 16778208.

43. Kiel MJ, Velusamy T, Betz BL, Zhao L, Weigelin HG et al. (2012) Whole-genome sequencing identifies recurrent somatic NOTCH2 mutations in splenic marginal zone lymphoma. J Exp Med 209: 1553-1565. doi:10.1084/ jem.20120910. PubMed: 22891276.

44. Rossi D, Trifonov V, Fangazio M, Bruscaggin A, Rasi S et al. (2012) The coding genome of splenic marginal zone lymphoma: activation of NOTCH2 and other pathways regulating marginal zone development. J Exp Med 209: 1537-1551. doi:10.1084/jem.20120904. PubMed: 22891273.

45. Trøen G, Wlodarska I, Warsame A, Hernández Llodrà S, De Wolf-Peeters C et al. (2008) NOTCH2 mutations in marginal zone lymphoma. Haematologica 93: 1107-1109. doi:10.3324/haematol.11635. PubMed: 18508802.

46. Hubmann R, Schwarzmeier JD, Shehata M, Hilgarth M, Duechler M et al. (2002) Notch2 is involved in the overexpression of CD23 in B-cell chronic lymphocytic leukemia. Blood 99: 3742-3747. doi:10.1182/blood. V99.10.3742. PubMed: 11986231.

47. Rosati E, Sabatini R, Rampino G, Tabilio A, Di Ianni M et al. (2009) Constitutively activated Notch signaling is involved in survival and apoptosis resistance of B-CLL cells. Blood 113: 856-865. doi:10.1182/ blood-2008-02-139725. PubMed: 18796623.

48. Park JT, Chen X, Tropè CG, Davidson B, Shih IeM et al. (2010) Notch3 overexpression is related to the recurrence of ovarian cancer and confers resistance to carboplatin. Am J Pathol 177: 1087-1094. doi:10.2353/ ajpath.2010.100316. PubMed: 20671266.

49. Dontu G, Jackson KW, McNicholas E, Kawamura MJ, Abdallah WM et al. (2004) Role of Notch signaling in cell-fate determination of human mammary stem/ progenitor cells. Breast Cancer Res 6: R605-R615. doi:10.1186/bcr920. PubMed: 15535842.

50. Farnie G, Clarke RB (2007) Mammary stem cells and breast cancer--role of Notch signalling. Stem Cell Rev 3: 169-175. doi:10.1007/s12015-007-0023-5. PubMed: 17873349.

51. Simmons MJ, Serra R, Hermance N, Kelliher MA (2012) NOTCH1 inhibition in vivo results in mammary tumor regression and reduced mammary tumorsphere forming activity in vitro. Breast Cancer Res 14: R126. doi:10.1186/bcr3321. PubMed: 22992387.

52. Wang J, Wakeman TP, Lathia JD, Hjelmeland AB, Wang XF et al. (2010) Notch promotes radioresistance of glioma stem cells. Stem Cells 28: 17-28. PubMed: 19921751.

53. Yan M, Plowman GD (2007) Delta-like 4/Notch signaling and its therapeutic implications. Clin Cancer Res 13: 7243-7246. doi:10.1158/1078-0432.CCR-07-1393. PubMed: 18094402.

54. Yen WC, Fischer MM, Hynes M, Wu J, Kim E et al. (2012) Anti-DLL4 Has Broad Spectrum Activity in Pancreatic Cancer Dependent on Targeting DLL4-Notch Signaling in Both Tumor and Vasculature Cells. Clin Cancer Res 18: 5374-5386. doi:10.1158/1078-0432. CCR-12-0736. PubMed: 22952347.

55. Koch U, Radtke F (2011) Mechanisms of T cell development and transformation. Annu Rev Cell Dev Biol 27: 539-562. doi:10.1146/annurev-cellbio-092910-154008. PubMed: 21740230.

56. Yan M, Callahan CA, Beyer JC, Allamneni KP, Zhang G et al. (2010) Chronic DLL4 blockade induces vascular neoplasms. Nature 463: E6-E7. doi:10.1038/ nature08751. PubMed: 20147986.

57. Phng LK, Gerhardt H (2009) Angiogenesis: a team effort coordinated by notch. Dev Cell 16: 196-208.

CHAPTER 17

IMMUNOHISTOCHEMISTRY AND IN SITU HYBRIDIZATION

Giovanni Anthony, Ju-Ahng Lee

INTRODUCTION

The advent of desktop publishing and personal printing devices in the 1980s fundamentally changed the way people create printed documents. Error-intolerant type writing and time-consuming cycles of sending documents to and from the professional printing service were replaced with user-friendly desktop publishing/word-processing and convenient printing from desktop printers. At the present time, equivalent or potentially even more significant changes are being introduced by the introduction of 3D printing technology: the social theorist Jeremy Rifkin predicts personal 3D printing as one of central driving forces for what he refers to as the third industrial revolution [1]. Indeed, early applications of this personal manufacturing technology have already demonstrated great promise in a bewildering array of fields, including rapid prototyping, parts manufacturing, education, robotics, pre-surgery simulation, organ fabrication, prosthetics, apparel design, paleontology, medicinal pill synthesis, material science, and art, to name just a few [2–6]. With the ever-increasing build resolution, some of today's 3D printers can print out devices with micrometer precision or even nanometer precision [7, 8]. Recently, 3D printing technology was also used to create an orientation device for zebrafish embryos[9, 10]. Another report relevant to the present study demonstrated 3D printed microfluidics devices [11], given that microfluidics devices have been used with live zebrafish embryos [12].

We built a custom tissue handling system with stereolithography-based 3D printing technology. Our system is particularly suited for handling multiple small tissue samples in parallel, using commercially available 6-well tissue culture plates. We have successfully tested this system for whole mount *in situ* hybridization of fixed zebrafish embryos. As this system was designed to be readily modified for fully automatic tissue handling in any XYZ machine, we believe that applications beyond histology could be envisioned according to the end user's needs.

Citation: Anthony G, Lee J-A (2016) Immunohistochemistry and In Situ Hybridization. PLoS ONE 11(8): e0159991. doi:10.1371/journal.pone.0159991.

RESULTS

Main Features of the 6-Well Chambers

Our original system contained individually detachable 6 cells for each liftable chamber core (data now shown). However, no significant benefit was obtained from this detachable design. On the contrary, occasional falling of cells made the entire system prone to sample loss. Thus, we altered the design to make the system simpler and more robust. We introduced 6 holes for each chamber. This was a strategic compromise between our desire to process as many samples as possible and the practical ease of tissue handling through small openings (Fig 1C and 1D). We found each well comfortably accommodates more than 3 dozen zebrafish larvae. During our test run, we encountered a problem when multiple different samples were used: namely, easy confusion between samples. To address this issue, we added surface engravings on top of chambers and lids (Fig 1C and 1D). Specifically, by generating 3D model files of 6 different chambers and their lids, each engraved with A to F, we could track each chamber separately. Moreover, separate numbers (1–6) were engraved next to each well. Thus, any well can be easily identified with a combination of a letter (A-F) and a number (1–6): 1A, 3C, 5F, etc. Although the labels were discernable from an oblique angle, it requires effort to clearly read them as the letters are shallow grooves on the transparent body. We could enhance the readability of the labels as follows. A small bit of non-drying modeling blue clay was applied on top of the letter grooves and then cleaned off by smudging with Kimwipes, leaving the grooves filled with the blue clay. A thin layer of superglue was uniformly applied to seal off the blue clay. Each lid-chamber pair was tested for smooth closing and opening: a quick filing with a triangular file was enough to ensure the proper closure of the lid through the cylindrical handle.

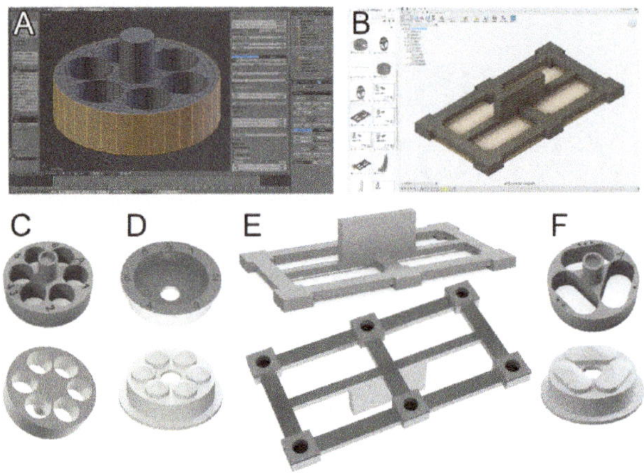

Figure 1: 3D modeling programs used in this study and image rendering of the devices.

Despite the transparent resin used for actual manufacturing, the images were created with a simulated opaque material for better visualization. Each device was rendered from top and bottom angles. (A) A chamber model shown in Blender 3D. (B) A lifter model shown in Fusion 360. (C) Rendered images of a chamber. Notice that the surface engraved labeling is visible on top of the chamber. A shallow hole for a magnetic disc is found at the top of the cylindrical handle. (D) Rendered images of a lid. Surface engraved labeling is shown on top of the lids. (E) Rendered images of a lifter. 6 holes at the bottom of the lifter would accommodate 5mm x 2mm magnet discs. The rendering of the lifter is not to scale in relation to the renderings of the chamber and lid. (F) Rendered images of a chamber and a lid with larger holes to accommodate more/larger samples.

Main Features of the Lids

Unlike IHC, *in situ* hybridization includes a high temperature (~70°C) treatment for a prolonged period of time (overnight probe hybridization). Our initial test showed that if we use a small amount of hybridization solution (~2ml) for each chamber, evaporation of the solution left the tissue dry even if the whole plate was kept in the humid chamber with the plate's lid closed. Thus, we designed a custom lid that fits our chamber. Our first attempt with a flat surfaced lid could not solve the problem, however, as the evaporated water remained as condensation on the lid. Our next model, equipped with a pointed end facing towards the bottom of the well, successfully prevented the evaporation and tissue from getting dried, as water condensation on the lid readily dripped.

Certain riboprobes for in situ hybridization work better when they are hybridized for an extended period of time, such as 3–4 days (personal observation). We encountered an unexpected problem with such a long incubation. Specifically, a large amount of water vapor from the humid chamber was condensed on the inner side of the plate's lid and trickled into the wells, which diluted the hybridization solution significantly—more than 100% dilution after 3 day incubation. Thus, we redesigned the lid to include a round side wall and a thin circular rim that seals off the well to prevent accidental water drip (Figs 2 and 3B). With the enhanced lid design, the volume of hybridization solution inside the well remained unchanged. For a long incubation at a high temperature, we found that it is better not to use the 6-well plate's lid as long as it is kept in the humid chamber. Additionally, a gabled (^ shaped) lid for the humid chamber (or water bath) helps prevent the condensed water from dripping into the plate.

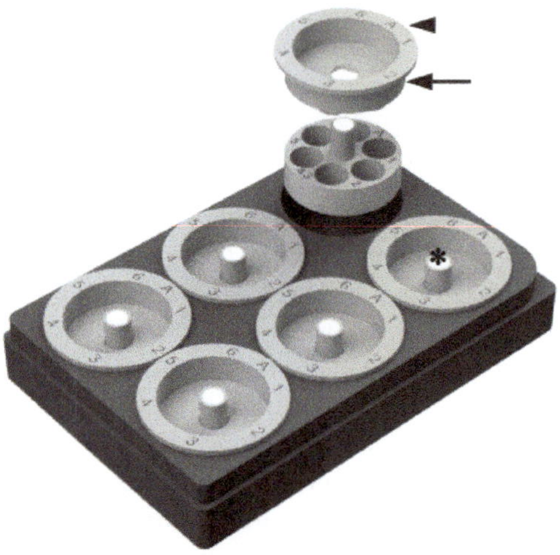

Figure 2: Arrangement of chambers and lids on a 6-well plate.

Notice that the flat rim (arrow head) and cylindrical side wall (arrow) of the lid prevent water from evaporating out of and dripping into the well. The rim makes direct contact with the top edge of the plate's well. The length of the chamber's handle was designed such that the magnet (asterisk) directly contacts the corresponding magnet of the lifter, even with the circular lid placed on the chamber.

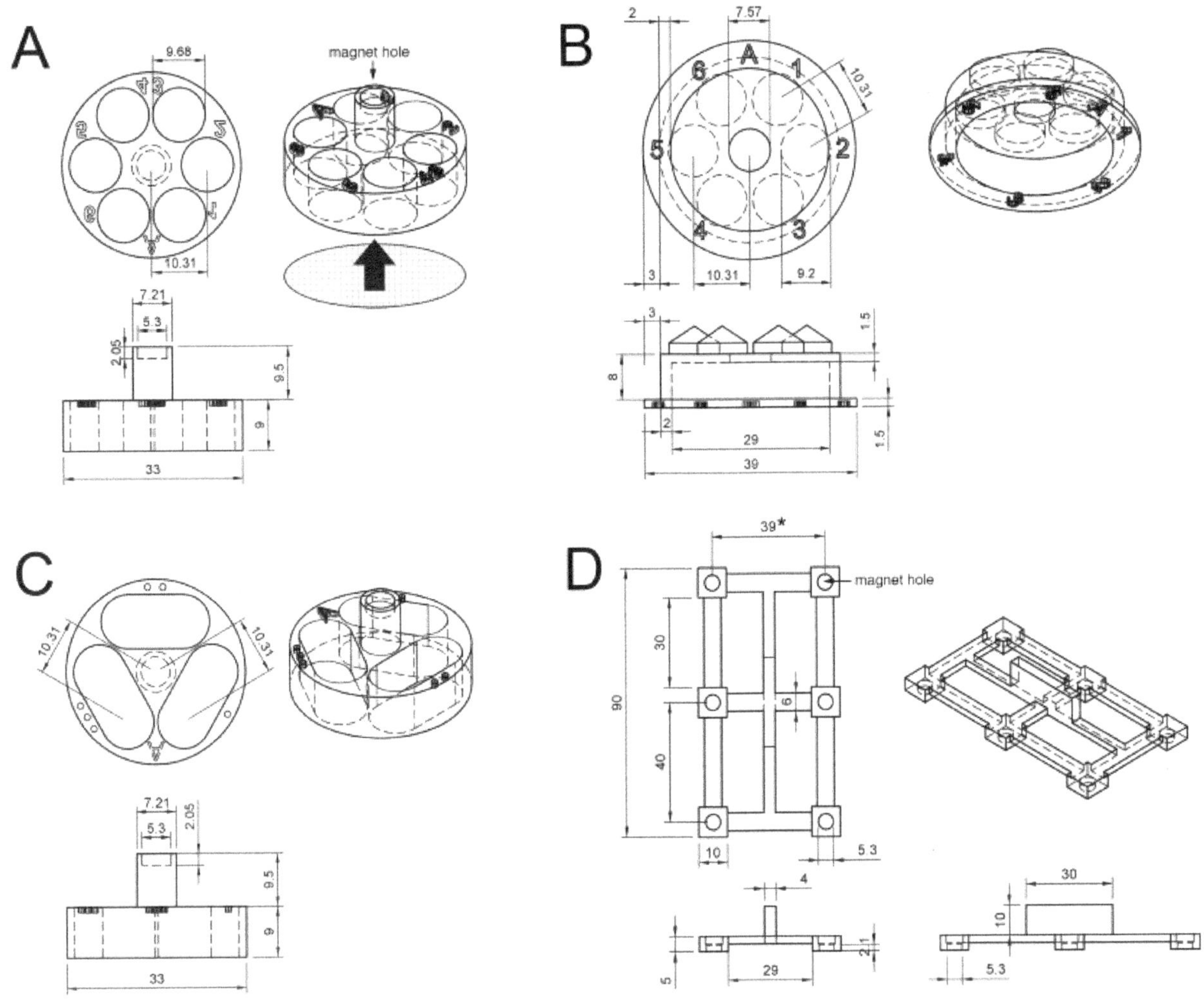

Figure 3: Detailed blueprints for each component.

(A) A blueprint for the 6-well chamber. A circularly cut piece of mesh (nylon or stainless) is glued on the bottom of the chamber, as shown with a meshed circle and a large arrow. (B) A blue print for the 6-well lid. Letters (A, 1–6) indicate the surface engraving. (C) A blueprint for the 3-well chamber. (D) A blue print for the lifter. Notice the width of 39mm (asterisk) is 1mm wider than the known dimension (38mm) of the standard 6 well plates (see text). The drawing of the lifter is not to scale in relation to the drawings of the chamber and lid. All units are in mm.

Magnetic Lifter

A small but functionally important point of our lifter design is noteworthy. Our initial model was built in accordance with the dimension of standard 6 well cell culture plates: the distances between the well centers are 38mm (width) and 40mm (length). However, when we made our lifter to this dimension, magnetically attached chambers were inserted into the 6 well plates with substantial friction. Two plates from different vendors yielded identical results, i.e., significant friction. Upon inspection, we noticed the friction was mainly caused because the distance between the neighboring chambers was slightly too close, only in the direction of width. Since the gluing of magnet discs can cause slight distortion of angles (our observation), we used a completely fluid form of instant adhesive and ensured the leveled adhesion of discs before the glue set. However, even the most careful installation of magnet discs did not solve the friction. Thus, we increased the distance between the neighboring centers of the discs on our lifter from 38mm to 39mm (Fig 3D, asterisk), which solved the problem instantly. To better reduce the potential mal-alignment problem, especially for the full automation—see below, we also reduced the diameter of the chambers and lids from 34mm to 33mm (Fig 3A and 3B).

After a few trials of different versions, the height of the chamber's cylindrical wall was lowered to 9mm to make the tissue handling easy but deep enough for stable transfer of samples through many washing steps (Fig 3A). The length of the handle was decided to make it easy to manually transfer the chamber (Fig 4D), as well as to be magnetically attached to the lifter, even with the chamber's lid in place. While it is convenient to leave the magnetic lifter attached to the chambers during liquid treatment steps, one can readily detach the lifter by holding three chambers in the 6-well plate with the free hand's index finger and gently detaching the lifter from the three chambers. One can then hold the remaining three chambers in the same manner while detaching the lifter from them.

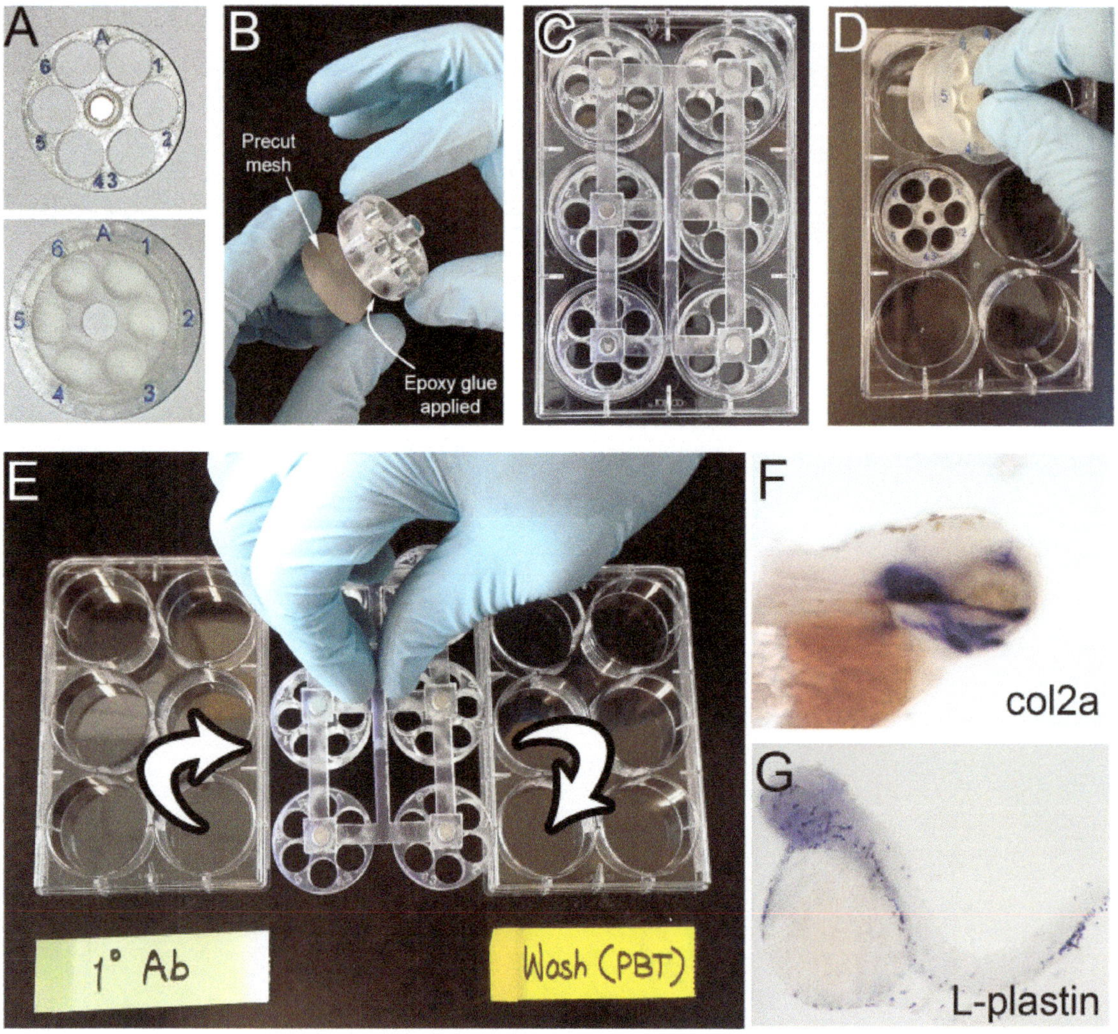

Figure 4: Actual photos of the system and its use for *in situ* hybridization.

(A) Enhanced labeling with artist's modeling clay and coating. (B) Mesh attachment with epoxy glue. (C) A fully loaded plate with a magnetic lifter attached. (D) With only a few samples, individual chambers can be conveniently transferred manually. Chamber A, with its lid closed, was picked up by hand, whereas the chamber B is shown without its lid in pace. (E) 6 chambers (36 samples) are handled simultaneously with a magnetic lifter. (F, G) Examples of whole mount *in situ* hybridization results.

DISCUSSION

Previously, attempts have been made to reduce the repetitive liquid handling time common to histology techniques such as immunohistochemistry and *in situ* hybridization. Notable early attempts include the use of plastic "baskets" which were hand-crafted by cutting readily available microcentrifuge tubes and attaching nylon or metal mesh at the bottom of the baskets [13, 14]. The benefit from these early hand-made devices was already apparent. First, simple transfer of baskets by forceps significantly saved time compared with repeated liquid exchange by pipetting. Secondly, the flat bottom mesh maximized the even exposure of tissue to the reagents, in contrast to the typical incubation at the bottom tip of the vertically positioned microcentrifuge tubes. However, these approaches left room for improvement. In particular, manual transfer with forceps of individual baskets still requires substantial time for each sample handling and is also vulnerable to accidental drop of the baskets. Moreover, cutting the hard plastic tubes into open cylinders involves sizable safety risk, whether the tubes are cut by cutters, blades, or saw. Our 3D printing-mediated devices offer benefits in these aspects. Specifically, our approach does not include risky plastic cutting. Most significantly, by assembling multiple holes into a chamber, even manual transfer of chambers without the lifter still significantly cuts down the time for repetitive steps, with much lower risk of accidental slippage. The time-saving achieved by our system is maximized when the magnet-mediated lifter is used to simultaneously handle up to six chambers (6x6 = 36 samples). Moreover, we believe that our system can be readily modified to be used with any standard, programmable XYZ robotic arms.

Though our laboratory seldom needs chambers with larger holes, the need for handling bigger tissue or more number of small tissues will necessitate the design change. Such changes in the pre-made 3D models may require substantial remodeling in mesh-based 3D modelers. However, Fusion 360's parametric modeling approach provided a powerful means to visit an old version in history and generate multiple different models without re-modeling the subsequent steps. For example, we could rapidly generate a modified 3D model of a chamber with 3 larger holes, which took just a few minutes

(Fig 1D). Moreover, as a tool specifically built for engineering CAD, Fusion 360 provides various forms of presentation of the finished models, including standard 3D rendering and interactive 2D blueprints as shown in Figs 1 and 3.

As we increased the number of samples for one round of experiment, we needed to develop a labeling system to distinguish different samples. Thus, we incorporated surface engraving on the top of both chambers and lids. We created 6 different 3D models of chamber-lid pairs. Thus, individual chambers and lids can be readily identified with a combination of A-F and 1–6: 1A, 3C, 5F, etc (Fig 1).

We tested magnet discs in two different sizes (4mm x 3mm and 5mm x 2mm), both of which were made of neodymium. For the final products, 5mm x 2mm magnet discs were used for more surface area to achieve better adhesion. Our decision to use magnets for lifting was based on our future plan to automate the entire process. We envision that the rectangular handle of the lifter designed for manual handling could be readily changed to adopt a bigger magnet (or a grid of magnets for better precision) and the corresponding magnetic frame could be readily printed out to be equipped on any standard programmable XYZ robotic arm. This would enable a full automation of the tissue handling.

SLA 3D printers, despite their distinct advantage of high resolution, have some drawbacks. Most notable are the lengthy printing time and rather involved post-print procedures. Some of the most recent innovations on SLA printing technologies markedly reduced the printing time [15]. However, the complete removal of sticky resin from the printed parts still requires the use of organic chemicals such as pure isopropyl alcohol, which is not only inconvenient and hazardous but also creates a problem of safe disposal of solvent containing the dissolved resin, particularly at home. We disposed leftover resin only after it is completely cured to become a hard block. Moreover, our access to chemical fume hood gave us an easy and safe means of disposal of the used isopropyl alcohol: simple evaporation of the isopropyl alcohol in the hood and curing of the remaining resin.

During our *in situ* hybridization test, we encountered one unexpected caveat, which limits the use of our devices, at least as produced in the way described here. At the end of color reaction in widely used digoxigenin-alkaline phosphatase *in situ* hybridization, tissues are sometimes cleared in organic solutions such as the mixture of benzyl benzoate and benzyl alcohol [16]. This solvent mix, however, melted the surface of the cured resin that we used for this work, leaving some of the fine structures disappeared: parts of the thin walls between wells were melted away. We have not tested if the same solvent mix dissolves other printing materials commonly used in other types of 3D printers. This result demonstrates the need for developing diverse 3D printer resins and for careful evaluation of particular 3D printing materials for specific usage. Encouraging in this regard is the current trend of rapid development of diverse functional resins, including the resins whose printout is either flexible or burns out cleanly without residue, ideal as a mold material (http://formlabs.com/company/press/formlabs-announces-new-suite-functional-resins/).

In conclusion, we developed a 3D-printed tissue handling system that provides numerous advantages such as significant time-saving, superior tissue preservation, minimal sample-to-sample variations, and readily modifiable design flexibility.

MATERIALS AND METHODS

3d Printer

We used Form1+ SLA 3D printer from FormLabs (http://formlabs.com/products/3d-printers/form-1-plus/). PreForm is an accompanied software that we used on iMac desktop computers (Apple Inc.) to send the 3D models to the Form1+ printer. We used the following settings: Clear Resin version 2, 0.05mm. It took about 5 hours to print 9 chambers/lids with the z axis resolution of 0.05mm and about 2.5 hours with the 0.1mm z resolution.

3d Modeling Softwares

For 3D modeling, we first used Blender 3D, a powerful and comprehensive open source 3D software package, widely used by motion graphics professionals and artists. Despite rather limited usage for precision CAD, this software could be readily used for our modeling (Fig 1A). Eventually, however, we switched our main modeling software to Fusion 360 (Autodesk Inc.) as this cloud-based software was primarily built for precision CAD and CAM applications (Fig 1B). Fusion 360 can be used as a free software with a 3-year free license for personal or educational purposes.

Resins for 3d Printing

We tested two different resins built by FormLabs: grey version 2 and clear version 2. Although both resins were compatible for our purpose, we decided to use clear resin due to its transparency that helps visually inspect samples within the chambers.

Post-Print Processing

For post-print cleaning, we used 99.5% isopropyl alcohol (VWR, BDH1133-4LP). Specifically, upon the completion of printing, the printed parts were carefully detached from the build platform and rinsed in the post-rinse tubs provided with the printer. For the first rinse, the tub with isopropyl alcohol and parts was vigorously shaken with its lid closed for two minutes. If printed parts include small crevices, we also used disposable plastic transfer pipettes (Fisher Scientific, 13-711-9D) to clear remaining uncured resin from the crevices with strong jets of isopropyl alcohol. Once the first rinse was finished, parts were transferred to the second tub with fresh isopropyl alcohol and rinsed for about 10 minutes on a wave motion shaker or by manual shaking. Used isopropyl alcohol from the first and second tubs was filtered with paper coffee filters and stored in separate bottles. Filtered alcohol from the first rinse was re-used up to 3 times and replaced with the alcohol from the second rinse. As the uncured resin for Form1 printers has been recently shown to be toxic in the zebrafish toxicity assay [17], we disposed all unused resin in readily available transparent plastic containers and thoroughly cured the resin in sunlight. In addition, the resin-containing used isopropyl alcohol was kept in a well-ventilated chemical fume hood overnight to evaporate the alcohol, leaving the dissolved resin at the bottom, which was subsequently cured in sunlight for disposal.

The rinsed parts were kept next to the sun-lit window for at least two days and the scaffolding supports were carefully removed using the provided flush cutters. Remaining support marks were removed and the area was smoothened using a triangular/three-square file (Grainger, 24N391).

Magnet Disks and Tissue-Collecting Mesh

5mmx2mm neodymium magnet discs (www.magnets365.com) were used for lifting chambers. To ensure the consistent angle of the glued magnets, we used liquid form of superglue (also known as krazy glue) to attach the magnet discs into the magnet holes. Before the glue sets, each magnet was evenly positioned to the casing.

For the tissue-collecting mesh, we used nylon mesh with 210μm opening size (Small parts, CMN-0210-C), 300μm opening size (Ted Pella, Inc. 41-X105), or stainless cloth with varied opening size (Grainger wire cloth). Circular meshes were initially made by drawing a circle on the mesh along an unused chamber and by cutting with a pair of scissors. We eventually selected 300μm opening mesh and cut out the circles using a laser cutter.

For chemical resistance and stable adhesion, we used epoxy adhesive (J-B Weld, 50112) to attach the mesh to the bottom of the chamber. Flat wooden coffee stirrers were used to apply the adhesive evenly and accurately, before the chamber was pressed down to the pre-cut circular mesh. It is important to keep the epoxy glue layer consistently thin in order to keep the height of the chambers consistent.

Support Editing

When resin-based 3D printers print, the objects are connected to the base platform by numerous support structures that need to be removed after the printing is finished. As the contact point of support and the main object slightly distorts the fine surface geometry, delicate surfaces that need precise geometry such as small engraved letters should avoid direct contact with supports. In the PreForm software, support positions can be edited: Supports > Edit Selected. By removing supports and adding others in the nearby non-critical area, one can maintain the print stability and avoid the misconfiguration of fine geometry where needed. In case problems such as friction between the lid and chamber arise, they can be fixed by simple filing using a triangular file.

Labeling

To enhance the label readability, non-drying modeling clay (Ultra blue, 10106, Van Aaken) was used to fill the lettering grooves (Fig 4A). Remaining clay debris was removed by simple smudging action with Kimwipes. The modeling clay in the grooves was fixed by a thin layer of superglue.

In Situ Hybridization

In situ hybridization was conducted according to the previously published protocol [18]. Col2a1 antisense riboprobe was made by RT-PCR and *in vitro* transcription using the following primers: forward primer 5' GTTGGACCTGCTGGTAAGGA 3', T7 reverse primer 5' TAATACGACTCACTATAGGGAGATTCTTGCGTGGGATTTTAGG 3'. L-plastin antisense riboprobe was made by T7 RNA polymerase reaction after a full-length L-plastin IMAGE clone 6794749 was digested with EcoRI.

Zebrafish Care

The AB* wildtype zebrafish were housed in automatic fish housing systems (Aquaneering, San Diego). All zebrafish procedures were approved by North Carolina Central University Insitutional Animal Care and Use Committee.

ACKNOWLEDGMENTS

The authors thank Dr. Gregory Cole for comments on the manuscript and NCCU animal facility for zebrafish care. This work was supported by NIAAA U54 AA019765-06 to J.-A.L.

REFERENCES

1. Rifkin J. The third industrial revolution: how lateral power is transforming energy, the economy, and the world. New York: Palgrave Macmillan; 2011.
2. Jones N. Science in three dimensions: the print revolution. Nature. 2012;487(7405):22–3. doi: 10.1038/487022a. pmid:22763531
3. Murphy SV, Atala A. 3D bioprinting of tissues and organs. Nat Biotechnol. 2014;32(8):773–85. doi: 10.1038/nbt.2958. pmid:25093879
4. Savage N. Technology: Building opportunities. Nature. 2014;509(7501):521–3. pmid:24860876 doi: 10.1038/nj7501-521a
5. Schubert C, van Langeveld MC, Donoso LA. Innovations in 3D printing: a 3D overview from optics to organs. Br J Ophthalmol. 2014;98(2):159–61. doi: 10.1136/bjophthalmol-2013-304446. pmid:24288392
6. Chia HN, Wu BM. Recent advances in 3D printing of biomaterials. J Biol Eng. 2015;9:4. doi: 10.1186/s13036-015-0001-4. pmid:25866560
7. Lee M, Kim HY. Toward nanoscale three-dimensional printing: nanowalls built of electrospun nanofibers. Langmuir. 2014;30(5):1210–4. doi: 10.1021/la404704z pmid:24471865.
8. Huang TY, Sakar MS, Mao A, Petruska AJ, Qiu F, Chen XB, et al. 3D Printed Microtransporters: Compound Micromachines for Spatiotemporally Controlled Delivery of Therapeutic Agents. Adv Mater. 2015;27(42):6644–50. doi: 10.1002/adma.201503095 pmid:26415002; PubMed Central PMCID: PMCPMC4669391.
9. Masselink W, Wong JC, Liu B, Fu J, Currie PD. Low-cost silicone imaging casts for zebrafish embryos and larvae. Zebrafish. 2014;11(1):26–31. doi: 10.1089/zeb.2013.0897. pmid:24237049
10. Wittbrodt JN, Liebel U, Gehrig J. Generation of orientation tools for automated zebrafish screening assays using desktop 3D printing. BMC Biotechnol. 2014;14:36. doi: 10.1186/1472-6750-14-36. pmid:24886511
11. Ho CMB, Ng SH, Li KHH, Yoon Y-J. 3D printed microfluidics for biological applications. Lab Chip. 2015. doi: 10.1039/c5lc00685f.

12. Rudin-Bitterli TS, Tills O, Spicer JI, Culverhouse PF, Wielhouwer EM, Richardson MK, et al. Combining motion analysis and microfluidics—a novel approach for detecting whole-animal responses to test substances. PLoS One. 2014;9(12):e113235. doi: 10.1371/journal.pone.0113235. pmid:25464030

13. Thisse C, Thisse B. High-resolution in situ hybridization to whole-mount zebrafish embryos. Nature protocols. 2008;3(1):59–69. doi: 10.1038/nprot.2007.514. pmid:18193022

14. Chitramuthu BP, Bennett HPJ. High resolution whole mount in situ hybridization within zebrafish embryos to study gene expression and function. J Vis Exp. 2013;(80):e50644. doi: 10.3791/50644. pmid:24192694

15. Tumbleston JR, Shirvanyants D, Ermoshkin N, Janusziewicz R, Johnson AR, Kelly D, et al. Additive manufacturing. Continuous liquid interface production of 3D objects. Science. 2015;347(6228):1349–52. doi: 10.1126/science.aaa2397. pmid:25780246

16. Nüsslein-Volhard C, Dahm R. Zebrafish: a practical approach. 1st ed. Oxford: Oxford University Press; 2002. xviii, 303 p. p.

17. Oskui SM, Diamante G, Liao C, Shi W, Gan J, Schlenk D, et al. Assessing and Reducing the Toxicity of 3D-Printed Parts. Environmental Science \& Technology Letters. 2016;3(1):1–6. doi: 10.1021/acs.estlett.5b00249.

18. Lee J-A, Anholt RRH, Cole GJ. Olfactomedin-2 mediates development of the anterior central nervous system and head structures in zebrafish. Mechanisms of development. 2007;125(1–2):167–81. doi: 10.1016/j.mod.2007.09.009. pmid:18037275

CHAPTER 18

META-ANALYSIS OF THE PROGNOSTIC VALUE OF SMAD4 IMMUNOHISTOCHEMISTRY

Yiping Du, Xin Zhou, Zebo Huang, Tianzhu Qiu, Jian Wang, Wei Zhu, Tongshan Wang, Ping Liu

INTRODUCTION

For many years, cancer has been the leading cause of death worldwide, making it a global health problem [1]. Newer diagnostic methods to detect cancer with improved sensitivity and specificity have been developed. However, because cancer is characterized by invasion and metastasis, which are the main factors contributing to its high mortality rate, the prognosis of cancer remains poor, with a disappointing five-year survival rate. Digestive system tumors, particularly gastric, colorectal and pancreatic cancer, are common malignancies and are the leading cause of cancer-related deaths worldwide. Clinicopathological characteristics—for example, tumor size and stage—do not fully predict individual clinical outcomes. Thus, molecular prognostic biomarkers to predict the progression of the disease, response to treatment, and survival were widely explored during the past decades.

Recently, the presence of certain proteins, such as matrix metalloproteinase 9 (MMP-9), C-reactive protein and vascular endothelial growth factor (VEGF), has been found to be associated with a poor prognosis in multiple cancers [2]–[4]. Among these biomarkers, Smad4 has attracted increasing research attention. Smad4, also termed DPC4, is a tumor suppressor gene that is recognized as a common intracellular mediator that can alter transforming growth factor β (TGF-β) signaling to promote tumor progression. Smad4-dependent TGF-β signaling is common during tumor development and progression and can modulate cell proliferation, affect cell motility, regulate the epithelial-mesenchymal-transition (EMT) process and affect sensitivity to clinical therapy [5]–[7]. Inactivation of the Smad4-induced deregulation of the TGF-β superfamily signaling is well established in some cancers. Moreover, it was found that Smad4 was associated with tumor invasion, metastasis and prognosis in different cancers [8]–[10]. However, the potential prognostic value of the immunohistochemical detection of Smad4 in various types of cancer is inconsistent. For instance, in pancreatic cancer, Milind Javle et al. [11] reported that the expression level of Smad4 was not associated with OS. However, it was found that the immunohistochemical detection of Smad4 was an independent and significant prognostic factor for overall and disease-free survival in the study of Hua et al. [12]. Regarding colorectal and gastric cancer, inconsistent results concerning the prognostic value of Smad4 were also found in different articles. Thus, an effective meta-analysis to explore the prognostic value of Smad4 in various cancers is urgently needed. To our knowledge, this study is the first comprehensive meta-analysis to explore the prognostic role of Smad4 in different types of cancer.

Citation: Du Y, Zhou X, Huang Z, Qiu T, Wang J, Zhu W, et al. (2014) Meta-Analysis of the Prognostic Value of Smad4 Immunohistochemistry. PLoS ONE 9(10): e110182. doi:10.1371/journal.pone.0110182.

MATERIALS AND METHODS

Publication Search and Inclusion Criteria

PubMed, EMBASE and ISI Web of Science were searched to collect potentially relevant published studies. Medical subheading (MeSH) terms related to Smad4 (or DPC4) in combination with words related to cancer (or tumor or neoplasms or carcinoma) and terms related to prognosis (or outcome or survival or prognostic) were used to retrieve eligible studies through February 2014. The article references and review articles were also examined to identify additional potentially relevant studies. Studies were considered eligible if they met the following criteria: (a) included cancer patients who were pathologically confirmed; (b) investigated the association between the immunohistochemical detection of Smad4 and overall survival (OS) or cancer-specific survival (CSS) or recurrence-free survival (RFS); and (c) were published as a full paper in English. Studies were excluded based on the following criteria: (a) letters, reviews, case reports or laboratory studies; (b) studies with duplicate data or a repeated analysis; (c) lack of key information for further analysis; and (d) non-human research.

Data Extraction

Data were evaluated and extracted independently by two investigators under the guidelines of the Dutch Cochrane Centre proposed by the Meta-analysis of Observational Studies in Epidemiology (MOOSE) [13]. For each study, the following information was recorded: first author, year of publication, country of origin, ethnicity, total number of cases, cancer type, stage, follow ups and hazard ratios (HRs) with their 95% confidence intervals (CIs) and *P*value. For discrepancies, a consensus was reached on each item among the authors.

Statistical Analysis

HRs with their 95% CIs obtained from studies were used to calculate pooled HRs. When the data were not directly reported, a mathematical estimation was performed by calculating the necessary data according to the methods published by Parmer et al. [14]. We investigated the heterogeneity of pooled results using Cochran's Q test and the Higgins I-squared statistic. If the result of the *Q* test revealed $P_{heterogeneity}>0.1$ and $I^2<50\%$, indicating the absence of heterogeneity, then a fixed-effects model (the Mantel–Haenszel method) was used to estimate the summary HRs/ORs [15]. Otherwise, the random-effects model (the DerSimonian and Laird method) was used [16]. Stratification and meta-regression analyses were used to detect the potential heterogeneity among studies. Begg's funnel plot and Egger's linear regression test were conducted to examine publication bias in the literature, and $p<0.05$ was considered significant. All statistical analyses were performed using the STATA software, version 12.0 (STATA Corporation, College Station, TX, USA). All P values were two-sided.

RESULTS

Study Characteristics

A total of 376 articles were identified by the initial search. Figure 1 shows the detailed screening process. After careful screening of the titles, abstracts, figures and key data, 26 articles were included in our meta-analysis according to the inclusion criteria [11], [12], [17]–[40]. Only two articles evaluated the prognostic value for RFS, and six evaluated the prognostic value for CSS. Considering that the number of studies for these two indicators was small, we combined the data for CSS with RFS. Thus, 20 studies involving 4247 patients and evaluating OS and 8 studies involving 3323 cases for RFS/CSS were analyzed in our meta-analysis. As shown in Table 1, the ethnicity background of patients was classified as Caucasian or Asian. The number of patients ranged from 34 to 1404. The patients were diagnosed with various carcinomas, among which digestive tumors accounted for most carcinomas, particularly pancreatic cancer (n=10), colorectal cancer (n=7) and gastric cancer (n=4). And the remaining 5 studies included other tumor types.

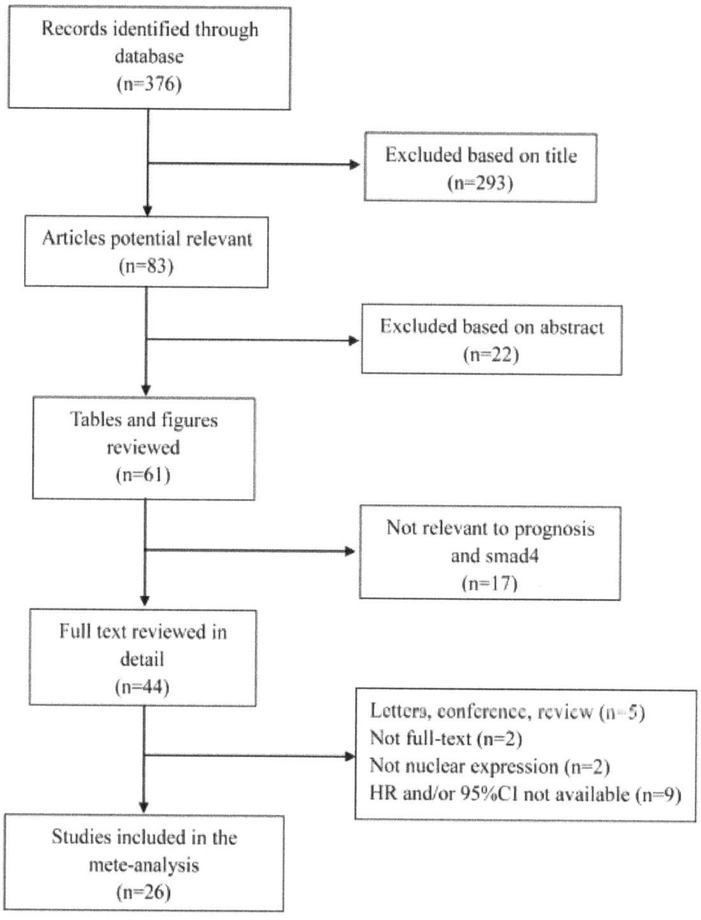

Figure 1: Methodological flow diagram of the meta-analysis.

Table 1: Main characteristics of the studies included in this meta-analysis

Author	Year	Country	Ethnicity	Type	Stage	Number	Follow up (months) (median and/or range)
Milind Javle	2014	Greece	Caucasian	Pancreatic	NA	81	NA
Jeong Hwan Park	2013	Korea	Asian	Renal	I–IV	637	74 (2–187)
Minoru Oshima	2013	Japan	Asian	Pancreatic	I–II	106	17.3 (2.8–124.8)
Arnaud D. Roth	2012	Switzerland	Caucasian	Colorectal	II–III	1404	69
Adriana Handra-Luca	2012	France	Caucasian	Pancreatic	NA	99	26 (1.2–95.5)
J. B. Bachet	2011	France	Caucasian	Pancreatic	I–II	444	54 (1.1–143.7)
Niki A. Ottenhof	2012	Netherlands	Caucasian	Pancreatic	I–III	78	NA
Pavlos Lampropoulos	2012	Greece	Caucasian	Colorectal	I–IV	195	56 (1–72)
Martin Isaksson	2011	Sweden	Caucasian	Colorectal	I–IV	441	NA
Philip W. Voorneveld	2012	Netherlands	Caucasian	Colorectal	NA	209	65 (1.5–257)
Maartje G. Noordhuis	2011	Netherlands	Caucasian	Cervical	I–II	255	66 (4–223)
Xuemei Li	2011	China	Asian	Colorectal	NA	147	NA
Hirokazu Okano	2004	Japan	Asian	Gastric	NA	166	48.8(1.8–136.2)
By Andrew V. Biankin	2002	Australia	Caucasian	Pancreatic	NA	114	3.5 (0–117)
Kyu Yeoun Won	2009	Korea	Asian	Osteosarcoma	I–IV	34	NA
Judith N Kloth	2008	Netherlands	Caucasian	Cervical	NA	117	NA
Li-HuiWang	2007	Korea	Asian	Gastric	I–IV	114	NA
Mesker We	2009	Netherlands	Caucasian	Colorectal	I–II	135	NA
Che Xiangming	2001	Japan	Asian	Gastric	NA	249	73.5 (54–76)
Y. H. Kim	2003	USA	Caucasian	Gastric	I–IV	304	67 (1–72)
Martin Isaksson-Mettavainio	2006	Sweden	Caucasian	Colorectal	NA	86	NA
Kiyokazu Hiwatashi	2009	Japan	Asian	Hepatocellular	I–IV	121	53
Metin Tascilar	2001	USA	Caucasian	Pancreatic	I–IV	249	17
Khorana AA	2005	USA	Caucasian	Pancreatic	NA	124	NA
Zhan Hua	2003	China	Asian	Pancreatic	I–IV	34	NA
Tomoko Toga	2004	Japan	Asian	Pancreatic	I–IV	88	NA

Main results

As shown in Table 2, we found that loss of Smad4 staining predicted a poor outcome with a pooled HR of 1.97 (95% CI: 1.55–2.51; $P_{heterogeneity}<0.001$) for 20 studies evaluating OS (Figure 2). Similarly, the prognostic role of Smad4-negative expression for RFS/CSS was also investigated with a combined HR of 1.81 (95% CI: 1.30–2.54; $P_{heterogeneity}<0.001$).

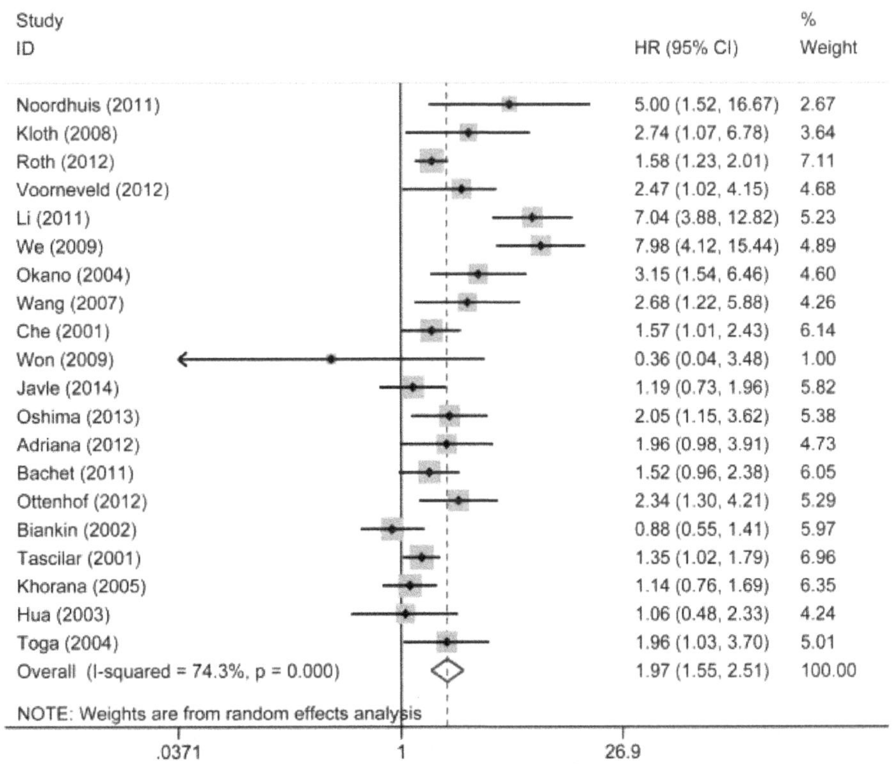

Figure 2: Forest plots of studies evaluating hazard ratios (HRs) of Smad4 for overall survival.

Table 2: Meta-analysis results

Outcome	Variables	Number of studies	Model	HR(95%CI)	Pheterogeneity
OS	ALL	20		1.97 (1.55–2.51)	<0.001
	Cancer type				
	Cervical	2	Fixed	3.43 (1.65–7.12)	0.436
	Colorectal	4	Random	3.76 (1.53–9.25)	<0.001
	Gastric	3	Fixed	2.02 (1.44–2.83)	0.197
	Pancreatic	9	Fixed	1.39 (1.19–1.61)	0.185
	Ethnicity				
	Asian	7	Random	2.24 (1.32–3.81)	<0.001
	Caucasian	13	Random	1.82 (1.39–2.37)	<0.001
	Participate number				
	Large	6	Fixed	1.56 (1.34–1.82)	0.277
	Small	14	Random	2.09 (1.42–3.06)	<0.001
CSS/RFS	ALL	8		1.81 (1.30–2.54)	<0.001
	Cancer type				
	Colorectal	5	Random	2.54 (1.46–4.39)	<0.001
	Others	3	Fixed	1.24 (0.95–1.61)	0.544
	Ethnicity				
	Asian	2	Fixed	1.34 (0.99–1.81)	0.647
	Caucasian	6	Random	2.12 (1.32–3.43)	<0.001
	Participate number				
	Large	4	Fixed	1.41 (1.19–1.67)	0.353
	Small	4	Random	2.89 (1.34–6.24)	<0.001

OS: overall survival; CSS: cancer-specific survival; RFS: recurrence-free survival; HR: hazard ratio; CI: confidence interval; Small: studies with less than 200 participants; Large: studies with more than 200 participants.

Regarding OS, subgroup analyses by cancer type showed that loss of Smad4 staining predicted an unfavorable prognosis in cervical carcinoma (HR=3.43, 95% CI: 1.65–7.12; $P_{heterogeneity}$=0.436), gastric cancer (HR=2.02, 95% CI: 1.44–2.83; $P_{heterogeneity}$=0.197), colorectal cancer (HR=3.76, 95% CI: 1.53–9.25; $P_{heterogeneity}$<0.001) and pancreatic cancer (HR=1.39, 95% CI: 1.19–1.61; $P_{heterogeneity}$=0.185). When ethnicity was considered, results revealed that negative Smad4 expression indicating poor OS was found both in Asian cases (HR=2.24, 95% CI: 1.32–3.81; $P_{heterogeneity}$<0.001) and Caucasian populations (HR=1.82, 95% CI: 1.39–2.37; $P_{heterogeneity}$<0.001). Subgroup analysis stratified by the number of participants (Since mean number of participants was close to 200, studies with more than 200 participants were classified as "large" and studies with less than 200 patients were classified as "small") revealed that inactivation of Smad4 was closely correlated with poor OS regardless of the number of patients (Large: HR=1.56, 95% CI: 1.34–1.82; $P_{heterogeneity}$=0.277; Small: HR=2.09, 95% CI: 1.42–3.06; $P_{heterogeneity}$<0.001).

Regarding RFS/CSS, when different ethnicities were considered, Smad4-negative expression was a negative prognostic marker for Caucasian patients (HR=2.12, 95% CI: 1.32–3.43; $P_{heterogeneity}$<0.001) than for Asian patients (HR=1.34, 95% CI: 0.99–1.81; $P_{heterogeneity}$=0.647). Subgroup analyses by cancer type showed that loss of Smad4 staining was associated with a worse outcome in colorectal cancer (HR=2.54, 95% CI: 1.46–4.39; $P_{heterogeneity}$<0.001). When performing subgroup analyses stratified by the number of participants, we found that inactivation of Smad4 predicted worse survival regardless of the number of participants (Large: HR=1.41, 95% CI: 1.19–1.67; $P_{heterogeneity}$=0.353; Small: HR=2.89, 95% CI: 1.34–6.24; $P_{heterogeneity}$<0.001).

The relationship between clinical parameters (reported in more than 2 studies) and Smad4 staining was explored in gastric cancer, colorectal cancer and pancreatic cancer (Figure 3). In gastric cancer, loss of Smad4 staining was found to be significantly associated with the rate of lymph node metastasis (OR=2.11, 95% CI: 1.03–4.34; $P_{heterogeneity}$=0.038) but not with tumor histology (OR=0.87, 95% CI: 0.45–1.69; $P_{heterogeneity}$=0.037). When colorectal cancer was analyzed, age (OR=1.69, 95% CI: 1.09–2.61; $P_{heterogeneity}$=0.648) and stage (OR=2.31, 95% CI: 1.71–3.10; $P_{heterogeneity}$=0.218) but not gender (OR=0.85, 95% CI: 0.30–2.44; $P_{heterogeneity}$=0.013) were positively associated with loss of Smad4 staining. However, no significant relationship was found between Smad4 staining and clinical parameters in pancreatic cancer, including tumor differentiation (OR=0.90, 95%CI: 0.48–1.68; $P_{heterogeneity}$=0.597), lymph node metastasis (OR=0.40, 95%CI: 0.09–1.81; $P_{heterogeneity}$<0.001) or tumor size (OR=1.21, 95%CI: 0.83–1.78; $P_{heterogeneity}$=0.458).

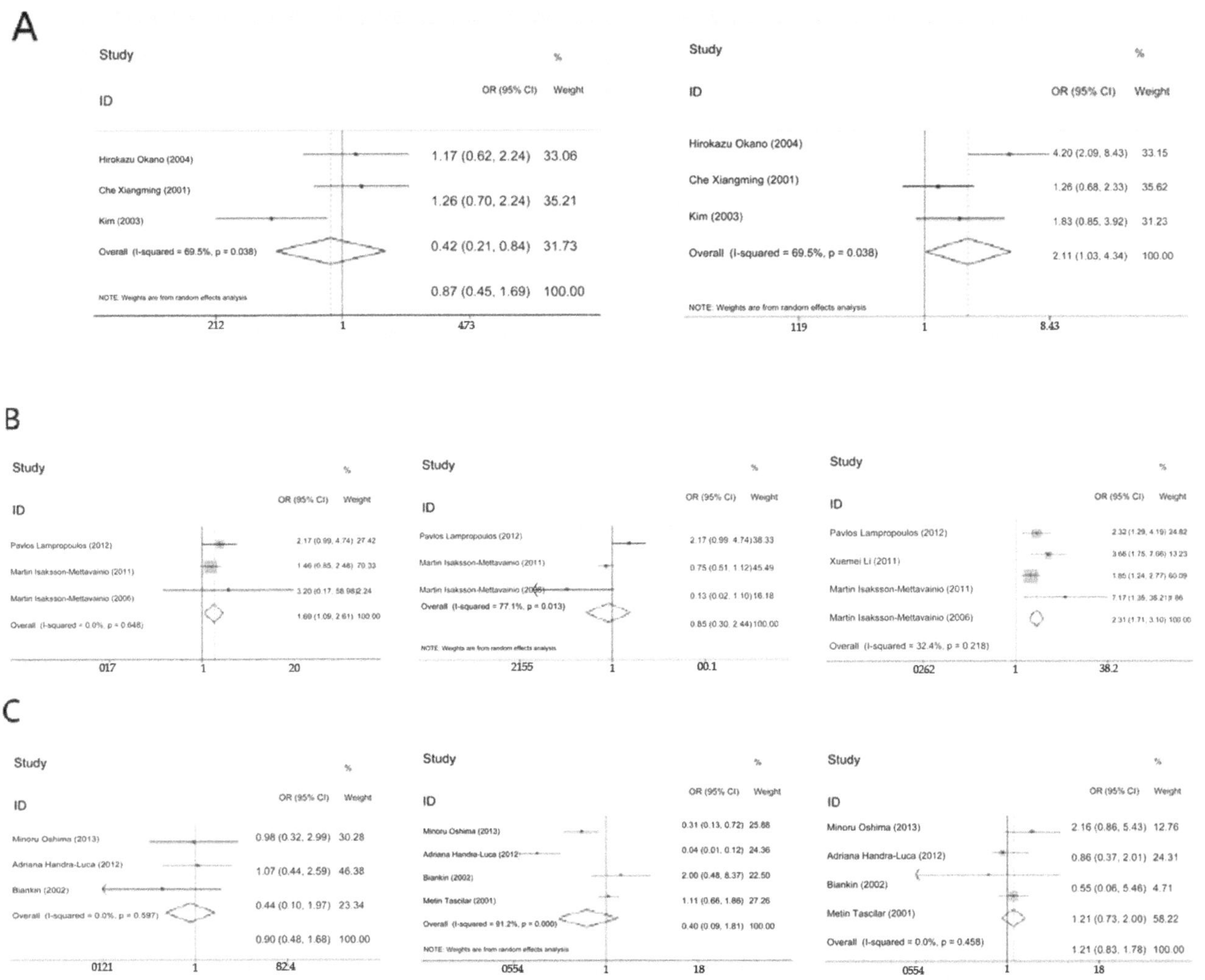

Figure 3: Forest plots of studies evaluating the association between Smad4 and clinical parameters.

In gastric cancer (A): histology (left; differentiated vs. undifferentiated); lymph node (right; absent vs. present). In colorectal cancer (B): age (left; old vs. young); gender (middle; male vs. female); TNM stage (right; advanced vs. early). In pancreatic cancer (C): differentiation (left; well/moderate vs. poor); lymph node (middle; absent vs. present); tumor size (right; small vs. large).

Heterogeneity

To explore the potential source of heterogeneity among studies, a meta-regression was conducted that utilized the following variables: year of publication, ethnicity, cancer type and number of participants (large vs. small). For OS, the results showed that year of publication, ethnicity and number of participants did not contribute to the source of heterogeneity. Cancer type was an exception (p=0.003), and this variable could explain 46.36% of the heterogeneity. For RFS/CSS, no variable included in the meta-regression appeared to be a source of heterogeneity.

Sensitivity analysis

We sequentially removed studies to investigate the influence of an individual study on the pooled results. As shown in Figure 4, pooled HRs were found to be stable, suggesting that no individual study significantly affected the pooled results.

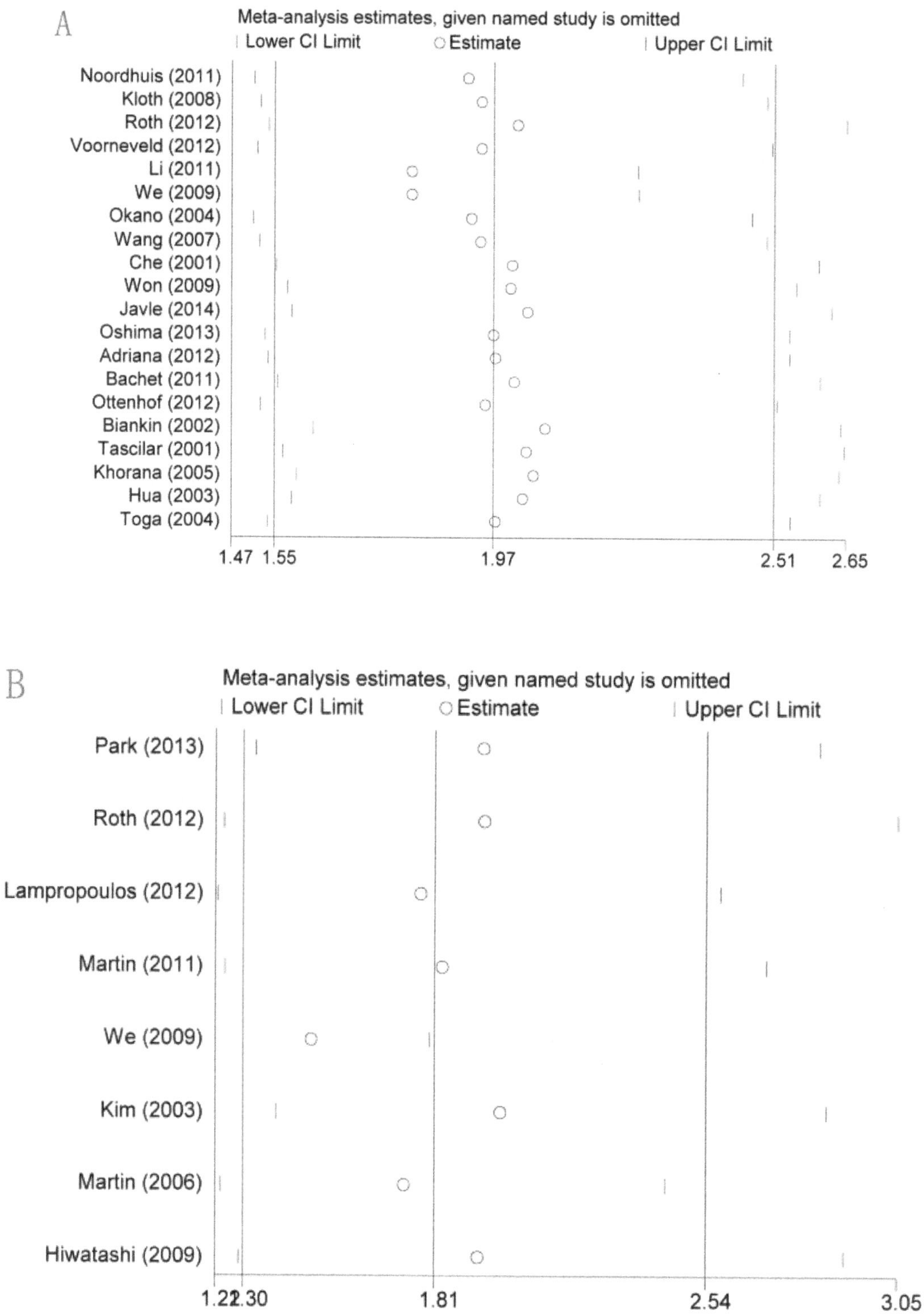

Figure 4: Effect of individual studies on the pooled hazard ratio (HR) for OS (A) and RFS/CSS (B).

Publication bias

Begg's funnel plot and Egger's linear regression test were used to assess publication bias. Begg's funnel plot for both OS (P=0.05) and RFS/CSS (P=0.108) revealed no obvious bias. Further confirmation using Egger's regression test also failed to find evidence of a publication bias for OS (P=0.088) and RFS/CSS (P=0.229). There was no evidence of a significant publication bias in the meta-analysis because the P values were not <0.05 (Figure 5).

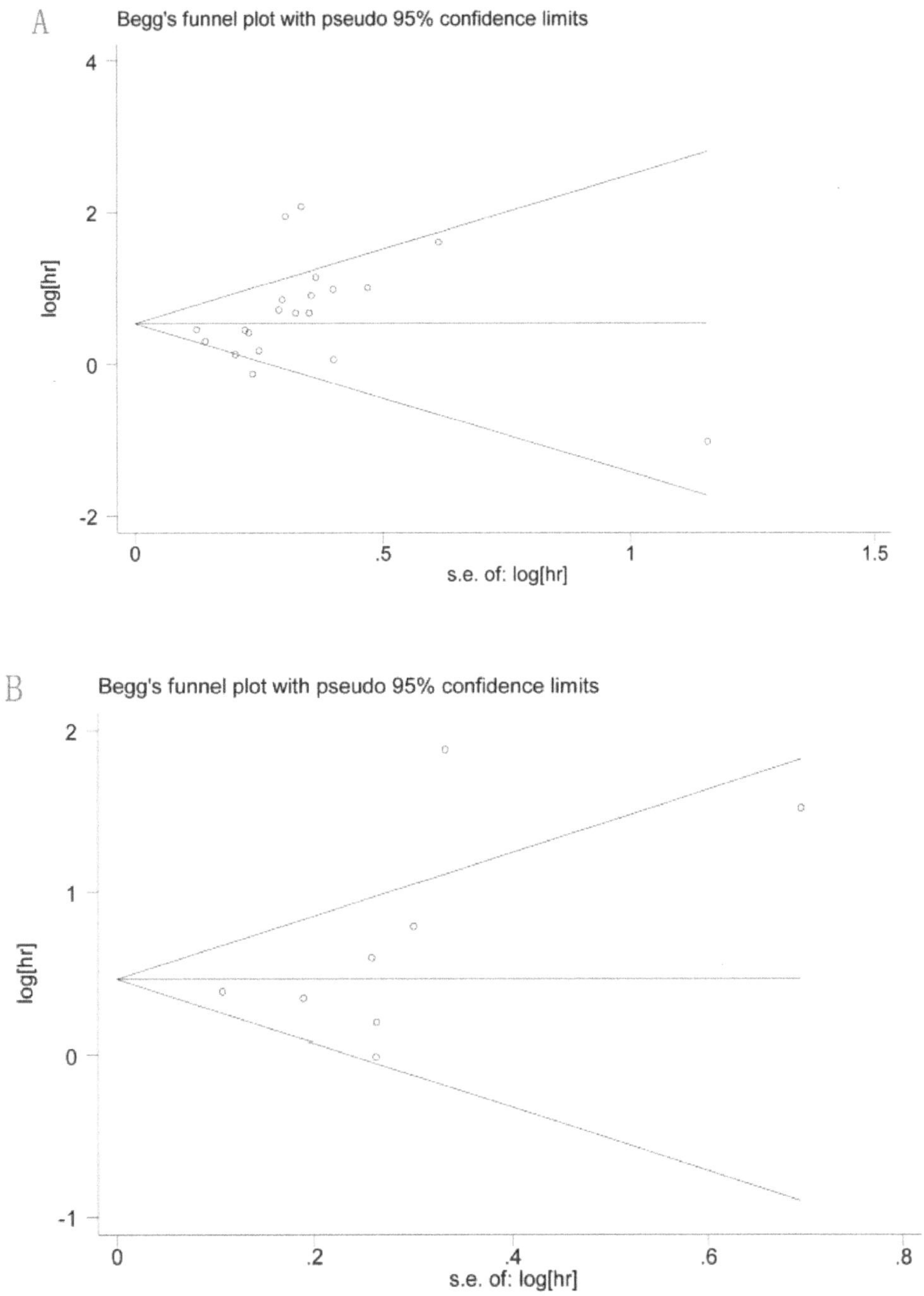

Figure 5: Begg's funnel plots for all of the included studies reported with OS (A) and RFS/CSS (B).

DISCUSSION

Cancer is a major public health problem worldwide and is a complex process resulting from environmental factors, genetics, and their interactions. Due to the lack of an early diagnosis and of effective treatment for various cancers, the prognosis of a cancer patient is often poor. Various predictors such as TNM stage, genetic factors, and inflammatory factors have been identified and applied for determining the prognosis of patients with various carcinomas. Some proteins that could act as tumor suppressors or oncogenes, such as p53 and EGFR, have also been reported to be effective biomarkers for providing a prognosis [41]–[43]. Smad4, a tumor suppressor gene located on chromosome 18q21.1, was recently reported to predict clinical outcomes in some cancers. However, the prognostic value of this marker in various cancers has remained inconclusive. Thus, we conducted a meta-analysis to evaluate the prognostic role of Smad4 in various cancers.

In our meta-analysis, which includes 26 studies involving 7570 patients, it is interesting to note that loss of Smad4 staining was strongly associated with a worse prognosis for OS and CSS/RFS. Subgroup analyses revealed that unfavorable OS with Smad4-negative expression could be found in both Asian and Caucasian cases. Additionally, loss of Smad4 staining was a significant prognostic marker for a poor outcome in different cancers (cervical carcinoma, colorectal cancer, gastric cancer and pancreatic cancer), regardless of the number of participants (small or large). Compared with the previous meta-analysis, the present study includes more studies and individuals and thus might produce a more comprehensive result than the study of RA et al. [44] that identified vascular endothelial growth factor (VEGF), bcl2, p16 and bax but not Smad4 as immunohistochemical prognostic markers in pancreatic cancer. Worse CSS/RFS with negative Smad4 could be found in Caucasian populations but not in Asian cases. Subgroup analyses revealed that unfavorable CSS/RFS with loss of Smad4 staining was also found in colorectal cancer, regardless of the number of participants. Meta-regression was performed to investigate the potential source of heterogeneity, and cancer type was found to explain most of the heterogeneity for studies evaluating OS in our meta-analysis. However, this type of heterogeneity is difficult to exclude because the recruitment of sufficient patients with a specific type of cancer is difficult. Future studies including more cancer types and a larger number of participants are needed to explore the prognostic value of Smad4 in specific cancers.

As a member of the Smad family, Smad4 plays an important role in the transforming growth factor β (TGF-β) signaling pathway from the cell surface to the nucleus. Activation of Smad4 under different conditions may result in apoptosis or growth arrest in the G1 phase of the cell, responses that are primarily associated with the development of several tumors [45], [46]. In addition, the inactivation of the Smad4 gene within an evolving neoplasm may indirectly influence the extracellular matrix to promote neoplastic growth and affect the prognosis. In our study, loss of Smad4 staining expression was associated with unfavorable outcomes for various cancers, a finding that was consistent with the results of previous studies. We also explored the association between Smad4 expression and clinico-pathological factors. In gastric cancer, patients with Smad4-nagative expression had high rates of lymph node involvement. It was interesting to determine that inactivation of Smad4 in patients with colon cancer was more likely to be found in older populations and in patients with a later tumor stage. However, in pancreatic cancer, no obvious relationship was found between Smad4 staining and clinical parameters. The results might suggest that the exact biology or mechanism of SMAD4 is likely different for divergent tumor types. Thus, more studies that include more cancer types are needed to assess the association of clinical parameters and Smad4 and explore the appropriate mechanisms in the future.

Some limitations exist regarding this meta-analysis. First, most of the enrolled studies were retrospective, making them more susceptible to some bias. Second, all of the included studies measured Smad4 expression by immunohistochemistry. Many factors, such as the primary antibody and antibody concentration, may affect the results. However, it was impossible to perform a subgroup analysis to investigate the potential effect of the technique on the combined result. Third, heterogeneity among studies due to cancer type was relative large in our meta-analysis. Many other factors may also contribute to heterogeneity. However, due to the lack of sufficient information, our analysis was limited. More related analyses are needed in the future. Moreover, although we tried to identify as many pertinent studies as possible, limited databases were searched, which might reduce the persuasive power of the pooled estimate to some extent.

In summary, this study demonstrated that loss of Smad4 staining was a poor predictor for survival in patients with various cancers. To make better use of Smad4 and apply the potential prognostic factor clinically, additional studies are needed to provide a more detailed picture of the clinical relevance and biological mechanism of Smad4.

Supporting Information

Checklist S1 PRISMA checklist

PRISMA 2009 Checklist

Section/topic	#	Checklist item	Reported on page #
TITLE			
Title	1	Identify the report as a systematic review, meta-analysis, or both.	1
ABSTRACT			
Structured summary	2	Provide a structured summary including, as applicable: background; objectives; data sources; study eligibility criteria, participants, and interventions; study appraisal and synthesis methods; results; limitations; conclusions and implications of key findings; systematic review registration number.	2
INTRODUCTION			
Rationale	3	Describe the rationale for the review in the context of what is already known.	3
Objectives	4	Provide an explicit statement of questions being addressed with reference to participants, interventions, comparisons, outcomes, and study design (PICOS).	3,4
METHODS			
Protocol and registration	5	Indicate if a review protocol exists, if and where it can be accessed (e.g., Web address), and, if available, provide registration information including registration number.	4
Eligibility criteria	6	Specify study characteristics (e.g., PICOS, length of follow-up) and report characteristics (e.g., years considered, language, publication status) used as criteria for eligibility, giving rationale.	4
Information sources	7	Describe all information sources (e.g., databases with dates of coverage, contact with study authors to identify additional studies) in the search and date last searched.	4
Search	8	Present full electronic search strategy for at least one database, including any limits used, such that it could be repeated.	4
Study selection	9	State the process for selecting studies (i.e., screening, eligibility, included in systematic review, and, if applicable, included in the meta-analysis).	4
Data collection process	10	Describe method of data extraction from reports (e.g., piloted forms, independently, in duplicate) and any processes for obtaining and confirming data from investigators.	4,5
Data items	11	List and define all variables for which data were sought (e.g., PICOS, funding sources) and any assumptions and simplifications made.	4,5
Risk of bias in individual studies	12	Describe methods used for assessing risk of bias of individual studies (including specification of whether this was done at the study or outcome level), and how this information is to be used in any data synthesis.	5
Summary measures	13	State the principal summary measures (e.g., risk ratio, difference in means).	5

PRISMA 2009 Checklist

Section/topic	#	Checklist item	Reported on page #
Risk of bias across studies	15	Specify any assessment of risk of bias that may affect the cumulative evidence (e.g., publication bias, selective reporting within studies).	5
Additional analyses	16	Describe methods of additional analyses (e.g., sensitivity or subgroup analyses, meta-regression), if done, indicating which were pre-specified.	5
RESULTS			
Study selection	17	Give numbers of studies screened, assessed for eligibility, and included in the review, with reasons for exclusions at each stage, ideally with a flow diagram.	6
Study characteristics	18	For each study, present characteristics for which data were extracted (e.g., study size, PICOS, follow-up period) and provide the citations.	7
Risk of bias within studies	19	Present data on risk of bias of each study and, if available, any outcome level assessment (see item 12).	8,9
Results of individual studies	20	For all outcomes considered (benefits or harms), present, for each study: (a) simple summary data for each intervention group (b) effect estimates and confidence intervals, ideally with a forest plot.	8,9
Synthesis of results	21	Present results of each meta-analysis done, including confidence intervals and measures of consistency.	8,9
Risk of bias across studies	22	Present results of any assessment of risk of bias across studies (see Item 15).	8,9
Additional analysis	23	Give results of additional analyses, if done (e.g., sensitivity or subgroup analyses, meta-regression [see Item 16]).	9
DISCUSSION			
Summary of evidence	24	Summarize the main findings including the strength of evidence for each main outcome; consider their relevance to key groups (e.g., healthcare providers, users, and policy makers).	9,10
Limitations	25	Discuss limitations at study and outcome level (e.g., risk of bias), and at review-level (e.g., incomplete retrieval of identified research, reporting bias).	11
Conclusions	26	Provide a general interpretation of the results in the context of other evidence, and implications for future research.	12
FUNDING			
Funding	27	Describe sources of funding for the systematic review and other support (e.g., supply of data); role of funders for the systematic review.	12

REFERENCES

1. Siegel R, Naishadham D, Jemal A (2013) Cancer statistics, 2013. CA Cancer J Clin 63: 11–30. doi: 10.3322/caac.21166
2. Li H, Zhang K, Liu LH, Ouyang Y, Bu J, et al.. (2014) A systematic review of matrix metalloproteinase 9 as a biomarker of survival in patients with osteosarcoma. Tumour Biol.
3. Yu Q, Yu XF, Zhang SD, Wang HH, Wang HY, et al. (2013) Prognostic role of C-reactive protein in gastric cancer: a meta-analysis. Asian Pac J Cancer Prev 14: 5735–5740. doi: 10.7314/apjcp.2013.14.10.5735
4. Ji YN, Wang Q, Li Y, Wang Z (2014) Prognostic value of vascular endothelial growth factor A expression in gastric cancer: a meta-analysis. Tumour Biol 35: 2787–2793. doi: 10.1007/s13277-013-1371-1
5. Lagna G, Hata A, Hemmati-Brivanlou A, Massague J (1996) Partnership between DPC4 and SMAD proteins in TGF-beta signalling pathways. Nature 383: 832–836. doi: 10.1038/383832a0
6. Papageorgis P, Cheng K, Ozturk S, Gong Y, Lambert AW, et al. (2011) Smad4 inactivation promotes malignancy and drug resistance of colon cancer. Cancer Res 71: 998–1008. doi: 10.1158/0008-5472.can-09-3269
7. Villanueva A, Garcia C, Paules AB, Vicente M, Megias M, et al. (1998) Disruption of the antiproliferative TGF-beta signaling pathways in human pancreatic cancer cells. Oncogene 17: 1969–1978. doi: 10.1038/sj.onc.1202118
8. Natsugoe S, Xiangming C, Matsumoto M, Okumura H, Nakashima S, et al. (2002) Smad4 and transforming growth factor beta1 expression in patients with squamous cell carcinoma of the esophagus. Clin Cancer Res 8: 1838–1842.
9. Alhopuro P, Alazzouzi H, Sammalkorpi H, Davalos V, Salovaara R, et al. (2005) SMAD4 levels and response to 5-fluorouracil in colorectal cancer. Clin Cancer Res 11: 6311–6316. doi: 10.1158/1078-0432.ccr-05-0244
10. Stuelten CH, Buck MB, Dippon J, Roberts AB, Fritz P, et al. (2006) Smad4-expression is decreased in breast cancer tissues: a retrospective study. BMC Cancer 6: 25. doi: 10.1186/1471-2407-6-25
11. Javle M, Li Y, Tan D, Dong X, Chang P, et al. (2014) Biomarkers of TGF-beta signaling pathway and prognosis of pancreatic cancer. PLoS One 9: e85942. doi: 10.1371/journal.pone.0085942
12. Hua Z, Zhang YC, Hu XM, Jia ZG (2003) Loss of DPC4 expression and its correlation with clinicopathological parameters in pancreatic carcinoma. World J Gastroenterol 9: 2764–2767.
13. Stroup DF, Berlin JA, Morton SC, Olkin I, Williamson GD, et al. (2000) Meta-analysis of observational studies in epidemiology: a proposal for reporting. Meta-analysis Of Observational Studies in Epidemiology (MOOSE) group. Jama 283: 2008–2012. doi: 10.1001/jama.283.15.2008
14. Parmar MK, Torri V, Stewart L (1998) Extracting summary statistics to perform meta-analyses of the published literature for survival endpoints. Stat Med 17: 2815–2834. doi: 10.1002/(sici)1097-0258(19981230)17:24<2815::aid-sim110>3.0.co;2-8
15. Mantel N, Haenszel W (1959) Statistical aspects of the analysis of data from retrospective studies of disease. J Natl Cancer Inst 22: 719–748.
16. DerSimonian R, Laird N (1986) Meta-analysis in clinical trials. Control Clin Trials 7: 177–188. doi: 10.1016/0197-2456(86)90046-2
17. Park JH, Lee C, Suh JH, Chae JY, Moon KC (2013) Nuclear expression of Smad proteins and its prognostic significance in clear cell renal cell carcinoma. Hum Pathol

44: 2047–2054. doi: 10.1016/j.humpath.2013.03.009

18. Oshima M, Okano K, Muraki S, Haba R, Maeba T, et al. (2013) Immunohistochemically detected expression of 3 major genes (CDKN2A/p16, TP53, and SMAD4/DPC4) strongly predicts survival in patients with resectable pancreatic cancer. Ann Surg 258: 336–346. doi: 10.1097/sla.0b013e3182827a65
19. Roth AD, Delorenzi M, Tejpar S, Yan P, Klingbiel D, et al. (2012) Integrated analysis of molecular and clinical prognostic factors in stage II/III colon cancer. J Natl Cancer Inst 104: 1635–1646. doi: 10.1093/jnci/djs427
20. Toga T, Nio Y, Hashimoto K, Higami T, Maruyama R (2004) The dissociated expression of protein and messenger RNA of DPC4 in human invasive ductal carcinoma of the pancreas and their implication for patient outcome. Anticancer Res 24: 1173–1178.
21. Handra-Luca A, Hammel P, Sauvanet A, Ruszniewski P, Couvelard A (2013) Tumoral epithelial and stromal expression of SMAD proteins in pancreatic ductal adenocarcinomas. J Hepatobiliary Pancreat Sci 20: 294–302. doi: 10.1007/s00534-012-0518-6
22. Bachet JB, Marechal R, Demetter P, Bonnetain F, Couvelard A, et al. (2012) Contribution of CXCR4 and SMAD4 in predicting disease progression pattern and benefit from adjuvant chemotherapy in resected pancreatic adenocarcinoma. Ann Oncol 23: 2327–2335. doi: 10.1093/annonc/mdr617
23. Ottenhof NA, Morsink FH, Ten Kate F, van Noorden CJ, Offerhaus GJ (2012) Multivariate analysis of immunohistochemical evaluation of protein expression in pancreatic ductal adenocarcinoma reveals prognostic significance for persistent Smad4 expression only. Cell Oncol (Dordr) 35: 119–126. doi: 10.1007/s13402-012-0072-x
24. Lampropoulos P, Zizi-Sermpetzoglou A, Rizos S, Kostakis A, Nikiteas N, et al. (2012) Prognostic significance of transforming growth factor beta (TGF-beta) signaling axis molecules and E-cadherin in colorectal cancer. Tumour Biol 33: 1005–1014. doi: 10.1007/s13277-012-0333-3
25. Isaksson-Mettavainio M, Palmqvist R, Dahlin AM, Van Guelpen B, Rutegard J, et al. (2012) High SMAD4 levels appear in microsatellite instability and hypermethylated colon cancers, and indicate a better prognosis. Int J Cancer 131: 779–788. doi: 10.1002/ijc.26473
26. Voorneveld PW, Jacobs RJ, De Miranda NF, Morreau H, van Noesel CJ, et al. (2013) Evaluation of the prognostic value of pSMAD immunohistochemistry in colorectal cancer. Eur J Cancer Prev 22: 420–424. doi: 10.1097/cej.0b013e32835e88e2
27. Noordhuis MG, Fehrmann RS, Wisman GB, Nijhuis ER, van Zanden JJ, et al. (2011) Involvement of the TGF-beta and beta-catenin pathways in pelvic lymph node metastasis in early-stage cervical cancer. Clin Cancer Res 17: 1317–1330. doi: 10.1158/1078-0432.ccr-10-2320
28. Li X, Liu B, Xiao J, Yuan Y, Ma J, et al. (2011) Roles of VEGF-C and Smad4 in the lymphangiogenesis, lymphatic metastasis, and prognosis in colon cancer. J Gastrointest Surg 15: 2001–2010. doi: 10.1007/s11605-011-1627-2
29. Okano H, Shinohara H, Miyamoto A, Takaori K, Tanigawa N (2004) Concomitant overexpression of cyclooxygenase-2 in HER-2-positive on Smad4-reduced human gastric carcinomas is associated with a poor patient outcome. Clin Cancer Res 10: 6938–6945. doi: 10.1158/1078-0432.ccr-0731-03
30. Biankin AV, Morey AL, Lee CS, Kench JG, Biankin SA, et al. (2002) DPC4/Smad4 expression and outcome in pancreatic ductal adenocarcinoma. J Clin Oncol 20: 4531–4542. doi: 10.1200/jco.2002.12.063
31. Won KY, Kim YW, Park YK (2010) Expression of Smad and its signalling cascade in osteosarcoma. Pathology 42: 242–247. doi: 10.3109/00313021003631288
32. Kloth JN, Kenter GG, Spijker HS, Uljee S, Corver WE, et al. (2008) Expression of Smad2 and Smad4 in cervical cancer: absent nuclear Smad4 expression correlates with poor survival. Mod Pathol 21: 866–875. doi: 10.1038/modpathol.2008.62
33. Wang LH, Kim SH, Lee JH, Choi YL, Kim YC, et al. (2007) Inactivation of SMAD4 tumor suppressor gene during gastric carcinoma progression. Clin Cancer Res 13: 102–110. doi: 10.1158/1078-0432.ccr-06-1467
34. Mesker WE, Liefers GJ, Junggeburt JM, van Pelt GW, Alberici P, et al. (2009) Presence of a high amount of stroma and downregulation of SMAD4 predict for worse survival for stage I-II colon cancer patients. Cell Oncol 31: 169–178.
35. Xiangming C, Natsugoe S, Takao S, Hokita S, Ishigami S, et al. (2001) Preserved Smad4 expression in the transforming growth factor beta signaling pathway is a favorable prognostic factor in patients with advanced gastric cancer. Clin Cancer Res 7: 277–282.
36. Kim YH, Lee HS, Lee HJ, Hur K, Kim WH, et al. (2004) Prognostic significance of the expression of Smad4 and Smad7 in human gastric carcinomas. Ann Oncol 15: 574–580. doi: 10.1093/annonc/mdh131
37. Isaksson-Mettavainio M, Palmqvist R, Forssell J, Stenling R, Oberg A (2006) SMAD4/DPC4 expression and prognosis in human colorectal cancer. Anticancer Res 26: 507–510.
38. Hiwatashi K, Ueno S, Sakoda M, Kubo F, Tateno T, et al. (2009) Strong Smad4 expression correlates with poor prognosis after surgery in patients with hepatocellular carcinoma. Ann Surg Oncol 16: 3176–3182. doi: 10.1245/s10434-009-0614-2
39. Singh P, Wig JD, Srinivasan R, Radotra BD (2011) A comprehensive examination of Smad4, Smad6 and Smad7 mRNA expression in pancreatic ductal adenocarcinoma. Indian J Cancer 48: 170–174. doi: 10.4103/0019-509x.82876
40. Khorana AA, Hu YC, Ryan CK, Komorowski RA, Hostetter G, et al. (2005) Vascular endothelial growth factor and DPC4 predict adjuvant therapy outcomes in resected pancreatic cancer. J Gastrointest Surg 9: 903–911. doi: 10.1016/j.gassur.2005.06.021

41. Fu HL, Shao L, Wang Q, Jia T, Li M, et al. (2013) A systematic review of p53 as a biomarker of survival in patients with osteosarcoma. Tumour Biol 34: 3817–3821. doi: 10.1007/s13277-013-0966-x

42. Malats N, Bustos A, Nascimento CM, Fernandez F, Rivas M, et al. (2005) P53 as a prognostic marker for bladder cancer: a meta-analysis and review. Lancet Oncol 6: 678–686. doi: 10.1016/s1470-2045(05)70315-6

43. Hong L, Han Y, Zhang H, Zhao Q, Yang J, et al. (2013) High expression of epidermal growth factor receptor might predict poor survival in patients with colon cancer: a meta-analysis. Genet Test Mol Biomarkers 17: 348–351. doi: 10.1089/gtmb.2012.0421

44. Smith RA, Tang J, Tudur-Smith C, Neoptolemos JP, Ghaneh P (2011) Meta-analysis of immunohistochemical prognostic markers in resected pancreatic cancer. Br J Cancer 104: 1440–1451.

45. Zhou S, Buckhaults P, Zawel L, Bunz F, Riggins G, et al. (1998) Targeted deletion of Smad4 shows it is required for transforming growth factor beta and activin signaling in colorectal cancer cells. Proc Natl Acad Sci U S A 95: 2412–2416. doi: 10.1073/pnas.95.5.2412

46. Dai JL, Bansal RK, Kern SE (1999) G1 cell cycle arrest and apoptosis induction by nuclear Smad4/Dpc4: phenotypes reversed by a tumorigenic mutation. Proc Natl Acad Sci U S A 96: 1427–1432. doi: 10.1073/pnas.96.4.1427

INDEX